Handbook of Early Language Impairment in Children

Assessment and Intervention

Linda R. Watson, Ed.D., CCC-SLP
Clinical Associate Professor
University of North Carolina at Chapel Hill

Elizabeth R. Crais, Ph.D., CCC-SLP
Associate Professor
University of North Carolina at Chapel Hill

Thomas L. Layton, Ph.D., CCC-SLP
Professor, Communication Sciences and Disorders
North Carolina Central University, Durham

Delmar
Thomson Learning™

Africa • Australia • Canada • Denmark • Japan • Mexico
New Zealand • Philippines • Puerto Rico • Singapore
Spain • United Kingdom • United States

NOTICE TO THE READER

Delmar Staff
Business Unit Director: William Brottmiller
Executive Editor: Cathy L. Esperti
Development Editor: Deb Flis
Executive Marketing Manager: Dawn Gerrain
Project Editor: Stacey Prus
Production Coordinator: John Mickelbank
Art/Design Coordinator: Mary Colleen Liburdi

Printed in Canada
1 2 3 4 5 6 7 8 9 10 XXX 05 04 03 02 01 00

For more information contact: Delmar, 3 Columbia Circle, PO Box 15015, Albany, NY 12212-0515; or find us on the World Wide Web at http://www.delmar.com

ISBN NO: 0 8273 7524 7

Contents

List of Illustrations

List of Tables

Preface

This book deals with the assessment and treatment of children with or at risk for specific language impairments. The chapters have been divided so that the first two address primarily assessment issues, the middle three link assessment and intervention, and the final four address specific intervention issues. As is apparent throughout the book, it is difficult to cover one area without the other; consequently, assessment and intervention have been interrelated throughout each chapter. In addition, this book does not attempt to provide comprehensive coverage of all aspects related to assessment and intervention nor of child language impairment. Instead, we have identified current theories and recent trends in working with children with language impairments and have developed a book to highlight these important areas. We feel fortunate to have contributions from many of the leading experts in the areas being addressed. They have contributed a wealth of knowledge to this book.

Chapters 1 and 2 set the stage for this book in identifying the importance of utilizing *ecologically valid* assessment procedures with infants, toddlers, and preschoolers. These types of assessments take into account the influence of sociocultural factors on the child and family and the need to individualize all aspects of the assessment process. Chapter 1 outlines the necessary components for assessing children from birth to 2 years of age and provides a case study illustrating the use of these components. Chapter 2 sets the stage by providing a brief case study related to assessment, then focuses on seven guiding principles and the important components for assessing children aged 2 to 5 years old.

Chapter 3 extends the discussion of ecologically valid assessment to children who are identified as culturally-linguistically different (CLD). Various issues and challenges for the valid assessment of these children are presented. The discussion of high- and low-context communication styles among various cultures should prove interesting and informative. The later sections of the chapter describe partnerships formed with family members to plan intervention goals and provide case studies to illustrate the issues that arise in assessment and intervention planning.

Chapter 4 provides a conceptual model for linking assessment and intervention. The chapter begins with a historical review of early communicative assessment and intervention, differentiates types and purposes of assessment, and concludes with an alternative to the traditional approach to early communicative assessment and intervention. The authors provide a description of an available model and a detailed case study to illustrate its application.

Empowering the family in the assessment and intervention process is the focus of Chapter 5. The framework used to illustrate this collaboration is the Ecological Communication (ECO) program, which is a system for guiding the development of interactions between children and their partners from play through conversation. This program was designed to assist professionals in providing suggestions to families as they enhance their communicative interactions with their children. The case study at the end of the chapter illustrates the ways in which families and professionals can work together to identify and implement interventions.

Chapter 6 describes a variety of language intervention approaches. These include approaches that incorporate peer models with typically developing language skills, and various parent-based treatment approaches. The chapter concludes with a discussion of the role of early language intervention, and two case studies demonstrating the effectiveness of language intervention.

The issues of emergent literacy for children with language impairments are discussed in Chapter 7. The chapter begins by describing reading and literacy in typically developing language learners, as contrasted with children who have language impairments. Guidelines for facilitating emergent readings are then presented, followed by a description of parent and child behaviors during storybook interactions and emergent readings. Case examples are provided to illustrate children's narrative language productions during emergent storybook elicitation and oral storytelling.

Chapter 8 contains a description of language intervention for prelinguistic and nonverbal preschool children who are severely physically and/or cognitively challenged. First, critical needs for early intervention and issues related to the use of augmentative and alternative communication (AAC) systems are identified. Then the chapter provides guidelines for assessment and practical strategies for implementing AAC systems with young children and their caregivers. Finally, four case studies are used to highlight assessment and intervention planning strategies.

The concluding chapter discusses sensory integration (SI) treatment. The authors first describe Ayres's model of sensory integration and its importance to communication development. Because sensory-processing problems comprise one of the many contributing factors to language disorders, understanding sensory processing is integral for understanding language development and disorders. This chapter provides various case studies and models for intervention to illustrate the potential usefulness of SI treatment. This book presents several important concepts and advancements in assessing and intervening with very young children who have or are at risk for language impairments. The theme throughout the chapters involves ecologically valid strategies, most particularly the inclusion of the family in both assessment and intervention practices and the need for culturally valid assessment and intervention procedures. Many models of intervention are presented, including clinician-oriented and parent-oriented approaches, along with a focus on the inclusion of emergent literacy, augmentative communication, and sensory integration techniques in the treatment programs.

We have done our best to bring together *cutting edge* information to inform current assessment and intervention practices. We now invite readers to explore the issues, learn from the experts, and begin to implement the many suggestions provided in order to better serve young children who have, or are at risk for, language impairments, along with their families.

The editors, authors, and Delmar Publishers would like to thank the following individuals for their valuable comments during the review process:

Mary Beth Armstrong, Ph.D., CCC-SLP
Assistant Professor
Department of Communication Science and Disorders
University of Montevallo
Montevallo, Alabama

Frances P. Billeaud, M.A., CCC-SLP
Director of Clinical Activities
Department of Communicative Disorders
University of Southwestern Louisiana
Lafayette

W. P. Cupples, Ph.D., CCC-SLP
Associate Professor of Special Education
Director, Speech and Hearing Clinic
Eastern Michigan University
Ypsilanti

Mavis Donahue, Ed.D.
Professor, Special Education
University of Illinois
Chicago

Ann Lee B. McKeehan, CCC-SLP
Speech-Language Pathologist
Private Practice and Anne Arundel Public Schools
Annapolis, Maryland

Contributors

Diane Bricker, Ph.D., Professor, Early Intervention Program, University of Oregon, Eugene

Elizabeth R. Crais, Ph.D., CCC-SLP, Associate Professor, Division of Speech and Hearing Sciences, University of North Carolina, Chapel Hill

Elise Davis-McFarland, CCC-SLP, Associate Professor, Department of Rehabilitation Sciences, Medical University of South Carolina, Charleston

Bonita Dowell, Ph.D., CCC-CLP, Associate Professor, South Carolina State University, Orangeburg

Yvonne Gillette, Ph.D., CCC-SLP, Associate Professor, School of Communicative Disorders, University of Akron

Mary Blake Huer, Ph.D., CCC-SLP, Professor, Department of Speech Communication, California State University, Fullerton

Joan N. Kaderavek, Ph.D., CCC-SLP, Assistant Professor, Department of Special Education, Eastern Michigan University, Ypsilanti

Sandra N. Kleinman, Ed.D., CCC-SLP, Executive Director, The Howard School, Atlanta

Thomas L. Layton, Ph.D., CCC-SLP, Professor, Communication Sciences and Disorders, North Carolina Central University, Durham

Angela Losardo, Ph.D., CCC-SLP, Associate Professor, Department of Language, Reading and Exceptionalities, Appalachian State University, Boone, North Carolina

Barry M. Prizant, Ph.D., CCC-SLP, Director, Childhood Communication Services, Cranston, Rhode Island

Sarah K. Scharfenaker, M.A., CCC-SLP, Children's Hospital, Denver

Tracy Murnan Stackhouse, M.S., OTR, Children's Hospital, Denver

Elizabeth Sulzby, Ph.D., Professor, School of Education, University of Michigan, Ann Arbor

Linda R. Watson, Ed.D., CCC-SLP, Clinical Associate Professor, Division of Speech and Hearing Sciences, University of North Carolina, Chapel Hill

Susan Ellis Weismer, Ph.D., CCC-SLP, Associate Professor, Department of Communicative Disorders, University of Wisconsin, Madison

CHAPTER 1

Ecologically Valid Communication Assessment of Infants and Toddlers

Elizabeth R. Crais, Ph.D., CCC-SLP
Associate Professor
Division of Speech and Hearing Sciences
University of North Carolina, Chapel Hill

Key Terms

communicative functions
communicative means
curriculum-based assessment (CBA)
ecologically valid assessment

Overview

CASE STUDY: STEVEN

When his parents first called the early intervention center they noted that Steven was born with cystic fibrosis and had a history of eating difficulties, hospitalizations, and respiratory treatments. They relayed that he was being followed by the local hospital's cystic fibrosis clinic and that his eating difficulties were diminishing, but they were concerned about his limited communication skills and wanted him evaluated. In a follow-up telephone call made by one of the early interventionists to further identify the parent's concerns, Steven's mother reported that he was 16 months old yet made very few sounds or attempts to communicate with others. She said that Steven had difficulty letting them know what he wanted and his communication skills lagged far behind other children his age. When asked about his other skills, she felt that his motor skills were good and that he enjoyed playing with toys. When asked about any other concerns, she reported that Steven was very afraid of strangers and new situations and that, consequently, she was unsure of how he would react to the professionals who would need to evaluate him. She related that whenever Steven realized he was the focus of attention, he would generally hide and refuse to interact with anyone.

This introduction to the case of Steven presents a number of challenges to professionals who may need to assess such a child for the presence of developmental delays, and it pinpoints the need to individualize assessments for each child and family. The term "assessment" is used broadly, to cover the entire assessment process including screening, diagnosis, assessment for intervention planning, and evaluation of the child's progress. The principles of ecological validity cover each of these activities, while recognizing their differences in purpose and scope. Indeed, the assessment of young children who have, or are at risk for, developmental delays is both a science and an art. The science comes from knowing and applying relevant research that informs both the theory and practice of child assessment. The art comes from studying and applying the practical, personal, and interactive aspects that make child assessment meaningful to both families and professionals. Child assessment is a universal process: all children with special needs and their families take part in assessment as part of the early intervention system. Sometimes it is a positive experience for families and professionals, as it serves to identify the child's strengths and needs and guide the planning for the child and family's immediate future. At other times, however, the process may be difficult for families and professionals, and as a result, it may not provide the kind of information needed by either group.

In an effort to influence the ways in which assessment practices are selected and applied, this chapter will focus on both the science and the art of assessing young children. First, a clarification of the terms *evaluation* and *assessment* is provided. Second, an overview of the issues related to the use of ecologically valid procedures and tools is presented. Third, the necessary components in assessing communication skills in young children and practical strategies to assess each component are provided. Finally, the initial case study is expanded to illustrate how to use the principles and components of an ecologically valid assessment.

EVALUATION VERSUS ASSESSMENT

The Individuals with Disabilities Education Act Amendments (IDEA, 1997) differentiated between the terms *evaluation* and *assessment* in this way: evaluation refers to procedures used to determine a child's initial and continuing eligibility and must include a determination of the status of the child across developmental areas, whereas assessment refers to the ongoing procedures used to identify the child's unique strengths and needs; the family's concerns, priorities, and resources regarding the child's development; and the nature and extent of early intervention services and supports needed by the child and family. Evaluations often are conducted within a structured format, utilize standardized instruments, conclude within a limited time frame, and may exclude caregivers. Assessment activities are typically less formal in structure, utilize multiple tools and methods (e.g., standardized, observational, and nonstandardized), last over a longer time frame, and may involve caregivers more actively.

These two sets of activities may be performed separately; for example, some states utilize centralized teams of professionals to "evaluate" children and determine eligibility and other community-based teams to "assess" the children over time in order to plan and provide intervention services. In contrast, in some states and with certain teams, evaluation and assessment activities overlap and the same professionals perform both types. In these instances, evaluation and assessment are typically interwoven and indistinguishable from one another. Thus, the federal definitions of the two terms may set up artificial boundaries between these activities when, in reality, they are often joined together and provided within a continuum of early intervention services.

Due to the author's belief that evaluation and assessment activities should be part of a continuous and coordinated process for both children and families, the term assessment will be used to describe the entire process, including the activities and tools used to establish eligibility and those used to plan intervention. This broadened use of the term does not downplay the need for professionals to determine eligibility, but it encourages the modification of the time spent determining eligibility in favor of activities that enhance intervention planning. As indicated by Kleinman and Prizant (Chapter 2) and Bricker and Losardo (Chapter 4), different terms are utilized for different aspects of the assessment process; however, the important issue is the need to select tools and techniques that fit the differing assessment purposes. In addition, to be useful for intervention planning, assessment must be representative of the child and provide a picture of how he or she functions on a day-to-day basis with his or her caregivers. Thus, a major challenge to current practitioners is the need to select tools and techniques that provide a representative and ecologically valid picture of the child and family. The following sections address several issues regarding ecological validity and provide helpful suggestions for making the assessment process more ecologically valid.

ECOLOGICALLY VALID ASSESSMENT

Bronfenbrenner's (1977) concept of the child nested within the family, which is, itself, embedded within a larger community system, serves as the basis for taking an ecological approach. From an ecological perspective, the child, family, and community are viewed as sources of mutual influence, and thus actions that influence one component may affect the others. In regard to assessment, Bronfenbrenner asserted that to understand behavior, one must go beyond limited observations including only one or two people and one setting. He urged that the individual be examined in interaction with multiple people and across multiple settings. Similarly, in considering the ecologies surrounding a child (e.g., home, day care, playground, assessment facility), professionals are urged to take into account the child's interactions across multiple settings and the facilitators and constraints inherent in each.

In outlining the components of an **ecologically valid assessment**, Bailey (1989) proposed that:

a. all caregivers must be included as significant partners in the assessment process;

b. a child's cultural background, economic status, and family value system must be taken into account to avoid cultural bias and the planning of activities that do not fit the family's value system;

c. the focus of assessment should be on the naturalistic observation of play and daily routines to ensure awareness of the child's use of skills within meaningful contexts;

d. the assessment should include a plan for the child's immediate and future placement and an analysis of the skills necessary for the child to function in these settings.

The following sections provide a brief discussion of these four components and strategies for addressing the components within the assessment process.

Caregivers as Partners in the Assessment Process

Within the area of communication disorders, a variety of professionals have advocated for increased participation of parents and other caregivers throughout the assessment and intervention process (Andrews & Andrews, 1990; Crais, 1993; McLean & Crais, 1996; Wetherby & Prizant, 1992). As collaborators in assessment, caregivers can play a vital role in planning, implementing, and following up on assessment activities. Active participation of parents throughout assessment can:

a. provide multiple contexts for information-gathering and -sampling opportunities;

b. facilitate professional-parent collaboration;

c. help parents pinpoint the child's strengths and needs and, thereby facilitate the choice of intervention targets;

d. promote consensus building between caregivers and family members regarding critical issues related to assessment and intervention;

e. reduce costs and increase efficiency (Crais, 1995).

By facilitating participation of the caregivers in each component of the assessment process, professionals can increase caregiver decision making, improve the ecological validity of assessment, and, as a result, increase the reliability of the results and the likelihood of caregiver satisfaction.

Increasingly, family members are being offered more varied roles within the assessment process, including such activities as helping with activities designed to elicit specific behaviors, interpreting the child's behaviors, describing the child's daily routines, and validating the professional's assessment results (Crais & Wilson, 1996). As indicated by Crais and Wilson, these activities are in contrast with activities used infrequently by professionals, including asking family members to record observations, providing them with a way to organize their observations to share with professionals, asking them to help identify strategies to use in assessment, eliciting positive comments from them about the child, or giving them the choice of reviewing the reports before they are finalized. Although these latter practices have been advocated in the literature as helpful to developing a family-centered assessment process (Bailey, McWilliam, Winton, & Simeonsson, 1992; Crais, 1993; Kjerland & Kovach, 1990), they are not routinely used by most practicing professionals (Crais & Wilson, 1996).

Sociocultural Awareness

Across service delivery settings and throughout the provision of early intervention services, professionals need to be aware of, and sensitive to, the social, cultural, linguistic, and ethnic characteristics of the children and families they serve (Bailey, 1989; Hanson & Lynch, 1992). Due to demographic and health-care trends, professionals are increasingly interacting with families whose backgrounds and values differ from their own. One of the challenges to professionals is the need to understand the effects of sociocultural influences on the child and family and how those influences may affect the assessment process. For example, the ways the family views the child and his or her strengths and needs are highly dependent on their own sociocultural beliefs and values and those of the people (e.g., relatives, friends, religious leaders) in the ecologies surrounding them. Moreover, a child and family's experiences and beliefs about professionals in general will influence their perceptions of the entire assessment process. In all cases, it is important for professionals to be familiar with the sociocultural beliefs and values of the child and family and to plan and conduct assessments that are sensitive to these issues.

Despite the federal mandate in the IDEA (1997) legislation that test materials and procedures be nondiscriminatory, few standardized instruments are available that are dialectally or culturally sensitive (Battle, 1993). Moreover, within any particular social, cultural, or ethnic group, each child and family is unique. Therefore, practitioners need to individualize each assessment relative to the particular child and family. One primary way to enhance ecological validity is through the active participation of caregivers in the assessment process. Caregivers can guide early intervention professionals in understanding their beliefs, values, and preferences regarding the child and determining possible assessment activities.

Assessment must also take place in the family's native language; therefore, for professionals who are not bilingual or do not represent the family's cultural group, an interpreter or cultural mediator may be necessary (Moore & Beatty, 1995). As suggested by Moore and Beatty, interpreters or cultural mediators may take many roles within the assessment process, such as liaison with the parents, communication link between the staff and parents, parental advocate, "cultural gauge" for what may or may not be relevant for the family, source of information for the parents, interpreter during assessment and pre- or postassessment meetings, translator of all written materials (e.g., tests, reports), and a referral source for the community.

Other ways to increase sociocultural awareness include immersing oneself in the child's culture by observing other members of the child's cultural group, being sensitive to the family members' styles of communicating, using familiar and culturally appropriate toys and materials, and asking the families themselves to plan and perform the assessment activities (Crais, 1993; Nelson, 1993; Westby, 1990). Additional ideas for culturally appropriate assessment can be found in Anderson and Goldberg (1991), Battle (1993), Davis-McFarland and Dowell (Chapter 3), Lynch and Hanson (1992), and Moore and Beatty (1995).

Naturalistic Observation of Play and Daily Routines

Increasingly, professionals are questioning whether current assessment tools and practices reflect the best means to gain information about young children (Crais, 1995; Wetherby & Prizant, 1992). One of the drawbacks to traditional assessment practices has been the limited number of tools available for naturalistic observation and assessment. However, one assessment approach used widely in recent years that does focus on the child's natural and elicited behaviors and responses during play activities is Transdisciplinary Play-Based Assessment (TPBA), developed by Linder (1993). TPBA includes a play interaction context for performing developmental observations and allows the team to focus on social-emotional, cognitive, language, communication, and sensorimotor skills. After gathering caregiver information on the child's developmental status, a play session is conducted with the child, the parents, a peer, and a play facilitator. Throughout the process, the team observes the interactions and a parent facilitator discusses the activities with the parents. The session typically begins with "child-directed" activities using developmentally appropriate toys and materials, in which the facilitator imitates, models, and expands the child's play. A peer is then brought into the session to facilitate child-child interaction, followed by the parents being asked to play with the child. Structured and unstructured motor play and a snack are also included. Other instruments that also include play assessment as a primary component of their overall activities are the Assessment and Evaluation Programming System (AEPS) (Bricker, 1993), Assessing Linguistic Behavior (ALB) (Olswang, Stoel-Gammon, Coggins, & Carpenter, 1987), Communication and Symbolic Behavior Scales (CSBS) (Wetherby & Prizant, 1993), and Infant-Toddler Language Scale (Rossetti, 1990b). In addition, the Symbolic Play Scale (Westby, 1988) continues to be a popular means used to observe play behaviors.

Additional strategies for gathering information about children within play and daily routines include performing observations in the child's home or other familiar settings (e.g., child-care setting or a relative's home), asking caregivers to include familiar toys or books and a favorite snack in the assessment, including familiar people in the assessment, and asking caregivers to perform typical routines with the child such as changing diapers, feeding, or playing social games (e.g., "peekaboo," "this little piggie"). Additional ideas for using daily routines for assessment and intervention planning can be found in Bricker and Cripe (1992), Gillette (Chapter 5), and McWilliam (1995).

The use of **curriculum-based assessment (CBA)**, which focuses on trying to identify the settings, conditions, and goals for parents and interventionists to use daily activities as a vehicle for teaching can also be helpful (Cripe, Slentz, & Bricker, 1993). Excellent resources regarding curriculum-based assessment include the work of Bricker and her colleagues (Bricker, 1993; Bricker & Cripe, 1992; Bricker & Losardo, Chapter 4) and that of Johnson-Martin, Jens, Attermeier, and Hacker (1991). These are just a few examples of ways to gain information about children in more naturalistic contexts, which can be viewed as alternatives or supplements to the use of standardized instruments.

Planning for Immediate and Future Placements

An additional challenge to professionals in achieving ecologically valid assessment is the need to use assessment information to guide current and future intervention efforts. As suggested by Bricker and Losardo (Chapter 4), most standardized tests were not designed to provide programming information for planning intervention. Therefore, attempts by professionals to utilize standardized assessment results to plan for an intervention that is both functional and relevant to the child's day-to-day ecology may be limited. As suggested by Simeonsson (1989), "The more ecologically valid an assessment is, the more immediate and obvious to intervention priorities are its findings" (p. 169). Neisworth, Bagnato, and Munson (1989) use the term "linked" assessment to indicate the need to connect assessment with intervention planning. Accordingly, it is necessary for clinicians to identify measures that can lead directly to intervention and can also be viewed as ecologically valid. Chapter 4, by Bricker and Losardo, provides an excellent review of these issues and offers an assessment approach that directly links assessment with intervention.

The importance of gaining an ecologically valid view of the child cannot be underestimated at any point in the assessment process, from the determination of eligibility through the intervention-planning activities. The ongoing challenge for professionals and families is to accomplish ecologically valid assessments within the confines of the available time and resources and that meet the needs of both families and professionals. The following section outlines parameters for assessment and provides strategies for assessing each component.

PARAMETERS OF ASSESSMENT

Although each assessment should be individualized for the particular child and family, there are components that may be common across a variety of assessments. In particular, each assessment should start with the family's concerns and priorities, focus on the components of concern to the family and professional members of the team, and conclude by addressing the issues raised and identifying the next steps for the child and family.

Family Concerns, Priorities, and Resources

To begin identifying the family's concerns and priorities, many professionals have found it useful to use open-ended questions to develop a general perspective about the child and family. Questions such as, "How are things going with [child's name] right now?", "What are your concerns about [child's name] at this time?", or "What brought you here today?" can begin the dialogue. As issues are raised, specific questions can be used to gather further information (e.g., "Can you tell me more about Jimmy's feeding difficulties?", "Can you describe how Sarah communicates at this time?"). Additional strategies to identify concerns of caregivers and others (e.g., teacher, child-care provider) may be to ask about the child's daily routines and to inquire about particularly problematic times or situations. Follow-up questions may focus on the circumstances surrounding the events or activities of concern, strategies that have been attempted, and alternatives for resolving the issues. Information about how the family views the child's strengths and needs is also useful in planning and conducting the assessment. In addition, information gained about previous assessments and the family's perceptions of which activities and results were useful to them can also guide the process.

To facilitate a match between what families hope to gain from assessment and what actually occurs, professionals also need to find out what each family wants from the assessment. For example, some families recognize that their child has a "problem," and therefore, what they primarily want are ideas on how to help their child progress. Other families may have been referred by other professionals and may not suspect any difficulties; they may even question the need for an assessment. Thus, identifying what the family hopes to gain from the assessment can help guide the process. In addition, professionals and families need to begin the process of prioritizing the concerns to be addressed by the assessment and those that may be addressed by other resources or means.

To help in identifying the family's concerns, priorities, and resources, informal interviews are common and are often the strategy of choice (Summers et al., 1990). Westby (1990) and Winton and Bailey (1993) provide guidelines for using interviewing to gather information about the family's concerns and priorities. Surveys or self-report instruments can also be used to supplement the interviews; common instruments include the Family Interest Survey (Cripe & Bricker, 1993), Family Information Preference Inventory (Turnbull & Turnbull, 1986), and Family Needs Survey-Revised (Bailey & Simeonsson, 1990). Regarding family resources, instruments are also available, such as the Family Resource Scale (Leet & Dunst, 1988) or the Family Support Scale (Dunst, Jenkins, & Trivette, 1988). As an alternative, some professionals gather this type of resource information informally during the intervention-planning process in order to help identify the informal and formal supports that surround the child and family. This is particularly useful in creating an intervention plan that builds on the family's available resources, supplemented when necessary by other community resources.

The identification of family concerns, priorities, and resources should become the heart of the assessment process and should guide the steps that follow. If a primary goal of the assessment is to address the family's concerns and priorities, the process and results should reflect what the family wants and needs from the assessment process. As indicated by Crais (1993, 1995) and Gillette (Chapter 5), the role of the family in identifying the parameters for assessment and outlining strategies to assess those areas should be paramount.

For additional ideas for identifying the family's concerns, priorities, and resources and for working collaboratively to plan and conduct the assessment, see Crais (1993); McGonigel, Kaufman, and Johnson (1991); and McWilliam, Winton, and Crais (1996).

Although the specific parameters to include in the assessment will change relative to the specific concerns and priorities of the family and professionals who surround the child, the following areas are among those that may be considered. The list of parameters assumes that detailed developmental and medical histories also will be gathered.

Sensory Functions

Due to the increased survival rate of premature and/or low birth weight infants and the inherent increase in major disabilities in these children, attention to the risk of sensory deficits is critical. Risk factors for hearing loss in neonates and infants are listed in Table 1-1. An audiological evaluation is recommended for infants manifesting any risk factor or where concerns are raised by caregivers or professionals. Because screening efforts are not universal in most states and are based on high-risk criteria, only half of children screened who have a congenital hearing loss are identified (National Institutes of Health, 1993). In addition, between 20 and 30 percent of infants with a hearing impairment will acquire this loss after birth, during early childhood. Thus, the average age of identification of a hearing loss remains close to 2 to 3 years. For optimal development, however, the diagnostic process for hearing loss should be completed by an audiologist and rehabilitation begun by 6 months of age (Joint Committee on Infant Hearing, 1994). Indeed, there is evidence of improved developmental outcomes with early identification and early intervention follow-up (Harrison & Roush, 1996; Yoshinago-Itano, 1995). For more detailed information on hearing screening for infants and toddlers, see Roush (1990).

The first 3 months of a child's life are the most critical to the development of the visual system and the presence of a visual impairment affects all aspects of development, most particularly early relationships and communicative functions (Langley, 1996). The American Academy of Pediatrics (1986) recommends that screening for eye problems occur in four stages (when the child is in the newborn nursery, and then at 6 months, 3½ years, and 5 years of age) and be performed by an eye-care professional or pediatrician in response to any behavioral signs or parental reports of visual difficulties.

Other sensory areas in need of attention include vestibular, tactile, and proprioceptive modalities. The integration of these basic sensory processes forms the foundation for emotional stability, cognitive and motor development, and organized learning of behaviors (Langley, 1996). As suggested by Langley, sensory deficits may result in either a lack of sufficient information for processing or in disorganization and defensive behaviors. These types of dif-

Table 1-1. Risk Criteria for Hearing Loss

A. Use with neonates (birth through 28 days) when universal hearing screening is not available.
   1. Family history of hereditary childhood sensorineural hearing loss.
   2. In utero infections such as cytomegalovirus, herpes rubella, syphilis, toxoplasmosis.
   3. Craniofacial anomalies, including malformations of the pinna and ear canal.
   4. Birth weight less than 1,500 grams (3.3 lbs).
   5. Hyperbilirubinemia at a serum level requiring exchange transfusion (levels are set by hospital).
   6. Ototoxic medications, including but not limited to aminoglycoside antibiotics used repeatedly or with loop diuretics.
   7. Bacterial meningitis.
   8. Apgar scores of 0–4 at 1 minute and 0–6 at 5 minutes.
   9. Mechanical ventilation lasting 5 days or longer.
   10. Stigmata or other findings associated with a syndrome known to include a sensorineural and/or conductive hearing loss.

B. Use with infants (29 days through 2 years) when health conditions develop that require hearing rescreening.
   1. Parent/caregiver concern regarding hearing, speech, language, and/or developmental delay.
   2. Bacterial meningitis or other infections associated with sensorineural hearing loss.
   3. Head trauma associated with loss of consciousness or skull fracture.
   4. Stigmata or other findings associated with a syndrome or association known to include a sensorineural and/or conductive hearing loss.
   5. Ototoxic medications including but not limited to chemotherapy agents, aminoglycoside antibiotics used in multiple courses or in combination with loop diuretics.
   6. Recurrent or persistent otitis media with effusion for at least 3 months.

C. Use with infants (29 days through 3 years) who require periodic monitoring of hearing. [Some infants may pass initial hearing screening but require periodic tests due to history of delayed onset of sensorineural and/or conductive hearing loss. These infants require a test every 6 months until age 3 and at appropriate intervals thereafter.]

   For sensorineural loss:
   1. Family history of hereditary childhood hearing loss.
   2. In utero infections such as cytomegalovirus, herpes, rubella, syphilis, or toxoplasmosis.
   3. Neurofibromatosis Type II and neurodegenerative disorders.

   For conductive loss:
   1. Recurrent or persistent otitis media with effusion.
   2. Anatomic deformities and other disorders that affect eustachian tube function.
   3. Neurodegenerative disorders.

Source: Joint Committee on Infant Hearing. (1994). 1994 position statement. *Asha, 36,* 38–41. Used by permission of the American Speech-Language-Hearing Association, Rockville, MD.

ficulties can affect the child's ability to take advantage of the sensory and interactive experiences necessary for learning (DiGangi & Greenspan, 1989; Sears, 1994). Typically, the assessment of sensory functions would be conducted by an occupational or physical therapist in conjunction with other early intervention professionals and the family. Determining a child's sensory-processing strengths and needs will help identify his or her primary avenues for learning as well as critical strategies to support development (Langley, 1996).

Gross and Fine Motor Skills

Impairments in motor skills compromise the integration of behaviors across other domains, such as cognition, social, and communication skills. In children with special needs, it is generally difficult to differentiate the influence of a motor impairment from other factors (Nelson, 1993). For some children with severe physical disabilities such as cerebral palsy, the ability to communicate may be impaired even though their underlying cognitive and linguistic abilities may be intact (Crais & Roberts, 1996). For children with motor impairments, it is important to consider the effect of the motor impairment on the conceptual development underlying their language production abilities, their speech production skills, and their ability to indicate needs through nonverbal means (e.g., gesture, eye contact, body posture). Examinations of motor skills will typically be completed by an occupational and/or physical therapist, although there are several multidomain instruments, such as the AEPS (Bricker, 1993) and the Batelle Developmental Inventory (Newborg, Stock, Wnek, Guidubaldi, & Svinicki, 1988), that include motor skills and may be administered by other early intervention personnel.

Oral-Motor Skills

With infants and toddlers, oral-motor skills play a significant role in both eating and communicating (Morris & Klein, 1987). A detailed history will include information about feeding, gagging, drooling, or swallowing difficulties; effects of postural tone and movement; types and textures of foods eaten; presence of abnormal reflexes or sensory reactions; respiration and sound-making abilities (speech and nonspeech sounds); imitative abilities; other fine motor skills (e.g., gestures, use of hands); other sequencing skills (e.g., hand motions for patty-cake); and for older toddlers, the ability to follow oral-motor commands (e.g., stick out tongue, open mouth). Much of the assessment will be performed by watching and listening to the child perform skills such as eating, communicating, and playing and by drawing associations between what he or she does currently and what the child appears capable of doing. Detailed assessment techniques can be found in Jaffe (1989), Morris and Klein (1987), and Sheppard (1987), and for material on children with motor speech disorders that can be adapted for infants and toddlers, see Crary (1995).

Interactive Readiness

An infant's or toddler's readiness for interaction is dependent on both physiologic and environmental factors, as well as the interaction of these factors. In identifying an infant's progression toward an organizational level that allows and facilitates social interaction, Als (1986) describes a hierarchy of tasks, or behavioral subsystems, that the infant must master. The five subsystems include physiologic stability and autonomic control; freedom and control in movemen; differentiation of, and control over, states of arousal; social interactive competence through attention and response to social stimuli; and self-regulation, or the ability to manage complex environmental demands with minimal expense to the lower subsystems (O'Donnell, 1996). These subsystems develop through transaction with each other and the environment; therefore, both the individual status of the subsystems and their interactive effects need to be examined. As illustrated by O'Donnell (1996), an infant may have achieved physiologic stability yet may still be struggling to control movements of the legs and arms when placed on his or her back. Thus, incomplete development in the motor area may compromise the infant's development of well-defined states of arousal and responses to social stimuli (O'Donnell, 1996).

As infants gain some control over these behavioral subsystems, they become more ready to interact with other people around them. In the early stages, infants indicate a readiness to interact by their ability to stay calm and alert when presented with stimuli (e.g., visual and/or auditory). If the stimuli become overwhelming, infants may communicate feelings of displeasure by crying or physically turning away, hiccuping, yawning, stretching their arms, splaying their fingers, placing a hand over their eyes, grimacing, or even falling asleep (Reinhartsen, Edmondson, & Crais, 1997). All these behaviors are signs that a baby may be receiving too much stimulation (Brazelton, 1982; Fogel, 1991). Throughout assessment and intervention planning, professionals and family members need to identify and adapt to the infant or toddler's signals and provide support for gaining control and organization over these early subsystems. For guidelines for conducting early behavioral assessments of neonates and infants in order to identify their readiness for interaction, see O'Donnell (1996) and Rossetti (1990a).

For older infants and toddlers, interactive readiness may be indicated by eye contact; tolerance of shared physical space or touch; giving, showing, or receiving objects; and/or vocalizations or verbalizations directed toward the family member or professional. It is common for young children to show hesitance or even avoidance of interaction with strangers (especially vocally or verbally); thus, the presence of people familiar to the child and the use of as natural an assessment setting as possible are critical. In addition, family members can often provide helpful tips for professionals in interacting with the child and facilitating interaction during assessment. Suggested strategies for facilitating interaction with older infants and toddlers appear in Table 1-2.

Table 1-2. Guidelines for Interactions With Children

1. Choose developmentally appropriate toys and materials.
2. Limit your own talking, especially questions. Pause often to encourage the child to initiate communication and take a turn.
3. Watch for, and encourage, any means of communication demonstrated by the child (e.g., eye gaze, point, shrug, vocalization, word).
4. Parallel play with the child, mimicking his or her actions. Play animatedly with a toy or other object and occasionally comment on an object or action.
5. Place a few items within eye gaze but out of reach, and partially hide a few others. If necessary, point to or comment on objects to encourage a comment or request by the child.
6. Let the child choose objects and/or activities, particularly in the beginning (and throughout the assessment if possible). Be prepared to watch and interact or comment when the child shows interest.
7. Include a parent, a sibling, or another child to help "break the ice." Stay in the background and then slowly join the interaction.
8. Begin the interaction with activities that require little or no talking and then gradually move to more vocal or verbal tasks.
9. Be genuine in your questions and stay away from asking what is obvious to both you and the child.
10. Follow the child's lead in the interaction by maintaining his or her focus on particular topics and meanings.
11. Show warmth and positive regard for the child and value for his or her comments.

Source: Crais, E., & Roberts, J. (1996). Assessing communication skills. In M. McLean, D. Bailey, & M. Wolery (Eds.), *Assessing infants and preschoolers with special needs* (2nd ed.), pp. 334–397. Upper Saddle River, NJ: Prentice-Hall. Used by permission.

Social Contingency Relationships

The infant's interactions with people and objects in the environment set the stage for the development of many behaviors considered to be antecedents of language (Carlson & Bricker, 1982; Seibert & Hogan, 1982). The development of communicative competence in the infant depends on the caregiver's social responsiveness, which in turn is influenced by the child's behaviors (Dunst, Lowe, & Bartholomew, 1990). Initially, the infant's communication is unintentional and refers to movements that are reflexive or involuntary and were not purposefully used by the child to communicate with others. These movements or behaviors are frequently interpreted by others to have meaning, and therefore evoke a response from the listener (Wetherby & Prizant, 1989; Wilcox, Kouri, & Caswell, 1990). These early signals may indicate the infant's physical or emotional state, such as a need to change position, hunger, or the need for attention or comfort. When a baby's caregivers learn to identify his or her signals, interpret them appropriately, and respond as quickly and consistently as possible, the baby learns that he or she can have an effect on the world (Dunst et al., 1990; Wilcox, 1992). Through this process, the child learns to become an effective communicator by gaining attention and having his or her needs met.

Some babies' early communication signals are difficult to interpret and their parents may have trouble learning how to read their cues (Field, 1987; Wetherby & Prizant, 1993; Wilcox, 1992). Due, for example, to cognitive or physical impairments, some children have difficulty expressing themselves either verbally or nonverbally (Beukelman & Mirenda, 1992; National Institute on Disability, 1992). Moreover, even those who use verbal means may be limited in their ability to be understood. In addition to children with established disabilities, infants with chronic illness or those born prematurely may send subtle and inconsistent communication signals, thus making it difficult for caregivers to determine what they need (Field, 1987; Wyley, 1995). Other children, in spite of their chronological age, remain at a preintentional level, and identifying their needs may be a complex process. Developing contingency relationships where the child learns to signal in a particular way to get his or her needs met, therefore, may be difficult for some infants and their parents.

Contingency relationships between infants with special needs and their caregivers may be compromised by: (a) the infant's medical involvement, which decreases the opportunity for social interaction, (b) parental attitudes and feelings that limit their provision of associated events, (c) the limited response repertoire of the infant, (d) the limited ability of some children to detect and remember co-occurrences, and (e) the complex interactions of the infant and the environment, which may reduce the frequency of social co-occurrences (Siegel-Causey, Ernst, & Guess, 1987). The following sections highlight several areas through which contingency relationships may be identified.

Intentionality

Between 8 and 12 months of age, children typically progress from using unintentional communicative behaviors to intentional behaviors that function to directly affect another's behavior (Dunst et al., 1990). Children in this stage communicate primarily to: (1) control someone else's behavior by making a request or protesting; (2) achieve and maintain social interaction by using greetings, playing social games such as peekaboo or patty-cake, gesturing, and showing off; and (3) draw joint attention to an object, event, or action shared by both the child and listener (Wetherby & Prizant, 1989). More detailed definitions of these **communicative functions** are found in Table 1-3. Later-developing intentions include requesting permission, acknowledging, clarifying, and requesting information; these may not emerge until the one-word or multiword stage (Wetherby & Prizant, 1989).

As infants develop intentionality, their early **communicative means** (e.g., limb movements, facial expressions, gestures, cries, and vocalizations) typically progress to more sophisticated means of communicating (Wetherby & Prizant, 1989). Gestures and gestures combined with vocalizations predominate from 8 to 12 months of age, and gestures are typically combined with wordlike vocalizations between 12 and 18 months (Chapman, 1981). For most children, these behaviors or signals eventually advance from speech-like sounds to words. Through observation, practice, and exploration of their environment, children develop more adult-like and easily recognized ways of communicating (Reinhartsen et al., 1997). Typically, between 11 to 15 months children begin to say a few words, and by their second birthday they have begun to put words together (Bates, Thal, & Janowsky, 1992).

For infants and toddlers, the focus in assessment will be on whether the child uses intentional communication, and if so, for what purposes and through what means. For preintentional children, the assessment may focus on working with caregivers to identify behaviors that could be interpreted and reinforced as intentional. For children who are clearly intentional, the issue involves identifying the range of communicative functions and means exhibited by the child and pinpointing ways to enhance or expand these means and functions. Helpful sources for identifying intentional or potentially intentional communication in young children and for evolving strategies to enhance intentionality include Crais and Roberts (1991), Paul (1995), Wetherby and Prizant (1989), and Wilcox (1992).

Cognitive Skills

As suggested by Neisworth and Bagnato (1992), most cognitive assessments measure the child's disability rather than his or her ability. For children with motor, sensory, and/or communication impairments, the task becomes one of separating out the contributing factors to identify their cognitive abilities. Often the child's cognitive level becomes the reference point to which other developmental domains are compared (i.e., cognitive referencing) and around which decisions about intervention are made (Cole, Dale, & Mills, 1990). As with other domains, assessment ranges from standardized testing using an instrument such as the Bayley Scales of Infant Development-II (Bayley, 1993) and performed by psychologists to observations of free play behaviors using multidomain worksheets completed by early intervention team members, such as the Transdisciplinary Play-Based Assessment (Linder, 1993). Midway between these types of assessment fall criterion-referenced instruments such as the AEPS (Bricker, 1993) and the Carolina Curriculum for Infants and Toddlers with Special Needs (Johnson-Martin et al., 1991), which are particularly helpful in intervention planning. In a move away from the sole use of standardized tests, many professionals are encouraging the use of multiple measures and sources of information to identify a child's cognitive skills, with a particular focus on functional skills (Neisworth & Bagnato, 1992). In recognizing the overlap of cognitive and play skills and their interrelatedness with communication skills, a thorough communication assessment can provide rich details regarding a child's cognitive capabilities.

Table 1-3. Definitions of Categories of Communicative Functions

BEHAVIOR REGULATION *Acts used to regulate the behavior of another person to obtain a specific result. The child's goal is to get the adult to do something or stop doing something.*

Examples include:

Request Object/Action Acts—used to direct another to give a desired object or to carry out an action

Protest Object/Action Acts—used to refuse an object that is not desired or to direct another to cease an action that is not desired.

SOCIAL INTERACTION *Acts used to attract or maintain another's attention to oneself. The child's goal is to get the adults to look at or notice him or her.*

Examples include:

Request Social Routine Acts—used to direct another to begin or continue carrying out a game-like social interaction

Request Comfort Acts—used to seek another's attention for comfort from wariness, distress, or frustration

Call Acts—used to gain the attention of another to indicate that a communicative act is to follow

Greet Acts: used to indicate notice of a person or object's presence or to signal the initiation or termination of an interaction

Show-Off Acts—used to attract another's attention to oneself by displaying a performance

Request Permission Acts—used to seek another's consent to carry out an action; involves carrying out or wanting to carry out the action

JOINT ATTENTION *Acts used to direct another's attention to an object, event, or topic of a communicative act. The child's goal is to get the adult to look at or notice an entity or event.*

Examples include:

Comment on Object/Action Acts—used to direct another's attention to an entity or event

Request Information Acts—used to seek out information, explanations, or clarifications about an entity, event, or previous utterance; includes *wh-* questions and other utterances with a rising intonation contour

UNCLEAR *Acts used for a communicative purpose but for which there is insufficient information to determine the category of function that they most appropriately fit. That is, it cannot be determined whether the child's goal is to communicate for behavior regulation, social interaction, or joint attention.*

Source: Wetherby, A., & Prizant, B. (1993). *Communication and symbolic behavior scales.* Chicago: Riverside.

Play Skills

Although there are a variety of taxonomies available for categorizing children's play behaviors, most fit into one, or a combination, of four types of measures. These include measures that examine the complexity and maturity of object play (e.g., how a child acts in relation to objects), social play (e.g., the extent to which others are incorporated in the child's play), affective motivational play (e.g., the child's affect in play, level of enthusiasm, persistence), and symbolic play (e.g., pretend play with objects). For any one sample of play behavior, different assessment results may be obtained based on the type of measure used.

A simple taxonomy created by Olswang and her colleagues as part of the ALB (Olswang et al., 1987) to document object and symbolic play is shown in Figure 1-1. Within this taxonomy, early object play includes looking at, mouthing, banging, and manipulating objects and bringing them close. Later, semiappropriate toy use begins as the child's understanding of the relationships of objects emerges. Examples could include the child brushing both his or her teeth and his or her hair with a toothbrush or using the back of a hairbrush to brush someone else's hair. As children develop more sophisticated play behaviors, they begin to nest and group similar objects (e.g., put smaller objects into larger ones), use toys appropriately, and act on multiple objects in the same way (e.g., child feeds stuffed animal, feeds doll, feeds parent). Later, different-action, multiple play episodes evolve where, for example, the child stirs a pot and then pretends to pour food out on a plate. Extended multiple play episodes include evidence that the child is sequencing three or more behaviors thematically (e.g., child pretends to put food in pot, stirs, and then pretends to put food on a plate).

Another type of object play includes constructive or combinatorial play, which involves the manipulation of materials to create a product. Constructive play activities could include the use of nesting cups, stacking blocks, stacking rings, modeling clay, or drawing materials. Infants and toddlers can be seen progressing from early behaviors, such as squeezing or patting modeling clay, putting blocks in a bowl, or marking with a crayon, to more elaborate behaviors, such as building small towers, doing one-piece puzzles, or nesting a few cups.

As part of the CSBS, Wetherby and Prizant (1993) provide a brief procedure for analyzing constructive play by engaging 9- to 24-month-old children in interactions with blocks, nesting cups, and stacking rings. First, they engage the child in a turn-taking game of building a tower of blocks, knocking it down, and then encouraging the child to build a tower unassisted. The stacking rings are then taken off the ring stacker, mixed up, and the child is encouraged to put them on. If the child stacks four blocks or rings (regardless of order), then three nesting cups are presented and a turn-taking game of nesting or stacking them takes place. After the child has had an opportunity to stack or nest unassisted and has succeeded in combining the three cups,

Play Behavior Checklist

On the grid, the left margin of each horizontal bar represents the point at which at least 15 percent of the normal subjects reached criterion; the right margin represents the point at which approximately 85 percent of the subjects reached criterion. The criterion for determining the existence of a play category is three exemplars, except for Grouping, for which the criterion is one exemplar. Check a box adjacent to a play category as that behavior is observed during play.

1. Mouthing Objects ( ) ( ) ( )
2. Banging Objects ( ) ( ) ( )
3. Visual Regarding ( ) ( ) ( )
4. Manipulating Objects ( ) ( ) ( )
5. Approximating Objects ( ) ( ) ( )
6. Semiappropriate Toy Use ( ) ( ) ( )
7. Nesting Objects ( ) ( ) ( )
8. Grouping Objects (n = 1) ( )
9. Appropriate Toy Use ( ) ( ) ( )
10. Same-action Multiple Play Episode ( ) ( ) ( )
11. Different-action Multiple Play Episode ( ) ( ) ( )
12. Extended Multiple Play Episode ( ) ( ) ( )

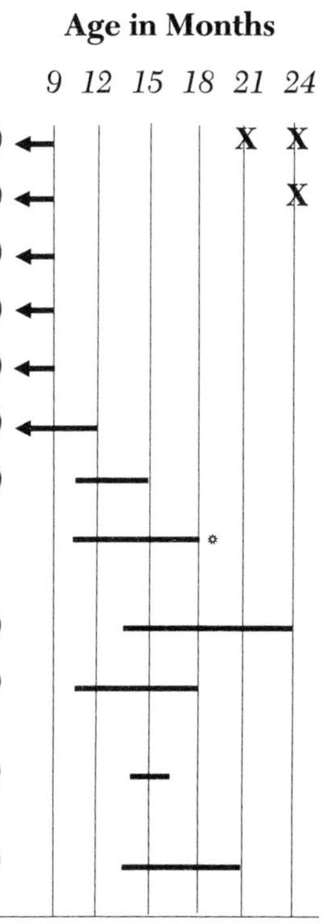

15% ——— 85%
* = Maximum value of 80%
x = Point at which occurrence of three or more behaviors can be viewed as atypical.

Figure 1-1. Play Scale. (From Olswang, L., Stoel-Gammon, C., Coggins, T., & Carpenter, R. [1987]. *Assessing prelinguistic and early linguistic behaviors in developmentally young children.* Seattle: University of Washington Press. Reprinted with permission.)

then he or she is given all six cups. Not only is the stacking or nesting ability of interest, so, too, are the ordering of objects, the child's persistence, the strategies used, and the child's frustration level. Thus, the opportunity to measure two play areas (i.e., object play and affective/motivational play) are included in this type of activity.

In regard to symbolic play, there is strong evidence that language and symbolic play are highly correlated and that during some stages of a child's development, they reflect common underlying cognitive processes (Kennedy, Sheridan, Radlinski, & Beeghly, 1991). As first words and consistent communicative gestures appear (12 to 20 months), single pretend schemes (e.g., child brushes teeth with toothbrush) are emerging during play (Kennedy et al., 1991). As children start to combine words (20 to 24 months), they commonly start to combine pretend schemes (e.g., child stirs in cup and feeds self). By 28 months, children are producing longer utterances and producing ordered play sequences (Kennedy et al., 1991; McCune-Nicholich & Bruskin, 1982). As suggested by Wetherby and Prizant (1993), symbolic play may be influenced by the child's social and cognitive abilities whereas constructive play may be a more direct measure of the child's mental representation abilities, with less social influence. Thus, both types of measures in infants and toddlers should be examined. See Westby (1988) for stages of symbolic play that correspond to stages of language development in young children.

As for affective/motivational aspects of play, developmental changes have been recognized in the way children sustain attention in play (Ruff & Lawson, 1990). As suggested by Ruff and Lawson, experimental results reflect developmental trends for more focused, effortful attention, and not just for attention generally. The increases in focused attention are associated with the increasing cognitive demands of more complex play and children's abilities to adapt their play to meet this complexity (Ruff & Lawson, 1990). Some aspects of affective/motivational play can be identified during examination of other types of play measures, which is a commonly occurring practice.

The final category of play, social play, is often exemplified by Parten's categories (1932) of unoccupied behavior, solitary play, onlooker behavior, parallel activity, associative play, and cooperative or organized play. Although these categories are not strictly developmental (children under 2 may exhibit all of the play behaviors), the more social categories do occur more frequently in older preschool children (Lifter, 1996; Parten, 1932). As suggested by Lifter (1996), Parten's taxonomy can be used along with other measures of play behaviors to gain a broader view of a child's play.

Two popular assessment tools focused on play are Linder's TPBA (1993) and Fewell's Play Assessment Scale (PAS) (1994). The TPBA includes six categories of play: three actions on objects (e.g., exploratory or sensorimotor, relational, and constructive play), plus symbolic (dramatic play), games with rules, and rough-and-tumble play. In terms of social play, there are planned opportunities throughout the TPBA to observe the child in play, both alone and with others (e.g., parent and peer). Within the TPBA chapter on cognitive development, there are also suggestions for attentional/motivational aspects. The PAS (Fewell, 1994) is a 45-item sequence of play behaviors from early infancy to 3 years. The items primarily represent acts on objects and symbolic behaviors, although some items attend to social and attentional/motivational aspects.

Language Production Skills

Language production includes behaviors such as producing sounds, words (word approximations or word equivalents, such as signs), and word combinations, as well as the ability to imitate others. Determining the child's ability to use sounds, words, or signs to get another's attention and to communicate needs is an essential component of a communication assessment.

Phonological Development. In order to make decisions regarding a child's overall communication level, an in-depth analysis of his or her capabilities for sound making must be performed. As suggested by Vihman (1992), phonological development is often a better predictor of developmental level than chronological age. Indeed, phonological development is interrelated with many other domains of development. For example, phonological development has a strong influence over the early words children produce (Bates et al., 1992; Ferguson & Farwell, 1975). Children often build their vocabulary with words with particular sounds, syllable structures, and sound classes or sound features (Lowe, 1994). Further, children as young as 18 months are more likely to learn new words that have sounds that are already in their inventories than words made up of sounds that are not (Schwartz & Leonard, 1982). In addition, children avoid the use of words they cannot produce and are selective in the words they will attempt. Phonological avoidance has also been shown to result in a delay in the emergence of two-word utterances and can limit the selection of words to be combined (Donahue, 1986; Matthei, 1989).

Lexical development also influences phonological development. A child's lexicon is predictive of phonological development, particularly in children with slow expressive language development (Paul & Jennings, 1992). As suggested by Paul and Jennings, it is difficult to determine whether these children's expressive language development is slow due to their poor phonological skills or their phonological skills are delayed because they have fewer words and, therefore, less opportunity to practice. The work of Rescorla and Ratner (1996), however, has indicated that children with specific expressive language impairment vocalize less than their typically developing peers, in addition to having proportionately smaller sound inventories and less-mature syllable shapes. In addition, Whitehurst and colleagues (Whitehurst, Smith, Fischel, Arnold, & Lonigan, 1991) noted a strong correlation between the amount of vocalizations with consonants and the language outcome in late talkers. The implications of these interrelationships for assessment are many, and to gain a full picture of the child's production skills, assessment must target both lexical/syntactic and phonological development.

In identifying delays in children's phonological development, it is first useful to identify critical milestones that serve as comparisons. Infants typically begin by producing reflexive sounds for the first few months, move on to comfort or cooing sounds between 2 and 4 months, begin to produce longer series of syllables and prolonged vowels and consonants with much vocal play between 4 and 6 months, produce reduplicated babbling between 7 and 9 months, and use more varied and complex babbling and their first words somewhere between 10 and 14 months (Smith, Goffman, & Stark, 1995). The most common early syllable types are consonant-vowel (CV), VC, and CVC; if CVCV syllables occur, they are typically reduplications (e.g., "wawa" for water) (Ferguson & Farwell, 1975; French, 1989). Although there is some variability across children, the most frequently used early consonants are nasals (/m/, /n/), labial stops (/p/, /b/), dental stops (/d/, /t/), velar stops (/k/, /g/), plus /h/, /w/, and /sh/ (Ferguson & Farwell, 1975; Vihman, 1992). The early vowels are typically /a/, /u/, and /i/ (Ingram, 1976). The number of sounds in the phonological inventory progresses from 3.4 phones (/b/, /d/, /h/ produced by 50 percent of children in the study) at 15 months, to 6.3 phones (/b/, /d/, /m/, /n/, /h/, /w/) at 18 months, 6.7 phones (/b/, /t/, /d/, /m/, /n/, /h/) at 21 months, and 9.5 phones (/b/, /d/, /t/, /k/, /g/, /m/, /n/, /h/, /w/, /f/, /s/) at 24 months (Stoel-Gammon, 1985).

Prosodic elements also develop in infants and toddlers. Young children use pitch variation and supersegmentals to indicate differences in meaning (Lowe, 1994). Between 8 and 10 months, infants begin to use prosodic contours and consonant-vowel babbling sounds that begin to approximate the linguistic input that surrounds them (Bates et al., 1992). Children also often use prosody to make a request or ask a question before acquiring the words to fill these slots (Dore, 1975). Prosodic units provide a social function (Lowe, 1994) and provide evidence for developing speech acts (Dore, 1975). Three parameters contribute to the perception of prosody—rate, intonational contour, and intensity changes—and these are used to signal word and sentence stress (Strand, 1995). The identification of the use of prosodic elements with children with expressive output disorders has been suggested by many (Dworkin, 1991; Strand, 1995).

For infants and toddlers, it is important to identify both the child's stage of phonological development (e.g., vocalizations, word approximations, words) and his or her breadth of sound-making capabilities at any one level. For example, a child may be producing words but with a very limited repertoire of syllable shapes or consonants and vowels. This child's prognosis would be quite different from that for a child who may not yet be producing words but who already has in vocal play a large range of consonants and vowels as well as varied syllable shapes. Thus, assessing phonological development serves as both a prognostic indicator and a later guide to choosing words to be included in the child's early lexicon (Paul, 1995).

For young children with no word approximations or recognizable words, parental report and observation of the child's sound production inventory can be compared with what might be expected at that chronological age. The child's use of prosodic elements, even in unintelligible strings, can signal the child's advancing development in sound and/or word-like combinations. For young children who are beginning to produce words or word approximations, Paul and Jennings's (1992) findings, that typically developing 18- to 24-month-old children produce an average of 14 different consonants in a 10-minute communication sample, can be used for a comparison. Parents can also be asked to list the child's words or word approximations, which can be categorized by individual sounds in terms of whether each sound occurs at the beginning, middle, or end of words.

Lexical Development. The acquisition of vocabulary has been argued to be the basis of learning in general and an indication of the child's ability to abstract from the environment the words and concepts that are important in the dominant culture (Sternberg & Powell, 1983). Vocabulary development is a window into his or her experiences, the input language, and the sociocultural influences that surround the child. Both comprehension and production vocabularies are important to ascertain, as is their relative development over time.

The acquisition of the first 50 words in production is a major milestone for many children and has been linked to an assortment of other developments. For example, by the end of this stage (between 18 and 20 months), the child is typically able to comprehend approximately 200 words (Ingram, 1989), indicating a major surge in comprehension vocabulary, from an average of 57.9 words at 10 months (Fenson et al., 1990). Acquisition of the first 50 words is fairly slow, especially compared to the "vocabulary burst" that frequently occurs after 50 words. Middle-class parents typically report that their children produce an average of 3.6 words or word-like sounds at 10 months, 11.9 at 12 months, 43.4 at 15 months, 79 at 16 months, 178.9 at 20 months, and 317 at 24 months (Fenson et al., 1990).

The first words typically refer to things and events in the "here and now," which are often things that move, act on other things, and are acted on by the child (Cairns, 1995). The largest proportion of early words consists of the names of people and things, followed by action words (Benedict, 1979). In examining a child's lexical development both the type of words used (e.g., object or person words, action words, possessives) and the range of words within types are important. For identifying emerging words and word approximations, parental report and observation can provide the data around which intervention planning can occur. As children acquire a larger set of words, from 9 to 30 months of age, parent report tools such as the MacArthur Communicative Development Inventories (Fenson et al., 1990) can be used to document production vocabularies. In addition, the 9- to 16-month form (Words and Gestures) allows a look at both production and comprehension vocabularies. The 16- to 30-month form (Words and Sentences) also documents some aspects of morphological and syntactic development.

Emergence of Word Combinations. Word combinations typically emerge between 18 to 24 months, but some typically developing children do not produce word combinations until after 24 months (Fenson, et al., 1990). An early red flag for a 24-month-old child is a failure to have a production vocabulary of 50 words and/or no two-word combinations (Rescorla, 1989). However, as indicated by the work of Rescorla and Schwartz (1990) and Paul, Looney, and Dahm (1991), by age 3, half of these "late talkers" will perform at age level on standardized measures. Thus, distinguishing between who will and who will not "outgrow" these early delays can be difficult (Paul, 1991). As suggested by Bates et al. (1992), the correlation between word combinations and vocabulary size is stronger than the correlation between word combinations and age. Most children begin to combine words when their cumulative vocabulary is between 50 and 100 words (Bates et al., 1992; Fenson et al., 1990); however, not all typically developing children do (Fenson et al., 1990). Thus, although vocabulary size can be predictive of the emergence of two-word combinations for some children, other factors, such as phonological, social, cognitive, and imitative skills, can help sort out the late talkers from children with expressive language disorders.

In examining a child's word combinations, it is important to identify the type of semantic relations (e.g., agent-action, action-object) and the range of relations used. Table 1-4 is a list of the most common semantic relations expressed in prelinguistic, one-word, and multiword utterances. Helpful sources for analyzing semantic complexity include Paul (1995) and Retherford (1993).

Development of Imitative Skills. In typical development, 8 to 10 months is often the turning point in becoming able to reproduce novel vocal and gestural patterns (Bates et al., 1992). Children begin the move toward full imitation through several stages (Piaget, 1954, 1962), starting with "pseudo-imitation" by neonates, who are able to reproduce a small set of innate motor patterns in response to an adult model (Meltzoff & Moore, 1979). Pseudo-imitation (repetition of adult models that already occur in the child's repertoire) continues through the 8th month until around the 9th month, when true imitation (repetition of novel motor patterns) appears. The stage of deferred imitation (reproduction of novel motor patterns from memory) typically occurs somewhere between 12 and 18 months (Bates et al., 1992), although it has been shown to occur in infants as young as 9 months (Meltzoff, 1988). This developmental progression highlights two important hierarchies in children's imitative abilities, from the use of patterns within the child's repertoire to the use of novel ones and from immediate to delayed imitations.

A continuum of difficulties has been reported to exist between the early indicators of phonological processing and imitative production and the later appearance of language-learning disabilities (Crary, 1993; Scarborough, 1990; Stackhouse, 1992; Stackhouse & Snowling, 1992; Tallal, 1980). Young children who fail to learn to imitate speech are also most likely to experience later disabilities in expressive formulation/language organization, developmental apraxia of speech, or language-learning disabilities (Velleman & Strand, 1994). Specific problems in early imitative ability include difficulty with speech/motor sequencing, limited expressive vocabulary, restricted length of

Table 1-4. Semantic Relations Expressed in Prelinguistic, One-Word, and Multiword Utterances

		Child Behavior		
General Relationship	Function/ Meaning	Prelinguistic	One-Word	Multiword
Agent	The individual performing the action	Throws ball to teacher and smiles proudly	Throws ball and says, "Me"	"Me throw."
Action	Requests action	Raises hands to be picked up	"Up," to indicate "Pick me up"	"Up Mommy."
Object	Comments on the object of action	Points to ball being pushed	"Ball," as ball is pushed	"Ball go."
Recurrence	Requests/ comments on repetition of activity/object	Drinks milk and holds up empty bottle	"More," to indicate more milk	"Me more milk."
Nonexistence	Comments on nonexistence/ disappearance of object or person	Points to missing wheel on car	"Wheel," while pointing to car	"No wheel."
Cessation	Comments on cessation of activity	Points to top that stopped spinning	"Stop," to indicate top is no longer spinning	"Top stop."
Rejection	Protests/ comments on undesired action or something forbidden	Turns head away from food	"No," in response to being offered peas	"No peas."
Location	Comments on spatial location	Holds truck and points to box	"Box," while pointing to toy box	"Put box."
Possession	Comments on possession of object	Reaches for own shoes among others' shoes and points	"Mine," while getting own shoes	"My shoes."
Agent-action*	Comments on agent and action			"Boy hit."
Action-object*	Comments on action and object			"Kick ball."
Agent-action object*	Comments on agent, action, and object			"Mommy throw ball."
Action-object-location*	Comments on agent, action, and location			"Put ball chair."

*These are more commonly used examples of relational combinations; many possibilities exist.

Source: Crais, E., & Roberts, J. (1996). Assessing communication skills. In M. McLean, D. Bailey and M. Wolery (Eds.), *Assessing infants and preschoolers with special needs* (2nd ed.). Upper Saddle River, N.J.: Prentice-Hall. Used by permission.

utterance, meager phonologic repertoire, inadequate organization of syllable structure, and problems in object naming and letter/sound association (Lund & Duchan, 1988; Parsons, 1984; Stackhouse & Snowling, 1992). Early assessment is a means to identify the risk for these later problems. The examination of imitative ability can be included in the oral-motor observations and activities noted previously.

Language Comprehension Skills

In assessing young children it is important to identify both their linguistic and their nonlinguistic comprehension. Chapman (1978) provides an excellent overview of infants' and toddlers' response strategies as utilized in comprehending their environment. Early nonlinguistic strategies, used between 8 and 12 months, include looking at objects looked at by others, acting on objects that are noticed, and imitating ongoing actions. Strategies used in the 12- to 18-month stage are typically based on some linguistic aspect and include attending to an object that was mentioned, giving evidence of notice to objects or actions, and doing what is usually done in a given situation (e.g., child goes to door when others do). In addition to those already mentioned, strategies used from 18 to 24 months include acting on objects as the agent (e.g., child brushes own teeth when asked to "brush the baby's teeth") and using conventional behaviors (e.g., combing hair with comb). Excellent techniques for assessing the comprehension skills of young children are provided in Miller and Paul (1995) and Paul (1995).

Parent-Child Interaction

The transactional model of development (Sameroff & Fiese, 1990) has had a profound impact on the way in which professionals view the early intervention process, and most particularly, parent-child interactions. The transactional model views parents as the primary influence on a child's development and suggests that the effects of intervention are mediated through the parent-child relationship (Dunst, 1993; Mahoney, Spiker, & Boyce, 1996). Within this model, the ability of parents to interact effectively with their children is seen as a complex process that is influenced by the economic, social, and familial supports available to parents (Mahoney et al., 1996). Given the strong influence parents have on their child's development, the inclusion of parent-child interaction as a key area within the assessment process has been recommended by many in the field (Greenspan & Meisels, 1994; McLean & McCormick, 1993).

The three primary means for examining parent-child interaction include the formal use of one or more parent-child interaction scales, the use of information from parent-child interaction scales to guide informal information gathering, and the use of evaluative judgment based on personal experiences and beliefs (see Mahoney et al., 1996, for a thorough review of each method). As indicated by Mahoney and his colleagues (1996), although each approach may be worthwhile, all three are influenced by problems with reliability and validity. For example, many of the parenting characteristics (e.g., enjoyment, praise, physical involvement) identified on parent/child interaction scales fail to be significant predictors of child functioning (Mahoney et al., 1996). In addition, across all three means of assessment, contextual issues such as the setting (e.g., home, clinic), familiarity of the observers, type of materials or toys available, type of interaction requested (e.g., completion of particular task, free play), and length of the observation can all influence how children and their parents interact. Moreover, sociocultural factors, such as culture, ethnicity, and socioeconomic level, as well as personality and interactive style strongly influence how various behaviors are exhibited and viewed. Thus, the problems with reliability and validity of most parent-child assessment methods indicate a need for care in their use.

An additional dilemma in assessing parent-child interaction is how to accomplish this task in a way that is family centered and therefore gives the family the key role in the decision-making process. One method, described by Gillette (Chapter 5), MacDonald (1989), and MacDonald and Gillette (1989), involves professionals and the family collaboratively identifying current parent-child interaction practices. These practices are then related to four primary outcomes: establishing a partnership between partner and child, developing routines together, acting and communicating in progressively matched ways, and sharing enjoyment. As parents and professionals identify desired modifications to parent-child interactions, they can use the guidelines and the child and partner strategies to enhance their interactions through play.

Another alternative in keeping with family-centered practices is to find out first what families want from the assessment (e.g., ideas for how to enhance their child's communication skills, ideas for ways to play with their child) and to begin working from the family's and child's strengths in their current interactions. Family members can be asked what things they already do that help the child communicate and the conditions or situations when the child communicates most effectively. Through this process, family members and professionals can build on skills and strategies that are already used and identify ways to make small refinements. The literature has also indicated a number of behaviors that facilitate communication, including providing contingent responses to what the child does, says, or looks at; providing positive models; imitating or expanding the child's actions or words; accepting and reinforcing the child's attempts; and providing the child with adequate time to initiate and respond to adults (Duchan, 1989; Dunst et al., 1990; Peck, 1989). Helping families gradually become aware of and learn to utilize some of these techniques intermixed with their current practices may also facilitate their children's communication skills. In this way, professionals scaffold the type and amount of support provided to parents without making every decision regarding how the parent-child interactions should, or could, be modified (McCollum & Yates, 1994).

Finally, as argued by Conti-Ramsden (1990), assessing and attempting to modify parental interactional behaviors may convey the message that the parents have somehow failed to provide what the child needed or, worse, that they may have contributed to the child's difficulties. Thus, in both examining and identifying strategies for modification, professionals need to be mindful of the message they send and respectful of the parents' individual style of communicating. Positive ideas for examining and influencing parent-child interactions within a family-centered context can be found in Gillette (Chapter 5 of this book) and McCollum and Yates (1994).

CASE STUDY: STEVEN

Once the basic referral information had been gained about Steven (reported in the Overview to this chapter), the service coordinator suggested that a preassessment planning meeting be held at the family's home. The suggested purposes of this meeting were to identify further Steven's parents' concerns, pinpoint his current strengths and needs, and set the parameters for the upcoming assessment. Due to Steven's reported hesitancy around strangers, the communications concerns expressed by his parents, and the lack of concerns in other major areas, it was agreed the speech-language pathologist and a psychologist would make up the initial team of professionals. Steven's parents were encouraged that these two professionals would work to keep the focus off Steven and to begin building some initial rapport with him and his older sister, Sarah. His parents were asked to complete a child history form and return it to the early intervention center before the first meeting.

During the preassessment planning meeting, the two professionals and Steven's parents talked around the kitchen table while Steven and Sarah played in the adjoining den. After confirming Steven's medical and developmental histories and the parents' immediate concerns, the professionals asked what the parents hoped to gain from the assessment. The parents related that they knew Steven's communication skills were delayed and that they were primarily looking for ideas on how to help him further develop his skills. They also suggested that they were concerned about his "shyness" and wanted ideas to help him "come out of himself more." The professionals then asked Steven's parents to describe his current skills, needs, and preferences for toys and activities. In discussing where the assessment should take place, everyone agreed that Steven would be most comfortable in his own home and, because his parents had no other concerns (e.g., medical, gross, or fine motor), that the two professionals currently in attendance would take part.

During this first meeting, the professionals listed for the parents various alternatives for assessment ranging from the use of standardized tools to primarily observation methods, with interactive/observational activities placed between the two ends of the continuum. After describing each type of assessment, the parents noted that the interactive/observational approach seemed best and that they felt Steven would be resistant if "pressed" for too much interaction, especially in the beginning. The professionals explained that if Steven were in need of intervention services he would have to be referred to, and determined eligible, by the local early intervention consortium. Therefore, his report would need to include some developmental estimates of his current skills and delays, since no formal test scores would be available. His parents said they would be interested in obtaining this type of information as well. When offered the option of documenting Steven's skills in the next week before his assessment, his parents seemed interested and wanted ideas of ways to do this. Since his parents were concerned about his overall communication skills, a parent report tool that would identify Steven's current comprehension skills and document some of his social and play skills was provided (MacArthur Communicative Development Inventory) (Fenson et al., 1990). In addition, his parents were encouraged to write down the different sounds he was currently making and to make note of any gestures, eye contact, or vocalizations that he used to communicate and the situation surrounding them. The professionals also asked if the parents would be willing to play with Steven and Sarah during the assessment to give them a better idea of how they themselves might interact with the children. They also suggested that the parents might provide for a snack during the visit so that they could gain an idea of Steven's oral motor skills while eating. Finally, they noted that since Steven had not had his hearing tested, audiological testing should be set up at the early intervention center to rule out a hearing loss.

When discussing the sequence of the assessment, the professionals asked Steven's parents how they thought things should begin. The parents suggested that they begin by playing with both children and then letting the professionals gradually begin to interact. The professionals noted they would use some portions of the Communication and Symbolic Behavior Scales (Wetherby & Prizant, 1993) and described the activities and materials that would be used (e.g., "communication temptations," constructive and symbolic play items). They suggested that these activities would highlight some of the ways in which and reasons why Steven communicates and would provide information on his level of play skills. Steven's parents seemed to like the idea of the temptations, which were designed to encourage Steven to interact with the professionals, and they also were pleased that they would sit next to their child during this part of the assessment. The professionals noted that throughout the assessment they would observe Steven's fine and gross motor, sound-making, social-emotional, imitation, and problem-solving skills to help identify further his strengths and needs.

For this first visit, the professionals brought a few toys in an open carrying bag in order to engage Steven and Sarah. When Sarah showed interest in one of the toys, she was encouraged to take it out and play with it. Later in the meeting, Steven actually moved toward the bag himself and began trying to get out a toy. He did not make eye contact with the professional or interact with her, but he whined and fussed when he was not easily able to get the toy out. The professional helped him, after which he took the toy to the den to play with; later he returned for another toy. His parents noted their surprise that he would even get in close proximity to the two professionals and felt encouraged by his "boldness."

In sum, the joint planning process allowed the resulting assessment to contain the major components of ecologically valid assessments (i.e., caregiver participation, sociocultural validity, naturalistic observation, and planning for the child's immediate and future settings). It also allowed the professionals to include the parameters of assessment that they and the family thought valid and useful for the particular child and family. The jointly gathered information and results confirmed the parents' concerns, provided a starting point for generating ecologically valid intervention strategies, and helped set the stage for collaborative efforts between these parents and the professionals, and also any future professionals the parents may encounter.

SUMMARY

Assessment that is not representative of the many social, physical, and cultural contexts that influence the lives of infants and toddlers cannot be seen as a valid estimate of a child's overall abilities. To be ecologically valid, assessment efforts must include more than just the use of standardized tests and must involve procedures individualized for each child and family. Moreover, if assessment is not meaningful to parents and other caregivers in ways that help them plan for the child, both immediately and in the future, then professionals have probably focused on the wrong things. If professionals and families are to develop comprehensive plans that meet the needs of both children and families, they must work together to identify what should be assessed, the specific assessment conditions, and what the implications of the results will mean for the child and family. This chapter has attempted to bring together the science and the art of assessing infants and toddlers and can serve as a guide to professionals and families who are seeking a more ecologically valid assessment process.

REFERENCES

Als, H. (1986). Assessing the neurobehavioral development of the preterm infant and the environment of the neonatal intensive care unit: A synactive model of neonatal behavioral organization. *Physical and Occupational Therapy in Pediatrics, 6,* 3–53.

American Academy of Pediatrics Committee on Practice and Ambulatory Medicine. (1986). Vision screening and eye examination in children. *Pediatrics, 77,* 918.

Anderson, M., & Goldberg, P. (1991). *Cultural competence in screening and assessment: Implications for services to young children with special needs ages birth through five.* Chapel Hill, N.C.: National Early Childhood Technical Assistance System.

Andrews, J., & Andrews, M. (1990). *Family based treatment in communicative disorders.* Sandwich, Ill.: Janelle Publications.

Bailey, D. (1989). Assessment and its importance in early intervention. In D. Bailey & M. Wolery (Eds.), *Assessing infants and preschoolers with handicaps* (pp. 1–21). Columbus, O.: Merrill.

Bailey, D., McWilliam, P., Winton, P., & Simeonsson, R. (1992). *Implementing family-centered services in early intervention: A team-based model for change.* Cambridge, Mass.: Brookline Books.

Bailey, D., & Simeonsson, R. (1990). *The Family Needs Survey–Revised.* Chapel Hill, N.C.: Frank Porter Graham Child Development Center.

Bates, E., Thal, D., & Janowsky, J. (1992). Early language development and its neural correlates. In I. Rapin & S. Segalowitz (Eds.), *Handbook of neuropsychology: Vol. 7. Child neurology* (pp. 693–110). Amsterdam: Elsevier.

Battle, D. (1993). *Communication disorders in multicultural populations.* Stoneham, Mass.: Andover Medical Publications.

Bayley, N. (1993). *Bayley Scales of Infant Development–II.* San Antonio: Psychological Corporation.

Benedict, H. (1979). Early lexical development: Comprehension and production. *Journal of Child Language, 6,* 183–200.

Beukelman, D., & Mirenda, P. (1992). *Augmentative and alternative communication: Management of severe communication disorders in children and adults.* Baltimore: Brookes.

Brazelton, B. (1982). Joint regulation of neonate-parent behavior. In E. Tronick (Ed.), *Social interchange in infancy* (pp. 7–35). Baltimore: University Park Press.

Bricker, D. (1993). *AEPS measurement for birth to three years* (Vol. 1). Baltimore: Brookes.

Bricker, D., & Cripe, J. (1992). *An activity-based approach to early intervention.* Baltimore: Brookes.

Bronfenbrenner, U. (1977). Toward an experimental ecology of human development. *American Psychologist, 32*(7), 513–531.

Cairns, H. (1995). *The acquisition of language* (2nd ed.). Austin, Tex.: Pro-Ed.

Carlson, L., & Bricker, D. (1982). Dyadic and contingent aspects of early communicative intervention. In D. Bricker (Eds.), *Intervention with at-risk and handicapped infants* (pp. 291–309). Baltimore: University Park Press.

Chapman, R. (1978). Comprehension strategies in children. In J. Kavanaugh & W. Strange (Eds.), *Speech and language in the laboratory, school, and clinic* (pp. 308–327). Cambridge, Mass.: MIT Press.

Chapman, R. (1981). Exploring children's communicative intents. In J. Miller (Ed.), *Assessing language production in children* (pp. 111–138). Baltimore: University Park Press.

Cole, K., Dale, P., & Mills, P. (1990). Defining language delay in young children by cognitive referencing: Are we saying more than we know? *Applied Psycholinguistics, 11,* 291–302.

Conti-Ramsden, G. (1990). Maternal recasts and other contingent replies to language-impaired children. *Journal of Speech and Hearing Disorders, 55,* 262–274.

Crais, E. (1993). Families and professionals as collaborators in assessment. *Topics in Language Disorders, 14*(1), 29–40.

Crais, E. (1995). Expanding the repertoire of tools and techniques for assessing the communication skills of infants and toddlers. *American Journal of Speech-Language Pathology, 4*(3), 47–59.

Crais, E., & Roberts, J. (1991). Decision making in assessment and early intervention planning. *Language, Speech, Hearing Services in Schools, 22*(2), 19–30.

Crais, E. & Roberts, J. (1996). Assessing communication skills. In M. McLean, D. Bailey, & M. Woolery (Eds.), *Assessing infants and preschoolers with special needs* (2nd ed.)(pp. 334–397). Upper Saddle River, N.J.: Prentice-Hall.

Crais, E., & Wilson, L. (1996). The role of parents in child assessment: Self-evaluation by practicing professionals. *Infant-Toddler Intervention, 6*(2), 125–143.

Crary, M. (1993). *Developmental motor speech disorders.* San Diego: Singular Press.

Crary, M. (1995). Clinical evaluation of developmental motor speech disorders. *Seminars in Speech and Language, 16*(2), 110–125.

Cripe, J., & Bricker, D. (1993). *Family Interest Survey.* In J. Cripe, K. Slentz, & D. Bricker (Eds.), *AEPS curriculum for birth to three years* (Vol. 2, pp. 315–319). Baltimore: Brookes.

Cripe, J., Slentz, K., & Bricker, D. (1993). *AEPS curriculum for birth to three years* (Vol. 2). Baltimore: Brookes.

DiGangi, A., & Greenspan, S. (1989). *Test of Sensory Function in Infants.* Los Angeles: Western Psychological Services.

Donahue, M. (1986). Phonological constraints on the emergence of two word utterances. *Journal of Child Language, 13*(2), 209–218.

Dore, J. (1975). Holophrases, speech acts and language universals. *Journal of Child Language, 3,* 22–39.

Duchan, J. (1989). Evaluating adults' talk to children: Addressing adult attunement. *Seminars in Speech and Language, 10,* 17–27.

Dunst, C. (1993). Implications of risk and opportunity factors for assessment and intervention practices. *Topics in Early Childhood Special Education,. 13,* 143–153.

Dunst, C., Jenkins, V., & Trivette, C. (1988). Family Support Scale. In C. Dunst, C. Trivette, & A. Deal (Eds.), *Enabling and empowering families* (p. 157). Cambridge, Mass.: Brookline Books.

Dunst, C., Lowe, L., & Bartholomew, P. (1990). Contingent social responsiveness, family ecology, and infant communicative competence. *National Student Speech, Language, and Hearing Association, 17*, 39–49.

Dworkin, P. (1991). *Motor speech disorders: A treatment guide.* St. Louis: Mosby.

Fenson, L., Dale, P., Reznick, S., Thal, D., Bates, E., Hartung, J., Pethick, S., & Reilly, J. (1993). *MacArthur Communicative Development Inventories.* San Diego: Singular Publishing.

Ferguson, C., & Farwell, C. (1975). Words and sounds in early language acquisition: English consonants in the first fifty words. *Language, 51*, 419–439.

Fewell, R. (1994). *Play Assessment Scale* (fifth revision). Mailman Center for Child Development, University of Miami School of Medicine, Miami, Fla.

Field, T. (1987). Affective and interactive disturbances in infants. In J. Osofsky (Ed.), *Handbook of infant development* (pp. 972–1005). New York: Wiley.

Fogel, A. (1991). *Infancy* (2nd ed.). St. Paul: West Publishing.

French, A. (1989). The systematic acquisition of word forms by a child during the first fifty-word stage. *Journal of Child Language, 16*, 69–90.

Greenspan, S., & Meisels, S. (1994). Toward a new vision of developmental assessment of infants and young children. *Zero to Three, 16*(6), 1–8.

Hanson, M., & Lynch, E. (1992). Family diversity: Implications for policy and practice. *Topics in Early Childhood Special Education, 12*(3), 283–306.

Harrison, M., & Roush, J. (1996). Age of suspicion, identification, and intervention for infants and young children with hearing loss: A national study. *Ear and Hearing, 17*, 55–62.

Individuals with Disabilities Education Act, Pub. L. No. 105-17 (1997). Washington, DC: Federal Register, June 4.

Ingram, D. (1989). *First language acquisition.* Cambridge, U.K.: Cambridge University Press.

Jaffe, M. (1989). Feeding at-risk infants and toddlers. *Topics in Language Disorders, 10*(1), 13–25.

Johnson-Martin, N., Jens, K., Attermeier, S., & Hacker, B. (1991). *Carolina Curriculum for Infants and Toddlers with Special Needs* (2nd ed.). Baltimore: Brookes.

Joint Committee on Infant Hearing. (1991). 1990 position statement. *American Speech-Language-Hearing Association, 33*(Suppl. 5), 3–6.

Kennedy, M., Sheridan, M., Radlinski, S., & Beeghly, M. (1991). Play-language relationships in young children with developmental delays: Implications for assessment. *Journal of Speech and Hearing Research, 34*, 112–122.

Kjerland, L., & Kovach, J. (1990). Family-staff collaboration for tailored infant assessment. In E. Gibbs & D. Teti (Eds.), *Inter-disciplinary assessment of infants: A guide for early intervention professionals* (pp. 287–298). Baltimore: Brookes.

Langley, M. (1996). Screening and assessment of sensory functions. In M. McLean, D. Bailey, & M. Wolery (Eds.), *Assessing infants and preschoolers with special needs* (pp. 123–164). Baltimore: Brookes.

Leet, H., & Dunst, C. (1988). Family Resource Scale. In C. Dunst, C. Trivette, & A. Deal, *Enabling and empowering families* (p. 141). Cambridge, Mass.: Brookline Books.

Lifter, K. (1996). Assessing play skills. In M. McLean, D. Bailey, & M. Wolery (Eds.), *Assessing infants and preschoolers with special needs* (pp. 435–461). Baltimore: Brookes.

Linder, T. (1993). *Transdisciplinary play-based assessment: A functional approach to working with young children* (revised edition). Baltimore: Brookes.

Lowe, R. (1994). *Phonology: Assessment and intervention applications in speech pathology.* Baltimore: Williams & Wilkins.

Lund, N., & Duchan, J. (1988). *Assessing children's language in naturalistic contexts.* Englewood, N.J.: Prentice-Hall.

Lynch, E., & Hanson, M. (Eds.). (1992). *Developing cross-cultural competence: A guide for working with young children and their families.* Baltimore: Brookes.

MacDonald, J. (1989). *Becoming partners: From play to conversation.* Chicago: Riverside Press.

MacDonald, J., & Gillette, Y. (1989). *The introduction to the ECO program.* Chicago: Riverside Press.

Mahoney, G., Spiker, D., & Boyce, G. (1996). Clinical assessments of parent-child interactions: Are professionals ready to implement this practice? *Topics in Early Childhood Special Education, 16*(1), 26–50.

Matthei, E. (1989). Crossing boundaries: More evidence for phonological constraints on early multiword utterances. *Journal of Child Language, 16*(1), 41–54.

McCollum, J., & Yates, T. (1994). Dyad as focus, triad as means: A family-centered approach to supporting parent-child interactions. *Infants and Young Children, 6*(4), 54–63.

McCune-Nicholich, L., & Bruskin, C. (1982). Combinatorial competency in play and language. In K. Rubin & D. Pepler (Eds.), *The play of children: Current theory and research* (pp. 30–45). New York: Karger.

McGonigel, M., Kaufman, R., & Johnson, B. (1991). *Guidelines and recommended practices for the individualized family service plan* (2nd ed.). Baltimore: Association for the Care of Children's Health.

McLean, M., & Crais, E. (1996). Procedural considerations in assessing infants and preschoolers with special needs. In M. McLean, D. Bailey, & M. Wolery (Eds.), *Assessing infants and preschoolers with special needs* (pp. 46–68). Columbus, Ohio.: Macmillan.

McLean, M., & McCormick, K. (1993). Assessment and evaluation in early intervention. In W. Brown, S. Thurman, & L. Pearl (Eds.), *Family-centered early intervention with infants and toddlers: Innovative cross-disciplinary approaches* (pp. 43–79). Baltimore: Brookes.

McWilliam, P., Winton, P., & Crais, E. (1996). *Practical strategies for family-centered early intervention.* San Diego: Singular Publishing.

McWilliam, R. (1995). *Family-centered intervention planning: A routines-based approach.* Tucson: Communication Skill Builders.

Meltzoff, A., (1988). Infant imitation and memory: Nine-month-olds in immediate and deferred tests. *Child Development, 59,* 217–225.

Meltzoff, A. & Moore, M. (1979). Interpreting "imitative" responses in early infancy. *Science, 205,* 217–219.

Miller, J., & Paul, R. (1995). *The clinical assessment of language comprehension.* Baltimore: Brookes.

Moore, S., & Beatty, J. (1995). *Developing cultural competence in early childhood assessment.* Boulder: University of Colorado at Boulder.

Morris, S., & Klein, M. (1987). *Pre-feeding skills: A comprehensive resource for feeding development.* Tucson: Communication/Therapy Skill Builders.

National Institute on Disability and Rehabilitation Research. (1992). Consensus statement on augmentative and alternative communication intervention, Washington, DC: Author.

National Institutes of Health. (1993). NIH consensus statement. Bethesda, Md.: Author.

Neisworth, J., & Bagnato, S. (1992). The case against intelligence testing in early intervention. *Topics in Early Childhood Special Education, 12*(1), 1–20.

Neisworth, J., Bagnato, S., & Munson, S. (1989). Linking developmental assessment and early intervention: *Curriculum-based prescriptions* (2nd ed.). Rockville, Md.: Aspen.

Nelson, N. (1993). *Childhood language disorders in context: Infancy through adolescence.* New York: Merrill.

Newborg, J., Stock, J., Wnek, L., Guidubaldi, J., & Svinicki, J. (1988). *The Battelle Developmental Inventory.* Allen, Tex.: DLM/Teaching Resources.

O'Donnell, K. (1996). Neurobehavioral assessment of the newborn infant. In M. McLean, D. Bailey, & M. Wolery (Eds.), *Assessing infants and preschoolers with special needs* (pp. 165–201). Columbus, Ohio.: Merrill.

Olswang, L., Stoel-Gammon, C., Coggins, T., & Carpenter, R. (1987). *Assessing prelinguistic and early linguistic behaviors in developmentally young children.* Seattle: University of Washington Press.

Parsons, C. (1984). A comparison of phonological processes used by developmentally dyspraxic children and nondyspraxic phonologically impaired children. *Australian Journal of Human Communication Disorders, 12*(2), 93–107.

Parten, M. (1932). Social participation among preschool children. *Journal of Abnormal and Social Psychology, 27,* 243–269.

Paul, R. (1991). Profiles of toddlers with slow expressive language development. *Topics in Language Disorders, 11*(4), 1–13.

Paul, R. (1995). *Language disorders from infancy through adolescence: Assessment and intervention.* St. Louis: Mosby.

Paul, R., & Jennings, P. (1992). Phonological behavior in toddlers with slow expressive language development. *Journal of Speech and Hearing Research, 35,* 99–107.

Paul, R., Looney, S., & Dahm, P. (1991). Communication and socialization skills at ages 2 and 3 in "late talking" young children. *Journal of Speech and Hearing Disorders, 34,* 858–865.

Peck, C. (1989). Assessment of social communicative competence: Evaluating environments. *Seminars in Speech and Language, 10,* 1–15.

Piaget, J. (1954). *The construction of reality in the child.* New York: Ballantine.

Piaget, J. (1962). *Play, dreams and imitation.* New York: Norton.

Reinhartsen, D., Edmondson, R., & Crais, E. (1997). Developing assistive technology strategies for infants and toddlers with communication difficulties. *Seminars in Speech and Language. 18*(3), 283–301.

Rescorla, L. (1989). The Language Development Survey: A screening tool for delayed language in toddlers. *Journal of Speech and Hearing Disorders, 54,* 587–599.

Rescorla, L., & Ratner, N. (1996). Phonetic profiles of toddlers with expressive language impairment (SLI-E). *Journal of Speech and Hearing Research, 39,* 153–165.

Rescorla, L., & Schwartz, E. (1990). Outcome of toddlers with expressive language delay. *Applied Psycholinguistics, 11,* 393–407.

Retherford, K. (1993). *A guide to analysis of language transcripts* (2nd ed.). Eau Claire, Wis.: Thinking Publications.

Rossetti, L. (1990a). *Infant-toddler assessment.* Boston: College-Hill.

Rossetti, L. (1990b). *Infant-Toddler Language Scale.* East Moline, Ill.: LinguiSystems.

Roush, J. (1990). Acoustic amplification for hearing impaired infants and young children. *Infants and Young Children,* 2(4), 59–71.

Ruff, H., & Lawson, K. (1990). Development of sustained, focused attention in young children during free play. *Developmental Psychology, 26,* 85–93.

Sameroff, A., & Friese, B. (1990). Transactional regulation and early intervention. In S. Meisels & J. Shonkoff (Eds.), *Handbook of early intervention* (pp. 119–149). Cambridge, U.K.: Cambridge University Press.

Scarborough, H. S. (1990). Very early language deficits in dyslexic children. *Child Development,* 61, 1728– 1743.

Schwartz, R., & Leonard, L. (1982). Do children pick and choose? Phonological selection and avoidance in early lexical acquisition. *Journal of Child Language, 9,* 319–336.

Sears, C. (1994). Recognizing and coping with tactile defensiveness in young children. *Infants and Young Children, 6,* 47–53.

Seibert, J., & Hogan, A. (1982). A model for assessing social and object skills and planning intervention. In D. McClowry, A. Guilford, & S. Richardson (Eds.), *Infant communication, development, assessment, and intervention* (pp. 21–53). New York: Grune & Stratton.

Sheppard, J. (1987). Assessment of oral-motor behaviors in cerebral palsy. *Seminars in Speech and Language, 8,* 57–70.

Siegel-Causey, E., Ernst, B., & Guess, D. (1987). Elements of nonsymbolic communication and early interactional processes. In M. Bollis (Ed.), *Communication development in young children with deafness/blindness: Literature review III* (pp. 57–102). Monmouth, Ore.: Oregon State System of Higher Education.

Simeonsson, R. (1989). Assessing family environments. In D. Bailey & R. Simeonsson (Eds.), *Family assessment in early intervention* (pp. 167–184). Columbus, Ohio.: Merrill.

Smith, A., Goffman, L., & Stark, R. (1995). Speech motor development. *Seminars in Speech and Language, 16*(2), 87–109.

Stackhouse, J. (1992). Developmental verbal dyspraxia: A longitudinal case study. In R. Campbell (Ed.), *Mental lives: Studies in cognition* (pp. 84–98). Oxford, U.K.: Basil Blackwell.

Stackhouse, J., & Snowling, M. (1992). Barriers to literacy development in two cases of developmental verbal dyspraxia: A longitudinal study. *European Journal of Communication Disorders, 27,* 35–54.

Sternberg, R., & Powell, J. (1983). Comprehending verbal comprehension. *American Psychologist, 38,* 878–893.

Stoel-Gammon, C. (1985). Phonetic inventories, 15-24 months: A longitudinal study. *Journal of Speech and Hearing Research, 28,* 505–512.

Strand, E. (1995). Treatment of motor speech disorders in children. *Seminars in Speech and Language, 16*(2), 126–139.

Summers, J., Dell'Oliver, C., Turnbull, A., Benson, H., Santelli, E., Campbell, M., & Siegel-Causey, E. (1990). Examining the individualized family service plan process: What are family and practitioner preferences? *Topics in Early Childhood Special Education, 10*(1), 78–99.

Tallal, P. (1980). Auditory temporal perception, phonics and reading disability in children. *Brain and Language, 9,* 182.

Turnbull, A., & Turnbull, H. (1986). Family Information Preference Inventory. In A. Turnbull & R. Turnbull (Eds.), *Families, professionals, and exceptionality: A special partnership* (pp. 368–373). Columbus, Ohio.: Merrill.

Velleman, S., & Strand, E. (1994). Developmental verbal dyspraxia. In J. Bernthal & .N Bankson (Eds.), *Child phonology: characteristics, assessment, and intervention with special populations* (pp. 110–139). New York: Thieme Medical Publishers.

Vihman, M. (1992). Early syllables and the construction of phonology. In C. Ferguson, L. Menn, & C. Stoel-Gammon (Eds.), *Phonological development: Models, research, implications* (pp. 393–422). Timonium, Md.: York Press.

Westby, C. (1988). Children's play: Reflections of social competence. *Seminars in Speech and Language, 9,* 1–14.

Westby, C. (1990). Ethnographic interviewing: Asking the right questions to the right people in the right ways. *Journal of Childhood Communication Disorders, 13*(1), 101–11.

Wetherby, A., & Prizant, B. (1989). The expression of communicative intent: Assessment guidelines. *Seminars in Speech and Language, 10,* 77–91.

Wetherby, A., & Prizant, B. (1992). Profiling young children's communicative competence. In S. Warren & J. Reichle (Eds.), *Causes and effects in communication and language intervention* (pp. 217–253). Baltimore: Brookes.

Wetherby, A., & Prizant, B. (1993). *Communication and Symbolic Behavior Scales.* Chicago: Riverside.

Whitehurst, G., Smith, M., Fischel, J., Arnold, D., & Lonigan, C. (1991). The continuity of babble and speech in children with specific expressive language delay. *Journal of Speech and Hearing Research, 34,* 1121–1129.

Wilcox, J. (1992). Enhancing initial communication skills in young children with developmental disabilities through partner programming. *Seminars in Speech and Language, 13,* 194–212.

Wilcox, J., Kouri, T., & Caswell, S. (1990). Partner sensitivity to communication behavior of young children with developmental disabilities. *Journal of Speech and Hearing Disorders, 55,* 679–693.

Winton, P., & Bailey, D. (1993). Communicating with families: Examining practices and facilitating change. In J. Paul & R. Simeonsson (Eds.), *Understanding and working with parents of children with special needs* (2nd ed.). New York: Holt, Rinehart, & Winston.

Wyley, V. (1995). *Premature infants and their families.* San Diego: Singular Publishing.

Yoshinago-Itano, C. (1995). Universal hearing screening for infants: Simple, risk-free, beneficial, and justified. *Audiology Today,* 7(1), 13.

CHAPTER 2

Ecologically Valid Assessment of Two- to Five-Year-Olds

Sandra N. Kleinman Ed.D., CCC-SLP
Executive Director
The Howard School
Atlanta
Clinical Assistant Professor
Emory University School of Medicine
Barry M. Prizant, Ph.D., CCC-SLP
Director
Childhood Communication Services
Cranston, Rhode Island
Adjunct Professor
Brown University
Providence

Key Terms

dynamic assessment
ecologically valid assessment
interdisciplinary team
multidisciplinary team
traditional assessment
transdisciplinary team

Overview

CASE STUDY: BRIAN

Brian, a boy aged 3 years, 3 months, was referred by his parents for a communication evaluation at the local hospital's speech and language clinic because of concerns about his language and behavior. Brian was able to communicate basic needs through one- to three-word utterances, but he frequently repeated others' speech and often preferred to play alone. Although his mother had suspected problems since Brian was 2, his pediatrician had told his parents to wait until he was 3. Brian's father denied anything was wrong on grounds that Brian had always been healthy, and delayed speech was common on his side of the family. His father agreed to seek an evaluation only on the insistence of Brian's preschool teacher. The developmental preschool, which Brian attended for four mornings a week, had 15 children plus a teacher and an aide. Brian had only been in the preschool for 2 weeks when his teacher expressed concern about his poor conversational skills, problems in paying attention in groups, and inability to play cooperatively with the other children. Although she noted that he was an enthusiastic and likable child, she believed that "he doesn't always use the language he has" and that "he acts out physically when he gets confused or too excited."

At the hospital clinic, the speech-language pathologist attempted to administer a number of standardized assessments, mostly requiring pointing to pictures or labeling pictures on pages. Brian showed little interest in the testing materials, and the speech-language pathologist became increasingly challenged as Brian wandered around the testing room and remained disinterested and disengaged. When she tried to intrude, he began to scream and push away the toys she offered to him. His parents, who were observing behind a one-way mirror, became increasingly frustrated because they knew that Brian behaved differently in other situations. They wondered why Brian could not be observed in more familiar activities with familiar people as part of the assessment. Following the unsuccessful evaluation, they asked the speech-language pathologist if she could observe him at home or at the preschool, but she said it was not possible given her schedule.

Two weeks later, the parents received a report indicating that Brian had speech and language delays and, in general, was noncompliant and 'unstable.' As a result of this experience, Brian's parents finally received confirmation that their child had a significant speech and language problem. However, they were dismayed that the report provided little insight as to the nature of his difficulties or how his speech and language problems might be related to his social and behavioral difficulties. They were most concerned that the report did not describe the child they knew, and they were afraid it could negatively influence other professionals' opinions of Brian.

The case study of Brian illustrates some of the difficulties encountered by children, their families, and professionals when more traditional assessment approaches are employed. These approaches can be contrasted with **ecologically valid assessment,** an approach described and illustrated within this chapter and in Chapter 1. A comprehensive, ecologically valid assessment of speech and language communication is an essential component in planning appropriate educational services for young children who are at risk or have disabilities and their families. It approaches speech, language, communication, and related abilities of young children as interdependent, rather than independent, processes. Ideally, caregivers are integrally involved in assessment by participating in activities, sharing their perceptions of their child's abilities, and prioritizing intervention needs. In this chapter, we will address ecologically valid assessment practices for 2- to 5-year-old children. Children within this age range are typically diverse in their language and communicative abilities, ranging from preintentional and prelinguistic communicators to those who use their language in conversations. For this range of abilities, we begin by addressing the purposes of assessment, with particular attention to the recent shift to ecologically valid assessments, rather than more formal and standardized evaluations. We then discuss the motivating events and theories that have kindled the shift to ecologically valid assessments, followed by a statement of the philosophy underlying the assessment domains and practices we espouse in this chapter. Various approaches and contexts for assessment are considered, as well as specific domains of child abilities. We conclude by considering the link between assessment and intervention, with specific attention to the roles of families and the family context in the assessment process.

PURPOSES AND GOALS OF ASSESSMENT

The most obvious goals of a communication assessment for a young child are to determine whether a problem exists and then to describe how it manifests itself. Table 2-1 provides a brief checklist of expected expressive and receptive communicative behaviors and may be used as a guideline for referral (Prizant, Wetherby, & Roberts, 1993).

Table 2-1. Checklist of Expected Communicative Behaviors

EXPRESSIVE	*RECEPTIVE*
By 18 months	
1. Produces a variety of sounds that may sound like words or short sentences	1. Responds to his or her name
2. Uses a variety of gestures and vocalizations to request objects and direct attention	2. Responds to names of objects within sight
3. Produces at least a few meaningful words	3. Responds to simple requests (e.g., "come here," "sit down," "stand up")
By 24 months	
1. Uses at least 10–15 words meaningfully	1. Responds consistently to many names of objects in the immediate environment
2. Uses two- to three-word sentences meaningfully	2. Retrieves some out-of-sight objects upon request
3. Speech is present and at least 50 percent intelligible to caregivers	3. Responds to 2-step requests (e.g., "get the ball and bounce it")
By 36 months	
1. Produces sentences of three–five words	1. Responds to "what," "who," and "where" questions
2. Talks about past and future events	2. On request, points to many different pictures in a book
3. Asks questions using "what," "who," and "where"	3. Responds to questions or comments about objects/events outside of immediate context
4. Has vocabulary of 100–200 words	4. Shows interest in other person's conversations
5. Speech is greater than 75 percent intelligible to caregivers	

Source: Prizant, B., Wetherby, A., & Roberts, J. (1993). Communication disorders in infants and toddlers. In C. Zeanah (Ed.), *Handbook of infant mental health* (pp. 260–279). New York: Guilford. Adapted by permission.

Note: Child should be referred for evaluation if most behaviors have not been observed by specified age (based on direct observation or caregiver report).

Although establishing a child's developmental level of communicative and language functioning helps to determine whether a problem exists and the child's eligibility for services, this information alone provides minimal direction for either intervention planning or working with caregivers. In this chapter, we focus on goals and strategies of assessment that contribute directly to intervention planning and the intervention process, specifically identifying the unique learning and communication style, strengths, and needs of the child and determining functional intervention targets.

Meisels and Provence (1989) present guidelines based on current best practice for the identification and assessment of young children. Accordingly, assessment in young children may be considered at three levels:

1. *developmental screening* to identify children who have a high probability of developmental delay or special needs and require further assessment;
2. *diagnostic assessment* to determine the existence of a delay or special needs and to identify a child's eligibility for services usually using formal assessment instruments;
3. *assessment for individual program planning* to determine a child's mastery of skills or tasks.

Developmental screening tools sample behaviors; they are designed to be used with large numbers of children. Diagnostic assessments are more comprehensive and draw from multiple sources of information. Diagnostic assessments are also administered as "second opinion" assessments when the nature of a child's special needs remains unclear following an initial assessment or if caregivers or professionals wish to obtain more information about the child. Both developmental screenings and diagnostic assessments typically include standardized, norm-referenced instruments which should be culturally unbiased. Current approaches to assessment are also characterized by including some of the more descriptive and qualitative assessments integrated with some of the more formal approaches.

Limitations of Available Instruments

Wetherby and Prizant (1992) reviewed characteristics of instruments that address communicative and related abilities of young children and were reported to be used most frequently in graduate programs in speech-language pathology (Crais & Leonard, 1990). From their review, they identified a number of limitations in these instruments. First, they tend to focus on the presence or absence of communicative milestones and linguistic forms (e.g., gestures, words), paying limited attention to the functions or purposes of communication. These instruments most typically provide developmental ages or quotients rather than a profile of a child's relative strengths and difficulties. Minimal attention is given to the wide range of preverbal communicative strategies available to young children (e.g., range of conventional gestures). Second, some instruments rely solely on either caregiver report or the direct assessment of a child. While caregiver reports are invaluable, some caregivers may have difficulty objectively judging their children's competence as communicators. However, caregiver involvement is nonetheless essential because multiple sources of information contribute to a more representative profile of a child's ability. Direct assessment typically places the child in a respondent role (e.g., responding to commands, naming objects), thus providing little opportunity to observe her or him in more natural, reciprocal interactions. Third, a child's use of social-affective signals (e.g., communicative gaze, expressions of positive and negative affect), which play an important role in regulating communicative interactions, are rarely considered when assessing communicative competence with these instruments.

FACTORS THAT HAVE MOTIVATED ECOLOGICALLY VALID ASSESSMENTS

The need for more ecologically valid assessments comes from many arenas including theory and current clinical experiences, as well as changes in the view of what are considered best practices in assessment. The following sections provide an overview of these motivating perspectives and beliefs.

A Developmental Perspective

In 1987, Howlin and colleagues wrote that "the nature of the relationship between language, cognitive, behavioral and emotional development is poorly understood" (p. 290). Despite the influences of developmental theorists such as Vygotsky and Piaget, who address that very relationship, understanding has remained limited due, at least in part, to the domain-specific manner in which each aspect of development has been studied, assessed, and described. For the most part, assessment has been based on maps of separate and distinct developmental trajectories. Over the past decade, however, both research and pedagogy across disciplines have shifted focus to an integrated view of language, communication, cognition, and socialization, and of how this relationship can be enhanced or minimized within treatment and educational programs. Specifically in the field of communication disorders, there has been a shift in attention from the specific structure of the child's utterances to her or his use of those utterances to convey intention or meaning for a variety of social purposes and in a variety of social contexts. This shift in focus has increased the demand for assessments of communicative abilities to better describe children's language, cognitive, and social-emotional profiles within natural contexts. For example, how does a child's language or speech disorder *impact* the ability to communicate needs, to seek attention, to express emotion? How do the child's communicative abilities *facilitate or restrict* opportunities to participate in play activities with peers? How might a child's communicative abilities *affect* her or his ability to benefit from a preschool or kindergarten curriculum?

Generalization

Over the last few decades, professionals and teachers working with young children with communication disorders have been increasingly concerned about their limited ability to generalize interventions to the child's day-to-day life. To address the problem of generalization, researchers and professionals have found some solutions by turning toward developmental psychology, which stresses:

1. the importance of describing the child's ecology to truly understand her/his development;
2. the manner in which knowledge of objects, events, and their relationships is acquired through this process.

Inherent within a child's ecology are a multitude of physical and social influences, cultural beliefs, and ideologies, as well as an increasingly complex set of relationships with parents, caregivers, teachers, siblings, and peers, all of which, directly or indirectly, affect the child's development (Bronfenbrenner, 1977; Cole & Cole, 1993; Harkness & Super, 1986 Heath, 1984). Nested in these contexts and relationships the child is portrayed not only by qualities unique to her or himself, but also within the broader context of her or his home, community, and cultures.

Language, communicative, cognitive, and social-emotional development occur as the child interacts within these contexts and relationships. Nelson (1986) suggests that as a result of their participation in routine, culturally organized events children acquire generalized event representations, or *scripts.* Scripts are schemas that identify the people who participate in an event, the roles they play, the objects that are used, and the sequence of actions that make up the event. As such, scripts link knowledge with specific events in the life of the child. These scripts play a variety of social, language, and cognitive functions (Cole & Cole, 1993):

1. they are "guides to action," allowing the child to anticipate what will happen next;
2. they facilitate the coordination of actions among people in a specific social context;
3. they allow the child to notice similarities and differences among events and relationships within those event contexts, or to generalize from one context to another.

Clearly, the child's social, language, communicative, and cognitive development is intimately linked to the people, settings, and cultural beliefs within her or his world and the opportunities for the child to develop generalized event representations. Therefore, the assessment of a child's language and communicative abilities must be functional, addressing the different manifestations of her or his abilities and difficulties with respect to the contexts of everyday events and routines, her or his relationships within those contexts, and the events and concurrent scripts that occur within her or his ecology. Otherwise, intervention programs will be contrived, reflecting a set of conditions within the assessment process that may not be the same conditions as those in the typical ecology of the child. One can then assume that the intervention procedures will yield results that are not generalizable to the child's day-to-day life. Given that assumption, the nature of the assessment of children's language and communicative abilities has shifted accordingly, toward more real-world, ecologically valid procedures. As part of the assessment process, ecologically valid assessment approaches consider the modifications and adaptations that may be necessary in the physical structure of the child's primary environments, the design of activities, the manner in which specific communication objectives can be met in those activities, and the interactions between caregivers and the child.

Principles of Assessment

Comprehensive communication and language assessments are guided by seven basic principles (Prizant & Bailey, 1996), each reflecting the inherent complexity, and the multidimensional and social nature of language and communication, as manifest in virtually all contexts of a child's life. These principles consider language development and, concurrently, the process of communication as highly transactional in nature, involving mutual influences between a child and the persons and events in that child's life over time (Sameroff, 1987; Sameroff & Fiese, 1990). As such, language and communication development must be assessed in the context of a child's cognitive and socioemotional profiles.

Principle 1. *Assessment is an ongoing process by which information is gathered about a child's communicative behavior across situational contexts and over time.* A child's communicative abilities vary considerably as a function of many factors, including, but not limited to, the environment or setting in which she or he is observed, the persons interacting with her or him, and the familiarity of the situation (Lund & Duchan, 1993). This is especially true for preschool children with language and communication disabilities (Fuchs, Fuchs, Power, & Daily, 1985). Thus, communication assessment must account for the typical variability observed in communicative functioning in young children across contexts. This is especially true for children with delays or identified disabilities in language and communication development: they may demonstrate significant variability across contexts because of a limited generalization of their abilities.

To address a child's performance variability, an assessment ideally involves gathering and coordinating information from persons who regularly interact with her or him in different contexts, such as direct care staff at a day-care center, parents, educational staff in an integrated preschool setting, and/or early interventionists (e.g., speech-language pathologists, occupational therapists, physical therapists, early intervention educators). This information gathering is, perforce, an ongoing process drawing on multiple sources as a child's communicative development and needs may change significantly over time. Consequently, formal and informal assessment must be consistently conducted over regular intervals.

Program planning should be dynamic, reflecting ongoing assessment that documents changes in a child's communication and language behavior. Both naturalistic observation and interviews are often used for ongoing assessments, with periodic direct assessments employed to more formally document a child's progress with respect to the aforementioned developmental framework. Ongoing documentation provides information with which to evaluate the effectiveness of approaches to enhance the child's communicative competence.

Principle 2. *A variety of strategies should be used for collecting information.* For a complete profile of a child's communicative strengths and needs, as well as the available learning opportunities, direct assessment, naturalistic observation, and interviews may be utilized. The use of a variety of strategies reflects currently recognized best practices in early childhood assessment for all assessment domains (Crais, 1995; Prizant & Bailey, 1996).

Direct assessment involves one-to-one interactions between a professional and the child, typically using standardized instruments, checklists, and relatively less structured play procedures to collect a language and communication sample for later analysis. Naturalistic observation is characterized by nonintrusive data collection through observing or videotaping a child interacting with familiar persons in familiar life routines and activities. Caregivers may also provide videotapes of their child in familiar activities and routines. Finally, information may be collected by interviewing significant persons in the child's life who have the opportunity to regularly observe and interact with the child (Schuler, Peck, Willard, & Theimer, 1989). Caregivers may also be interviewed in the context of their indirect or direct involvement in an assessment by providing feedback as to whether a child's communicative behavior is representative of her or his behavior in other contexts.

Direct assessment, naturalistic observation, and interviews have the potential to provide qualitatively different information about a child's communicative abilities, which may ultimately be integrated to construct a more holistic picture of a child's communication system. For example, for some preschool or clinic-based professionals, interviewing caregivers may be the only efficient means available to gather information about a child's communication abilities at home. The information provided by caregivers, along with more structured, direct assessment procedures and observation of caregiver-child interactions, may be sufficient to obtain an initial picture of a child's communicative strengths and needs. In addition to providing a more complete profile of a child, combining a variety of assessment strategies allows for cross-validation of the findings. That is, one can be more confident in the assessment findings if similar communication patterns have been observed across different contexts.

Principle 3. *A variety of instruments or tools may be used in assessment; these should be selected based upon a child's developmental level, the purpose of the assessment, and the assessment strategies used.* For example, a communication interview protocol or developmental checklist focusing on milestones in development may be used when interviewing caregivers or other familiar persons, when providing information to determine eligibility for services, and also for intervention planning. An observational checklist may be used, during naturalistic observation or during direct assessment, to provide information regarding eligibility for services and intervention planning. Standardized instruments are used primarily to determine eligibility for services and general developmental levels.

In general, direct, formal communication assessment strategies, such as standardized tests, are most appropriate for developmentally more sophisticated preschool children (e.g., children with conversational language abilities) and chronologically older preschoolers. Indirect, naturalistic observational approaches are most appropriate for developmentally and chronologically younger children. Videotaping is being used as an assessment tool with increasing regularity during communication and language assessment, as it provides an opportunity to observe vocal, verbal, and nonverbal communicative behaviors. Videotaping children across contexts affords several additional advantages, such as:

1. observing a child's behavior in many contexts without actually being there;
2. using videotapes as an educational tool for caregivers;
3. documenting a child's progress over time.

For example, reviewing and discussing videotapes of interactions over time may help parents to more clearly notice their child's emerging communicative behaviors, providing positive feedback and motivation for professionals as well as caregivers.

Principle 4. *Communication assessment must account for conventional as well as unconventional communicative behavior.* For some young children with language or communication difficulties, the acquisition of conventional verbal or nonverbal means of communication is especially difficult or challenging. These children may develop idiosyncratic, and even socially unacceptable means to communicate their intentions. Idiosyncratic means may include subtle or difficult-to-read behaviors that can only be understood by those who know the child well. Such behavior has been documented in children with multiple handicaps (Yoder, 1987) and children with social-communicative disorders such as autism (Prizant & Wetherby, 1987). Socially unacceptable forms of communication, including aggression and throwing tantrums, have been observed in children and adolescents with developmental disabilities (Carr et al., 1994; Wetherby & Prutting, 1984). Observational frameworks and instruments are available to document intentional, but idiosyncratic or socially unacceptable, forms of communication (Donnellan, Mirenda, Mesaros, & Fassbender, 1984; Schuler, Prizant, & Wetherby, 1997) as well as conventional forms, and can provide a more complete picture of a child's communication system than would be otherwise obtained.

Principle 5. *Parents or primary caregivers should be considered as expert informants about the child's communicative competence.* Often caregivers report that they observe different patterns or levels of communication in their young children than are observed directly by professionals during an assessment. Unfortunately, these differences in observations of a child's abilities have the potential to lead to misunderstandings, restricting the development of mutual respect and trust. To some professionals, for example, caregivers who report significantly higher abilities than they themselves observe may be characterized as denying the extent of their child's special needs or "overestimating" her or his abilities. Similarly, caregivers who report significantly lower abilities may be seen as "burned out" or unable to perceive their child's strengths or potential. On the other hand, caregivers may observe professionals who, in their opinion, underestimate their child's abilities, leaving the impression that the latter are overly focused on pathology. These differences in observations by professionals and caregivers, however, can be productive if the focus shifts from the reliability of the observer to the range of the child's communicative behaviors across a variety of social contexts. From the latter perspective, one would assume that the child's communicative patterns would naturally vary. Differences in observations, therefore, can be appreciated as reflecting the influence on the child's behavior of the various contexts in which she or he lives.

Thus, it is generally accepted that communication development and competence naturally vary across contexts. Caregivers have opportunities to observe and interact with the child far more frequently and in far more familiar and emotionally secure situations than do professionals. Positive effects of caregiver observation and participation have been documented in early neurobehavioral assessment (Brazelton & Cramer, 1990) and are now being advocated for communication assessment (Prizant & Wetherby, 1993). Thus, a general underlying principle in communication assessment is that the caregivers are most knowledgeable about the child's abilities. Early childhood educators also are a potential source of information about a child's communication and language abilities. Therefore, professionals must refine their interviewing skills (see Westby, 1990; Winton, 1988) and use appropriate communication assessment interview tools and strategies to tap the knowledge held by, for example, caregivers and early childhood educators (see Schuler et al., 1989). Different observations, therefore, are considered as opportunities to broaden the profile of a child's communicative development rather than as discrepancies between observers.

Principle 6. *Developmental research on the sequence and processes of language and communication development should provide the framework for assessing a child's communicative abilities.* For professionals working with preschool children, familiarity with the sequences and processes of communication and language development is essential for several reasons.

First, although clear individual differences exist in some aspects of language acquisition, 30 years of research has documented relatively invariant sequences and stages of development (Bates, O'Connell, & Shore, 1987). These sequences provide a broad framework with which to document major developmental transitions (e.g., movement from gestures to single-word utterances) (Lahey, 1988), as well as a more narrow focus on small increments in development within these major stages.

Second, an intervention plan should be based on a child's current level of ability, with targeted short- and long-term goals cast within a developmental framework. Although a child's functional needs and caregiver priorities are essential considerations in intervention planning, they must be understood with respect to the child's complete developmental profile. For example, parents of a 3-year-old nonspeaking child who uses conventional gestures and undifferentiated vocalizations (e.g., "uh") may indicate that it is important for their child to say, "I want potty," because she or he is nearly toilet trained and only loses control when there is no bathroom in sight. While this functional goal is clearly a priority for the family, the targeted communicative means are not appropriate to the child's developmental level. For this child, a picture symbol or sign plus vocalizations, rather than a multiword utterance (although appropriate for the child's chronological age), are clearly more consistent with the child's developmental abilities.

Third, developmental sequences and processes provide a specific reference from which professionals and caregivers can model language and communication in daily interactions to facilitate a child's communicative growth. Providing information about processes and sequences in language and communication development is often a first step in helping caregivers to support their child's communicative growth (MacDonald, 1989; Mahoney, 1988; Manolson, 1992).

Principle 7. *Assessment should be viewed as a potential form of intervention.* Caregivers' active involvement and participation in assessment activities may contribute to their understanding of their child's communicative strengths and needs and influence the ways in which they interact with her or him. Thus, assessment may serve as one form of intervention. During the assessment process, caregivers may become more aware of their child's communicative signals and, as a result, develop interactive strategies that are conducive to sustaining social and communicative exchange.

ASSESSMENT APPROACHES: DEVELOPING A PORTRAIT OF THE CHILD

There are two broadly defined approaches to assessment, **traditional assessment** and **dynamic assessment**. A traditional approach to assessment typically focuses on the presence or absence of a circumscribed set of communication skills at the time of the testing, according to the child's chronological and/or mental age. A dynamic approach, on the other hand, considers the child's demonstration of those skills in a variety of familiar and unfamiliar contexts that more or less replicate actual events or tasks in her or his life and include a variety of familiar and unfamiliar people. Dynamic assessment thus takes into account the manner in which a child's behavior may change across tasks, settings, and people and the manner in which her or his behavior changes over time.

The distinction between traditional and dynamic assessment may be likened to the distinction between evaluation and assessment as stated in the Individuals with Disabilities Education Act (see Crais, Chapter 1). An evaluation considers the range of skills and abilities of the child at a specific point in time for purposes of determining service eligibility. An assessment is a proactive, continuous process for purposes of planning and providing services to a child with respect to her or his evolving abilities and needs.

In the following section, we take a closer look at traditional and dynamic approaches to assessment, keeping in mind the relationship between a child's communicative abilities and her or his particular ecology and considering the need for intervention designed to generalize to the specific contexts, tasks, persons, and cultures relevant to the child's life.

Traditional Assessment

Traditional or static assessment (Wetherby & Prizant, 1992) is most typically designed around standardized measures: The assessment is guided by the measurement tool rather than by the child. These measures are designed to provide comparative, norm-referenced information across developmental areas, under a specified set of conditions, and as compared to a "typical" population. Neither the relevance of the child's performance to her or his daily life nor information about her or his potential performance are available from these measures. Furthermore, the tasks, although designed to simulate tasks that the child would likely perform relative to her or his chronological age, are more typically designed to assess hypothetical language and cognitive constructs such as "following directions" and "listening skills." Typically, responses are judged within a dichotomous paradigm (e.g., correct or incorrect; present or absent), without consideration of emerging behaviors (Kublin, Wetherby, Crais, & Prizant, 1998). Static assessments are characteristically professional-centered such that the child plays a passive or recipient role. Any deviation from the established protocol is considered to violate assumptions of standardization, consequently prohibiting reference to the established norms for the procedures.

Within traditional assessment, test results yield numerical scores for individual subtests, which are often collapsed into more general scores representing language and/or developmental ages based on comparisons of scores to those expected at the child's chronological and/or mental age (Peña & Iglesias, 1993). The latter may be estimated from a test protocol drawn from a previously administered test or estimated from a behavioral checklist. On some tests, a receptive language age, for example, may be generated from several subtests identified as assessing comprehension rather than expression. Specific areas of ability are often obfuscated as they are collapsed into the more general scores.

Traditional or static assessment measures bind the professional to a specific set of descriptors when providing feedback to the family. Often, these descriptors have little or no relevance to caregivers as they reveal no obvious, direct application to situations within the child's life. Furthermore, while information may emerge relative to the child's measurable abilities within the dimensions of the test measures, the emphasis is clearly on her or his disabilities; that is, on what the child is *unable* to do. Consequently, descriptions of the child's performance—be it developmentally typical or not—are diluted by the focus on disordered or developmentally atypical behaviors. The overall profile of the child, therefore, will be skewed toward a negative model of attribution. In addition, traditional assessments use responses to test items, rather than self-motivated communicative acts, as a unit of analysis.

Conditions within the testing paradigm are designed to approximate tasks that the child might do, but often, the relationship between those conditions and conditions in the child's natural ecology are not obvious. The professionals who must extrapolate from the hypothetical set of conditions to the actual contexts in the child's life, are, therefore, challenged when drawing pedagogical relevance from the standardized test data.

Dynamic Assessment

In contrast to a traditional approach, a dynamic approach is designed to maximize opportunities to elicit information that is directly applicable to a child's life at the time of the assessment, as well as throughout the period of intervention. This approach closely approximates the goals of the ecologically valid assessment of communicative abilities, as opposed to traditional assessment. Its purpose is to obtain a profile of the range of the child's communicative behaviors as they manifest in a variety of contexts. Furthermore, drawing from the seminal writings of Vygotsky (1978, 1986), Rogoff and Wertsch (1984), and Feuerstein, Rand, and Hoffman (1979), dynamic assessment provides a means to explore the potential of the child to learn new behaviors and/or expand on currently manifest behaviors within a familiar social context. Learning, as Vygotsky (1978, 1986) describes, is a social event unfolding as the child interacts within a particular environment with people and objects within that environment (see also Kublin et al., 1998).

Three influences converge to undergird the "dynamic" element in dynamic assessment. First is the ecology of the child, specifically, the importance of considering the effects of ongoing *interactions* between the child and the relevant people, settings, and activities within those settings, and particularly how those interactions affect the child's ability to perform tasks (Rogoff & Wertsch, 1984). As such, a dynamic assessment can account for the variability of performance of the child as a function of external factors describing the conditions in which she or he may be more or less successful at the same task. Second, the young child is in the process of developing, with her or his knowledge continually being shaped and reshaped. Consequently, the child's performance will continue to change over time, and therefore, an assessment of her or his communicative abilities must also be ongoing to reflect that development. Dynamic assessment, therefore, begins, but does not end, with the initial assessment.

The third influence comes from the work of Vygotsky (1978, 1986) and Feuerstein et al. (1979). Vygotsky proposed a theoretical "zone of proximal development," which has since been used to guide assessment, research, and pedagogy with respect to children's learning. The zone is defined as the distance between a child's demonstrated independent abilities in performing a task and that child's performance on the same task with assistance from an adult or peer. Feuerstein and his colleagues (1979) adapted Vygotsky's zone of proximal development to create a dynamic assessment model in which the focus was on the change and modifiability of the performance rather than the accuracy of the response. Based on the child's ability to change her or his performance, one can determine how generalizable that altered performance is to other tasks.

Dynamic assessment offers opportunities to explore the upper limits of the child's demonstrated abilities, providing information not only about the child's present abilities, but also about her or his potential for growth. To explore the child's potential, dynamic assessments are child centered, whereas traditional assessments are professional centered and test material centered. The child's behavior uniquely determines what will happen during the assessment, and the help or support that are given depend on what the child does (Burns, Vye, Bransford, Delclos, & Ogan, 1987; Kublin et al., 1998; Rogoff & Wertsch, 1984). The professional or caregiver draws on the child's actual performance as observed under a variety of conditions. The child attempts different approaches to facilitate her or his ability to complete a task that cannot be performed independently, and to elaborate on or improve (under a variety of conditions) her or his performance with the support of the adult. This type of facilitation is variously described in cognitive, learning, oral, and written language literatures as "scaffolding," "mediated learning," "interactive teaching," and "reciprocal teaching" (see Kublin et al., 1998, for a more complete review; see also Bruner, 1985; Rogoff, Malkin, & Gilbride, 1984).

In summary, rather than simply identifying developmental levels or considering a dichotomous (correct or incorrect) response as in traditional approaches, dynamic assessment considers multiple factors that influence the quality of the child's performance and examines how that performance might develop into a more elaborated, functional, or advanced response.

DESIGNING CHILD-SPECIFIC, DYNAMIC ASSESSMENTS

Outlining child-specific, dynamic assessment focuses on three components: the design of the assessment, the inclusion of familiar communicative participants, and the utilization of a collaborative team approach. These three components are described in the following sections.

Design

Ecologically valid, dynamic assessment is guided by an intervention design (Barnett, Macmann, & Carey, 1992; Crais, 1995). Specifically, the selection of the activities presented to the child during the assessment, as well as the settings and participants, are all motivated by the need to translate assessment information directly into intervention plans. Accordingly, the purpose of the assessment is threefold:

1. To describe the child's communicative and language abilities as manifest in key settings, with key caregivers, under a variety of conditions (e.g., routines, materials, activities). The setting, communicative partners, specific content of the interactions, and other influences external to the child are observed as they may impact on the child's communicative behaviors. Those behaviors are then compared across multiple settings, communicative partners, routines, and activities to describe how they may change, if at all.

2. To identify specific intervention objectives to elicit target behaviors by using the presented activities to explore the child's potential performance under adult-supported conditions.

3. To evaluate the specific environments themselves with respect to their ability to facilitate these intervention objectives, to identify modifications that may be made within those environments (both in physical structure and in the curriculum itself), and to explore the possible roles of caregivers, family members, and peers within those environments.

Participants

Familiar communicative partners are integral to the dynamic assessment process. They may elicit behaviors demonstrating a more complete range of the child's communicative abilities in both natural and novel settings than may be demonstrated if the child is working with an unfamiliar professional (Barnett et al., 1992; Crais, 1995; Olswang, Bain, & Johnson, 1992). Communicative partners also take the role of observer, commenting on the child's behavior as being "typical" or "atypical" of a particular behavior in other settings or with other caregivers.

The style of a child's communicative partners may facilitate or hinder communicative transactions (Prizant & Bailey, 1996). For example, responding contingently to children's initiations and expanding or elaborating on their comments typically supports further communicative interactions. However, an excessive use of test questions or directives may limit successful communicative exchange. Therefore, an assessment of the caregivers' communicative styles as they may enhance or inhibit the child's communicative development is an important part of the assessment process. Assessment of the child's familiar communicative partners should include a variety of dimensions of partner style, including degree of acceptance of a child's communicative attempts; use of directive rather than facilitative styles of interaction; contingency of responses to child behavior; provision of communicative models; maintenance of the topics of the child's initiations; and expansion or elaboration of the communicative attempts (Duchan, 1989; Marfo, 1990; Peck, 1989; Prizant & Bailey, 1996). These styles must be considered in the context of a variety of factors, including, but not limited to, cultural and familial influences, context and setting, and attentional abilities.

Collaborative Team Models

The assessment of a child's communicative abilities is a collaborative process including primary caregivers as well as participating specialists. The involvement of, and interaction among, these specialists and caregivers may take a variety of forms, which can be described as ranging from most collaborative to least collaborative.

The **transdisciplinary team** includes primary caregivers plus one or more specialists with expertise in more than one discipline, although one discipline may be identified as a primary area of need for the child. Assessments are driven by the understanding that a child's development reflects the simultaneous acquisition of different social and communicative abilities. Members of the transdisciplinary team are able to assess the child from a variety of perspectives, and thus comment on the relationship between the child's communicative abilities and social development. Typically within this approach, one professional is the primary interactant with the child and family.

The **interdisciplinary team** includes primary caregivers and several specialists, each with their own specific area of expertise. As a team, each specialist and caregiver compares and contrasts observations of the child during the assessment process, ideally moving toward a single, coherent profile.

The **multidisciplinary team** also includes primary caregivers and several specialists, each with a particular expertise. Their assessments are discipline driven. The specialists and caregivers independently present their observations and the final profile is a collection of observations specified within the separate domains (e.g., communication, emotional development, medical and home history, literacy) with little if any reference to the manner in which the specified behaviors or abilities are related. Furthermore, while observations may be included about the variability of the child's performance across settings, contexts, and communicative partners, that variability is also understood within the specific domain of each specialist rather than as a reflection of the whole child.

Settings and Interactive Contexts

Like the presence of familiar communicative partners, observation in familiar settings (e.g., day- or home-care centers, preschools, and home) and contexts (e.g., familiar routines) facilitates the process of assessing young children. Furthermore, these settings and contexts themselves are assessed as they facilitate or inhibit the child's communicative development.

Facilitative contexts include joint activity routines (Prizant & Bailey, 1996; Snyder-McLean, Solomonson, McLean, & Sack, 1984), social routines (McCormick, 1990), and special activities. In each case, the professional and the caregivers follow the child's lead in the activity, elaborating on her or his initiation or modeling behaviors as needed. Play-based approaches include the use of enticing developmentally appropriate toys and activities (e.g., blowing bubbles), as well as the child's favorite toys. These routines and activities provide opportunities for communicative exchanges focusing on a common theme or goal, and for reciprocal and exchangeable roles centered around a mutual focus of attention. They may include simple social games such as "peekaboo," as well as more complex activities such as dressing, preparing food, and singing songs including actions and gestures. In addition to routines and activities, the setting and contexts are assessed for their potential to provide situations that invite the child to communicate, thus creating a communicative need (Peck, 1989; Prizant & Schuler, 1987).

Alternatively or concurrently, unfamiliar settings typically are used in the assessment process, the most common of which is the diagnostic clinic. These may be made more familiar by the presence of caregivers or peers and the introduction of familiar routines, activities, and toys.

DOMAINS OF ASSESSMENT: DEVELOPING A PORTRAIT OF THE CHILD

A portrait or profile of a child's communicative strengths and needs evolves from an assessment of specific content areas or domains of a child's communicative behavior. This includes both developmental information (e.g., level of linguistic comprehension or understanding) and qualitative information (e.g., use of nonverbal signals, such as communicative gaze, in interactions).

Tables 2-2 and 2-3 present two generic frameworks delineating specific content areas for children at prelinguistic and early language levels (Table 2-2) (Prizant & Bailey, 1996), and for children beyond emerging levels (Table 2-3). The specific type of information assessed within each area varies according to a child's specific developmental level of communicative functioning. The major domains are listed in the two tables.

Expressive Language and Communication

The primary focus in this domain is the documentation of communicative means (i.e., specific behaviors with which information is communicated) and communicative functions (i.e., the purposes for the communication attempt) (Prizant & Bailey, 1996). Communicative means of preintentional preschool children may include nonverbal and vocal behaviors such as body posture, facial expression, limb extension, hand gestures, directed gaze and gaze aversion, cry and cooing vocalizations, and intonated vowel and/or babbling vocalizations. These behaviors may function to inform an observer of the child's physiological and emotional state, such as level of alertness, focus of attention, interest in interacting or receiving comfort from other persons, interest in obtaining objects, or desire to have events continue or cease. While a young child may not produce signals with the intention of affecting other persons' behavior in specific ways, it has been documented repeatedly that caregivers respond to such signals as if they were intentional (McLean; 1990; Wetherby & Prizant, 1989). Caregivers' responses to early communicative signals are considered to be important in fostering communicative development (Bruner, 1981). Thus, not only are a child's communicative means considered in the assessment, observations of caregivers' *responses to these signals* are equally important in the assessment of expressive language and communication.

For developmentally more advanced children who communicate through prelinguistic means, the intentional use of idiosyncratic and conventional gestures, as well as vocalizations and emerging word forms, should be documented. For children using language-based systems including speech, sign language, or graphic systems (e.g., communication boards), range of vocabulary and semantic and syntactic complexity, as well as communicative functions, should be documented. For range of vocabulary, the number of different words and word classes (e.g., object words, action words, modifiers

Table 2-2. Social-Communication Assessment Framework for Children at Prelinguistic and Early Language Levels

A. Expressive Language and Communication
   1. Communicative Means
      a. Gestural means—Idiosyncratic vs. conventional gestures; contact vs. distal gestures
      b. Vocal means—Syllabic structure and complexity
      c. Coordination of gestural and vocal acts
      d. Verbal means —Expressive lexicon, word combinations, linguistic complexity
   2. Communicative Functions
      a. Range of communicative functions—Proportion of joint attention, proportion of behavioral regulation
   3. Rate of Communicative Acts
   4. Persistence and Repair Strategies
B. Articulation and Phonology
   1. Perception
   2. Syllabic Shapes
   3. Phonetic Inventory—Consonants
   4. Vowel Inventory
   5. Syllable Sequences (monosyllables; multisyllables)
   6. Developmental and Idiosyncratic Processes
   7. Judgment of Intelligibility
   8. Oromotor
      a. Structure
      b. Function
      c. Volitional movements
      d. Repeated sequences
      e. Alternating sequences
   9. Prosody
C. Receptive Language
   1. Language Comprehension
   2. Nonlinguistic Response Strategies
D. Language-Related Cognitive Skills
   1. Symbolic Play
   2. Combinatorial/Constructive Play
   3. Imitation
   4. Attentional Abilities
E. Social-Affective and Socioemotional Behavior
   1. Use of Gaze and Gaze Shifts for Social Referencing and to Regulate Interactions
   2. Display of Affect—Sociability of Positive Affects
   3. Display of Affect—Episodes of Negative Affects
   4. Other Socioemotional Dimensions (see Table 2-4)

Source: Prizant, B., & Bailey, D. (1996). Facilitating the acquisition and use of communication skills. In D. Bailey & M. Wolery (Eds.), *Teaching infants and preschoolers with disabilities* (2nd ed.), pp. 299–361. New York: Merrill. Reprinted by permission.

Table 2-3. Social-Communication Assessment Framework for Children Beyond Emerging Language

A. Expressive Language and Communication
   1. Simple Sentence Development
      a. MLU-M (general index of development)
      b. Grammatical morphemes
      c. Sentence types
      d. Noun phrase (NP) development
      e. Verb phrase (VP) development
      f. Negative forms
      g. Question forms—*Wh*- question; yes-no
   2. Beyond Simple Sentence Development
      a. Embedding—Subordination, relativization
      b. Coordination
   3. Discourse
B. Speech Production
   1. Oral Motor Structure and Function
      a. Evidence of dyspraxia and/or dysarthria
   2. Phonological Processes
   3. Fluency
   4. Voice
   5. Prosody
C. Receptive Language (use of informal and standardized procedures)
   1. Vocabulary
   2. Grammatical Morphemes
   3. Sentence Types
      a. Negative forms
      b. Question forms—*Wh*- question, yes-no
D. Language-related Cognitive Skills
   1. Play—Level of Imaginative /Symbolic Play
   2. Attention
E. Emergent Literacy
   1. Phonological Awareness
   2. Invented Spelling
F. Social Use of Language
   1. Discourse Functions/Conversational Acts
   2. Presuppositional Skills—Knowledge of Adjustments According to Speakers and Situations
   3. Conversational Skills/Discourse Skills
   4. Narrative Development

or descriptors) used meaningfully are documented. *Semantic complexity* refers to the types of semantic functions or meaning categories expressed in language-based systems (see Retherford, 1993, for examples of analytic systems useful for assessing semantic complexity). To evaluate syntactic complexity in children beyond the earliest language stages, the structural or grammatical complexity of multiword forms is documented. Concurrently, in all these cases, communicative functions are assessed. It is important to note that as children become better able to regulate conversational interactions, the purposes for which they communicate may change. Several assessment protocols have been developed to document communicative intentions and functions. (See Chapman, 1981; Retherford, 1993, for reviews.)

Some preschool children, especially those with social-communicative disabilities, may develop unconventional verbal means to communicate (Prizant & Rydell, 1993). Echolalia, for example, is the most common form of unconventional verbal behavior and the most frequently discussed characteristic of children with autism and pervasive developmental disorder (Prizant, 1987). Based on Peters's (1983) work on typical language acquisition, echolalia has been described as composed of "gestalt language forms" (Prizant, 1983), and echolalic speech has been characterized as primarily composed of unanalyzed, whole units of speech that may be repeated immediately (i.e., immediate echolalia) or at some time after an utterance was heard (i.e., delayed echolalia). Some individuals who demonstrate primitive and noncommunicative echolalic behavior are not truly functioning at a specific linguistic level of communication (Schuler & Prizant, 1985). Others, however, evidence progressive changes in their echolalic utterances, ultimately leading to the emergence of flexible, rule-governed linguistic behaviors. For the latter group, assessment must include a profile of how their echolalic patterns may function in communicative interactions and the role echolalia may play in their acquisition of language. Procedures for the functional analysis of echolalia are summarized by Prizant and Rydell (1993) and Rydell and Prizant (1995).

Articulation and Phonology

Assessment of the child's speech production is completed in the context of both continuous speech—ideally spontaneous and topic-elicited—as well as with standardized tests of single-word and sentence production. According to Stoel-Gammon (1991), both independent and relational analyses should be completed. An independent analysis includes both an inventory of phonemes and an inventory of syllable shapes. Paul and Jennings (1992) developed a measure of syllable structure level (SSL) that accounts for both intelligible and unconventional forms (see also Paul, 1995). Using a relational analysis, a child's productions are compared to the corresponding adult form and identified as correct or incorrect. These productions are then characterized as developmentally appropriate (i.e., with respect to chronological age) or idiosyncratic phonological processes. The child's ability to imitate syllables and words, as well as stimulability to produce speech sounds in isolation, in syllables, and in words, are included in the assessment. Overall intelligibility may be judged formally, based on, for example, the percentage consonants correct (PCC) within the speech sample (Shriberg & Kwiatkowski, 1982).

Some young children, such as those with specific neuromotor speech disorders, may not be able to acquire and use speech as a primary mode of communication during early development. Their disorders may include dysarthria, a paralysis or paresis (i.e., weakness) in the oral musculature often observed in children with cerebral palsy or other identified neurological disorders, and developmental dyspraxia, a dysfunction in the ability to plan the coordinated movements to produce intelligible sequences of speech sounds. Dysarthria and dyspraxia may co-occur in young children; these range from conditions mildly affecting speech intelligibility to those rendering speech unintelligible or precluding speech development.

A complete oral function assessment should be conducted, including information about past or recent history of problems in chewing or swallowing, presence of abnormal reflexive patterns (e.g., hyperactive gag reflex), and informal observations of vocal control for speech and of patterns of chewing and swallowing. This assessment is augmented with developmental information, including interest in speech, motivation to use speech, and patterns of early babbling.

Receptive Language and Communication

A child's ability to comprehend and respond to others' communicative signals is the third domain that should be addressed in assessment. For developmentally young children, the perception of, and response to, environmental and speech sounds is assessed. Initially, a full audiological assessment appropriate for a child's chronological age and developmental level should be conducted by an audiologist to assess hearing status (Roush, 1991). With young children, informal behavioral observation and parental report may also contribute information about functional hearing. For developmentally young children, relevant behavioral observations would include the following: startle responses to loud environmental sounds; localization or orientation to speech or environmental sounds; and ability to be soothed or comforted by a caregiver's voice. Preverbal children's ability to approximate sounds or intonation patterns by imitation provides additional informal evidence of receptive status.

At higher prelinguistic levels of ability, children are able to respond to communicative gestures and vocalizations of others and, with the support of situational cues, to demonstrate their comprehension of words used in highly routinized and familiar activities. Chapman (1979) identified response strategies in young children beginning at approximately 8 months of age.

True linguistic comprehension is evidenced when children can comprehend words without situational or nonverbal cues, especially when words refer to persons, objects, or events outside the immediate environment. The ability to comprehend more complex utterances with a wider range of vocabulary referring to spatially and temporally distant events is assessed for children who are more developmentally advanced. Miller and Paul (1995) provide a more detailed discussion and provide informal procedures for the assessment of receptive language and communication.

Language-Related Cognitive Abilities

There are a number of reasons why communication and language abilities should always be considered in the context of a child's cognitive abilities. First, communication and language development are highly correlated with many aspects of cognitive development, including the development of symbolic play and the understanding of cause-effect relations (Bates, Benigni, Bretherton, Camaioni, & Volterra, 1979). Therefore, profiling a young child's communicative abilities relative to cognitive abilities and capacities provides information about the impact of a communication or language delay on cognitive development, and vice versa.

Second, communication is the means by which children express their knowledge and understanding of other persons and events in their world. Thus, language use is a reflection of, as well as dependent on, a child's knowledge of the world. Finally, the choice of augmentative communication systems, which may be influenced by levels of cognitive/representational ability, requires some estimation of cognitive abilities. Westby (1988) and Linder (1993) provide guidelines for assessing language-related cognitive abilities in young children.

Emergent Literacy and Phonological Awareness

Emergent literacy experiences have been described as "those in which children begin to develop ideas about how written language works and what it is for, before they actually begin decoding print" (Paul, 1995, p. 378). Literacy emerges incidentally, through exposure to print in daily life and through interactions between children and adults in which the adults read books aloud and/or tell stories. The manner in which stories are told or read may vary according to the culture of the adults in the child's life. In this way, children are introduced to "literary language" (Paul, 1995) as they learn about the associations between print and stories and the structure of stories. According to Cullinan (1989), children who have had experiences hearing written language read aloud or listening to stories told in the oral tradition are at a distinct advantage later when they begin to learn to read.

To assess emergent literacy in the 3- to 5-year-old period, naturalistic observation and interviewing approaches are most informative. Obviously, considering the interactive nature of emergent literacy, the caregiver's behaviors, as well as those of the child, with respect to books and storytelling routines are important. Observed behaviors would include interest in books, book looking, storytelling (with specific reference to story cohesion as created through the use of story grammar structures), story-listening behaviors, interest in writing words, and drawing pictures to represent stories.

Phonological awareness skills are often described as the ability to identify, analyze, and manipulate sound structures in language and typically include tasks such as phoneme analysis, synthesis, deletion, and rhyming (Catts, 1991a). Deficits in phonological awareness (and other skills such as syntactic skills, narration, and rapid naming) have been found to account for some difficulties in reading (Kamhi, Catts, Mauer, Apel, & Gentry, 1988; Kamhi & Keonig, 1985; Snyder & Downey, 1997). Concrete ideas for assessing phonological awareness skills can be found in Blachman (1991) and Catts (1991a, 1991b).

Social-Affective Behavior and Socioemotional Functioning

Communicative interactions are regulated by social-affective signaling (Prizant & Wetherby, 1990a). These signals may include facial expression, vocalizations, and other observable behavior reflecting emotional and physiological states. Young children also use gaze for social reference or to monitor the attention of others and signal attention to them. Some children with social and communicative impairments may demonstrate limited use of gaze shifts to regulate interactions, and their emotional states may be difficult to read due to a limited range of affect expression (Prizant & Wetherby, 1990b). Because social-affective signals influence communicative interactions, communication assessment should go beyond the sole consideration of intentional nonverbal and verbal behaviors. This domain of assessment is especially crucial for children who are developmentally young and who demonstrate limited intentionality or conventionality in their communicative signaling.

Additional dimensions of socioemotional abilities related to communicative competence include communicative and social motivation, emotional expression and relatedness, sociability of communicative functions, social-affective signaling, emotional regulation, and expression of emotion in language and play (Prizant & Meyer, 1993). Table 2-4 identifies dimensions of socioemotional functioning related to communication that may be addressed in assessment.

APPLYING INFORMATION FROM THE ASSESSMENT PROCEDURES TO CREATE INTERVENTION PROGRAMS

Within the context of a collaborative team model, the profile of relative abilities and difficulties observed throughout the assessment (including those

Table 2-4. Socioemotional Dimensions in Communication Assessment for Young Children

I. Social Relatedness
   A. *Social and communicative motivation*
      1. Does child prefer to be in proximity of others?
      2. Does child bring attention to self for social engagement?
      3. Does child respond to and initiate social games and routines?
      4. Does child visually orient to others (face-to-face gaze)?
      5. Does child regularly use gaze shifts to reference the attention of others?
      6. Frequency of communicative acts directed to adults and other children?
   B. *Joint attention*
      1. Does child follow adults' visual line of regard or observe adults' or other childrens' activities?
      2. Does child communicate to establish joint attention verbally or preverbally by commenting, requesting information, or providing information?
      3. Is child able to respond to the preverbal or verbal signals of others to establish shared attention?
      4. Is child able to maintain and follow up on topics introduced by others (for older preschoolers)?
   C. *Social imitation*
      1. Does child imitate actions, vocalizations, and/or verbalizations with some evidence of social orientation (e.g., gaze checks, sharing of affect, verbal communication)?
II. Emotional Expression and Relatedness
   A. *Attachment*
      1. Does child use caregivers as a base for security and emotional "refueling"?
      2. After a reasonable period of time, does an older preschool child see other adults (e.g., preschool teacher, grandparents) as a base of security?
   B. *Emotional Expression*
      1. Does child express different emotions through facial expression, vocalization, and/or verbalization that are appropriate to the situational and interpersonal context?
      2. Does child share emotional states by directing affect displays to others?
      3. Does the child understand and respond appropriately to the emotional expressions of others?

(continues)

Table 2-4. Socioemotional Dimensions in Communication Assessment for Young Children (continued)

C. *Empathy*
   1. Does older preschool child demonstrate concern for, or actively attempt to soothe, another child who has been hurt or is otherwise in distress?

III. Sociability in Communication
   1. Does child communicate for the function of:
      a. behavioral regulation (i.e, requesting objects/actions, protesting)?
      b. social interaction (i.e., greeting, calling, requesting social routine, requesting comfort)?
      c. joint attention (i.e., commenting, requesting and providing information)?
      d. Does child communicate for all three general functions or primarily for behavioral regulation, which may be indicative of a limited social profile?

IV. Emotion Regulation and Communicative Competence
   1. Does communicative competence vary significantly as a function of situational or relationship context?
   2. How does the degree of emotional arousal (positive or negative) influence communicative competence?
   3. Does the child demonstrate self-regulatory strategies to modulate arousal?
   4. Does the child demonstrate mutual regulatory strategies?
   5. What are the most effective means to modulate extreme states of arousal?

V. Expression of Emotion in Language Use and Play
   1. Does child use vocabulary to talk about emotional states (self or other)?
   2. Do emotional themes emerge consistently in play, and are they an attempt to understand stressful life events?

VI. Clinician's (parent's, educator's) Subjective Reactions
   1. Was the child fun to be with?
   2. Do you have to do most of the work to keep the interaction going?
   3. Do you find the child's communicative and affective signals easy to read?

Source: Prizant, B., & Meyer, E. (1993). Socioemotional aspects of language and social-communication disorders in young children and their families. *American Journal of Speech-Language Pathology, 2,* 56–71. © American Speech-Language-Hearing Association. Rockford, Md. Reprinted by permission.

obtained from interviews of the child's communicative partners) are documented and described as they manifest across settings, interactive contexts, and communicative partners. These behavioral patterns are merged and consolidated as they reflect functional, developmentally-referenced categories (e.g., communicative intent, emergent literacy) to create a single, coherent portrait of the whole child.

If the child's profile indicates eligibility for intervention services, the target settings, interactive contexts, and communicative partners are identified as the *intervention ecology.* Then, modifications for each setting are established. Specific objectives for communication, socialization, and learning are developed for each target setting, based on the child's independent behaviors as well as those elicited under "dynamic," adult-facilitated conditions. Finally, the interactive contexts and suggested materials with which each objective will be met (e.g., getting ready for bed; bathtime; group music time; independent play; snack time), and the communicative partners who will address these objectives, are specified. Evolving a list of objectives to be addressed across settings, contexts, and communicative partners provides the necessary redundancy to maximize the child's learning, offers a procedure to maximize generalization as the child acquires new behaviors, and creates a focused, rather than fragmented, plan for the child.

SUMMARY

The ecological validity of assessment of children ages 2 to 5 relies on the collaborative efforts of parents and professionals who are focused on observing and documenting the child's strengths and needs in naturalistic settings, conducting assessments intertwined with intervention planning, and including assessment strategies and activities that are meaningful to the child and family. This chapter has provided an overview of various approaches and contexts for assessment that may help professionals make the transition to using more ecologically valid assessment practices.

REFERENCES

Barnett, D., Macmann, G., & Carey, K. (1992). Early intervention and the assessment of developmental skills: Challenges and directions. *Topics in Early Childhood Special Education, 12*(1), 21–43.

Bates, E., Benigni, T., Bretherton, I., Camaioni, L., & Volterra, V. (Eds.). (1979). *The emergence of symbols: Cognition and communication in infancy.* New York: Academic.

Bates, E., O'Connell, B., & Shore, C. (1987). Language and communication in infancy. In J. Osofsky (Ed.), *Handbook of infant development* (2nd ed., pp. 149–203). New York: Wiley.

Blachman, B. (1991). Phonological awareness and word recognition: Assessment and intervention. In A. Kamhi & H. Catts (Eds.), *Reading disabilities: A developmental language perspective* (pp. 133–158). Boston: Allyn & Bacon.

Brazelton, B., & Cramer, B. (1990). *The earliest relationship.* New York: Addison Wesley.

Bronfenbrenner, U. (1977). Toward an experimental ecology of human development. *American Psychologist, 32*(7), 513–531.

Bruner, J. (1981). The social context of language acquisition. *Language and Communication, 1,* 155–178.

Bruner, J. (1985). Vygotsky: A historical and conceptual perspective. In J. V. Wertsch (Ed.), *Culture, communication and cognition* (pp. 21–35). Cambridge, U.K.: Cambridge University Press.

Burns, M. S., Vye, N. J., Bransford, J. D., Delclos, V., & Ogan, T. (1987). Static and dynamic measures of learning in young handicapped children. *Diagnostique, 12,* 59–73.

Carr, E. G., Levin, L., McConnachie, G., Carlson, J. I., Kemp, D. C., & Smith, C. A. (1994). *Communication-based intervention for problem behavior: A user's guide for producing positive change.* Baltimore: Brookes.

Catts, H. (1991a). Facilitating phonological awareness: Role of speech-language pathologists. *Language, Speech and Hearing in the Schools, 22,* 196–203.

Catts, H. (1991b). Phonological processing deficits and reading disabilities. In A. Kamhi & H. Catts (Eds.), *Reading disabilities: A developmental language perspective* (pp. 101–132). Boston: Allyn & Bacon.

Chapman, R. (1979). Comprehension strategies in children. In J. Kavanagh & W. Strange (Eds.), *Speech and language in the laboratory, school and clinic.* Cambridge, Mass.: MIT Press.

Chapman, R. (1981). Exploring children's communicative intents. In J. Miller (Ed.), *Assessing language production in children.* Baltimore: University Park Press.

Cole, M., & Cole, S. R. (1993). *The development of children* (2nd ed.). New York: Freeman.

Crais, E. R. (1995). Expanding the repertoire of tools and techniques for assessing the communication skills of infants and toddlers. *American Journal of Speech-Language Pathology, 4*(3), 47–59.

Crais, E., & Leonard, C. (1990). P.L. 99-457: Are speech-language pathologists prepared for the challenge? *American Speech-Language Hearing Association Journal, 32,* 57–61.

Cullinan, B. E. (1989). Literature for young children. In D. S. Strickland & L. M. Morrow (Eds.), *Emerging literacy: Young children learn to read and write* (pp. 35–51). Newark, Del.: International Reading Association.

Donnellan, A., Mirenda, P., Mesaros, R., & Fassbender, L. (1984). Analyzing the communicative functions of aberrant behavior. *Journal of the Association for Persons with Severe Handicaps, 9,* 201–212.

Duchan, J. (1989). Evaluating adults' talk to children: Assessing adult attunement. *Seminars in Speech and Language, 10,* 17–27.

Feuerstein, R., Rand, Y., & Hoffman, M. (1979). *The dynamic assessment of retarded performers: The Learning Potential assessment device, theory, instruments and techniques.* Baltimore: University Park Press.

Fuchs, D., Fuchs, L., Power, M., & Dailey, A. (1985). Bias in the assessment of handicapped children. *American Educational Research Journal, 22,* 185–197.

Harkness, S., & Super, C. M. (1986). The cultural context of gender segregation in children's peer groups. *Annual Progress in Child Psychiatry and Child Development,* 187–196.

Heath, S. B. (1984). *Ways with words: Language, life, and work in communities and classrooms.* Cambridge, U.K.: Cambridge University Press.

Howlin, P., Rutter, M., Berger, M., Hemsley, R., Hersov, L., & Yule, W. (1987). *Treatment of autistic children.* Chichester, U.K.: Wiley.

Kamhi, A., Catts, H., Mauer, D., Apel, K., & Gentry, B. (1988). Phonological and spatial processing abilities in language and reading impaired kids. *Journal of Speech and Hearing Disorders, 53,* 316–327.

Kamhi, A., & Koenig, L. (1985). Metalinguistic awareness in normal and language disordered children. *Language, Speech and Hearing Services in Schools, 16,* 199–210.

Kublin, K., Wetherby, A., Crais, E., & Prizant, B. (1998). Using dynamic assessment within collaborative contexts. In A. Wetherby, S. Warren, & J. Reichle (Eds.), *Transitions in prelinguistic communication: Preintentional to intentional and presymbolic to symbolic* (pp. 285–312). Baltimore: Brookes.

Lahey, M. (1988). *Language disorders and language development.* New York: MacMillan.

Linder, T. (1993). *Transdisciplinary play-based assessment* (2nd ed.). Baltimore: Brookes.

Lund, N., & Duchan, J. (1993). *Assessing children's language in naturalistic contexts* (3rd ed.). Englewood Cliffs, N.J.: Prentice-Hall.

MacDonald, J. (1989). *Becoming partners with children.* Chicago: Riverside Publishers.

Mahoney, G. (1988). Enhancing the developmental competence of handicapped infants. In K. Marfo (Ed.), *Parent-child interaction and developmental disabilities.* New York: Praeger.

Manolson, A. (1992). *It takes two to talk* (2nd ed.). Toronto, Canada: Hanen Early Language Resource Centre.

Marfo, K. (1990). Maternal directiveness in interactions with mentally handicapped children: An analytical commentary. *Journal of Child Psychology and Psychiatry, 31,* 531–549.

McCormick, L. (1990). Intervention processes and procedures. In L. McCormick & R. Schiefelbusch (Eds.), *Early language intervention* (pp. 215–260). Columbus, Ohio.: Merrill.

McLean, L. (1990). Communication development in the first two years of life: A transactional process. *Zero to Three, 11,* 13–19.

Meisels, S., & Provence, S. (1989). *Screening and assessment: Guidelines for identifying young disabled and developmentally vulnerable children and their families.* Washington, D.C.: National Center for Clinical Infant Programs.

Miller, J., & Paul, R. (1995). *The clinical assessment of language comprehension.* Baltimore: Brookes.

Nelson, K. (1986). Event knowledge and cognitive development. In K. Nelson (Ed.), *Event knowledge: Structure and function in development* (pp. 1–19). Hillsdale, N.J.: Erlbaum.

Olswang, L., Bain, B., & Johnson, G. (1992). Using dynamic assessment with children with language disorders. In S. Warren & J. Reichle (Eds.), *Causes and effects in communication and language intervention* (pp. 187–216). Baltimore: Brookes.

Paul, R. (1995). *Language disorders from infancy through adolescence: Assessment and intervention.* St. Louis: Mosby.

Paul, R., & Jennings, P. (1992). Phonological behavior in toddlers with slow expressive language development. *Journal of Speech and Hearing Research, 35,* 99–107.

Peck, C. (1989). Assessment of social communicative competence: Evaluating environments. *Seminars in Speech and Language, 10,* 1–15.

Peña, E. D., & Iglesias, A. (1993). *Dynamic assessment: The model and its application to language assessment.* Short course presented at the American Speech-Language-Hearing Association Annual Convention, Anaheim, Calif., November 20.

Peters, A. (1983). *The units of language acquisition.* Cambridge, U.K.: Cambridge University Press.

Prizant, B. (1983). Language acquisition and communicative behavior in autism: Toward an understanding of the "whole" of it. *Journal of Speech and Hearing Disorders, 48,* 296–307.

Prizant, B. (1987). Clinical implications of echolalic behavior in autism. In T. Layton (Ed.), *Language and treatment of autistic and developmentally disordered children* (pp. 65–88). Springfield, Ill.: Thomas.

Prizant, B., & Bailey, D. (1996). Facilitating the acquisition and use of communication skills. In D. Bailey & M. Wolery (Eds.), *Teaching infants and preschoolers with disabilities* (2nd ed., pp. 299–361). New York: Merrill.

Prizant, B., & Meyer, E., (1993). Socioemotional aspects of language and social-communication disorders in young children and their families. *American Journal of Speech-Language Pathology, 2,* 56–71.

Prizant, B., & Rydell, P. (1993). Assessment and intervention strategies for unconventional verbal behavior. In S. Warren & J. Reichle (Eds.),

Communicative approaches to challenging behavior (pp 263–297). Baltimore: Brookes.

Prizant, B., & Schuler, A. (1987). Facilitating communication: Theoretical foundations. In D. Cohen & A. Donnellan (Eds.), *Handbook of autism and pervasive developmental disorders* (pp. 289–300). New York: Wiley.

Prizant, B., & Wetherby, A. (1987). Communicative intent: A framework for understanding social-communicative behavior in autism. *Journal of the American Academy of Child and Adolescent Psychiatry, 26,* 472–479.

Prizant, B., & Wetherby, A. (1990a). Incorporating a socioemotional perspective in early communication assessment. *Zero to Three, 11,* 1–12.

Prizant, B., & Wetherby, A. (1990b). Toward an integrated view of early language and communication development and socioemotional development. *Topics in Language Disorders, 10,* 1–16.

Prizant,. B., & Weatherby, A. (1993). Communication and language assessment for young children. *Infants and Young Children, 5,* 20–34.

Prizant, B., Wetherby, A., & Roberts, J. (1993). Communication disorders in infants and toddlers. In C. Zeanah (Ed.), *Handbook of infant mental health* (pp. 260–279). New York: Guilford.

Retherford, K. (1993). *A guide to analysis of language transcripts* (2nd ed.). Eau Claire, Wisc: Thinking Publications.

Rogoff, B. (1990). *Apprenticeship in thinking: Cognitive development in social context.* Oxford, U.K.: Oxford University Press.

Rogoff, B., Malkin, C., & Gilbride, K. (1984). Interaction with babies as guidance in development. In B. Rogoff & J. V. Wertsch (Eds.), *Children's learning in the "zone of proximal development": New directions for child development* (pp. 1–6). San Francisco: Jossey-Bass.

Rogoff, B., & Wertsch, J. V. (1984). Editor's notes. In B. Rogoff & J. V. Wertsch (Eds.), *Children's learning in the "zone of proximal development": New directions for child development* (pp. 2–3). San Francisco: Jossey-Bass.

Roush, J. (1991). Early intervention: Expanding the audiologist's role. *ASHA, 33,* 47–49.

Rydell, P., & Prizant, B. M. (1995). Assessment intervention strategies for children who use echolalia. In K. Quill (Ed.), *Methods to enhance communication and socialization in children with autism and PDD* (pp. 105–129). Albany: Delmar Publishers.

Sameroff, A. (1987). The social context of development. In N. Eisenburg (Ed.), *Contemporary topics in development* (pp. 273–291). New York: Wiley.

Sameroff, A., & Fiese, B. (1990). Transactional regulation and early intervention. In S. Meisels & J. Shonkoff (Eds.). *Handbook of early childhood intervention* (pp. 119–149). Cambridge, U.K.: Cambridge University Press.

Schuler, A., Peck, C., Willard, C., & Theimer, K. (1989). Assessment of communicative means and functions through interview: Assessing the communicative capabilities of individuals with limited language. *Seminars in Speech and Language, 10,* 51–61.

Schuler, A., & Prizant, B. (1985). Echolalia. In E. Schopler & G. Mesibov (Eds.), *Communication problems in autism.* New York: Plenum.

Schuler, A., Prizant, B., & Wetherby, A. M. (1997). Enhancing communication: Prelanguage approaches. In D. Cohen & A. Donnellan (Eds.), *Handbook of autism and pervasive developmental disorders* (2nd ed., pp. 539–571). New York: Wiley.

Shriberg, L., & Kwiatkowski, J. (1982). Phonological disorders II: A conceptual framework for management. *Journal of Speech and Hearing Disorders, 47,* 242–256.

Snyder, L., & Downey, D. (1997). Developmental differences in the relationship between oral language deficits and reading. *Language, Speech and Hearing Services in Schools, 17,* 27–40.

Snyder-McLean, L., Solomonson, B., McLean, J., & Sack, S. (1984). Structuring joint action routines: A strategy for facilitating communication and language development in the classroom. *Seminars in Speech and Language, 5,* 213–228.

Stoel-Gammon, C. (1991). Normal and disordered phonology in two-year olds. *Topics in Language Disorders, 11*(4), 21–32.

Vygotsky, L. (1978). *Mind in society: The development of higher psychological processes.* Cambridge, Mass.: Harvard University Press.

Vygotsky, L. (1986). *Thought and language.* (A. Kozulin, Ed. & Trans.). Cambridge, Mass.: Harvard University Press.

Westby, C. (1988). Children's play: Reflections of social competence. *Seminars in Speech and Language, 9,* 1–13.

Westby, C. (1990). Ethnographic Interviewing: Asking the right questions to the right people in the right ways. *Journal of Childhood Communication Disorders, 10,* 101–111.

Wetherby, A., & Prizant, B. (1989). The expression of communicative intent: Assessment guidelines. *Seminars in Speech and Language, 10,* 77–91.

Wetherby, A., & Prizant, B. (1992). Profiling young children's communicative competence. In S. Warren & J. Reichle (Eds.), *Causes and effects in communication disorders.* Baltimore: Brookes.

Wetherby, A., & Prutting, C. (1984). Profiles of communicative and cognitive-social abilities in autistic children. *Journal of Speech and Hearing Research, 27,* 364–377.

Winton, P. (1988). Effective communication between parents and professionals. In D. Bailey, Jr,. & R. Simeonsson (Eds.), *Family assessment in early intervention* (pp. 207–208). Columbus, Ohio.: Merrill.

Yoder, P. (1987). Relationship between degree of infant handicap and clarity of infant cues. *American Journal of Mental Deficiency, 91,* 639–641.

CHAPTER 3

Sociocultural Issues in Assessment and Intervention

Elise Davis-McFarland, Ph.D., CCC-SLP
Associate Professor, Medical University of South Carolina
Charleston
Bonita Dowell, Ph.D., CCC-SLP
Associate Professor
South Carolina State University
Orangeburg

Key Terms

AAEV (African American English vernacular)
code switching
criterion-referenced assessments
cultural competence
culturally-linguistically different (CLD)
cultural sensitivity
curriculum-based intervention
dialect
dynamic assessment
ethnographic assessment
norm-referenced tests
Standard English vernacular (SEV)

Overview

America is moving closer to becoming a multicultural society. By the year 2000 the majority of the population will be persons of non-European ancestry. Latin Americans, African Americans, Asian Americans, Native Americans, and other nonmainstream cultural groups will constitute 52 percent of America's population. The impact of these demographic changes will be felt across society. Americans will be forced to acknowledge and accommodate sociocultural diversity as never before. The awareness of sociocultural differences brings with it the requirement to view people within the context of their culture. Culture, which is the sharing of a common language, worldview, values, and mores, is the glue that binds people into a community.

One of the most important aspects of culture is language. Aside from one's physical features, it is language and communication style that most clearly mark sociocultural group membership. Not only is it the currency of human interaction, language and communication style also support and underpin educational achievement. Children must be able to communicate and compete academically with others from diverse socioeconomic backgrounds. Therefore, it becomes necessary for speech-language pathologists, teachers, and other professionals to differentiate between culturally determined language styles and true disorders of communication. They must also be able to use culturally valid assessment and intervention strategies to assist children in achieving communicative competence and academic success.

The purpose of this chapter is to discuss sociocultural issues related to language assessment and intervention with children from nonmainstream cultures. Although the focus is on assessment and intervention with preschoolers, much of the information is also applicable to school-aged children.

LANGUAGE AND CULTURE

Language is developed within a cultural context. Indeed, culture and language are reflections of one another and reciprocally influence each other (Gudykunst & Ting-Toomey, 1988). Both are intertwined, much like a French braid, with strands of each inseparably woven into one another. Hilliard (1983) stated that "language . . . is a prime source of cultural identity" (p. 27). It is also a cognitive structuring of the world that is linked to one's worldview, identity, self-concept, and self-esteem. Heath (1986a) made the point that all language learning is cultural learning. Children do not only learn the sounds, words, and expressions of language, they also learn how language is used to negotiate the demands of the immediate environment and life in general. They learn to use language to acquire their desires, influence others, and interact with others in their own behalf. Cultural learning includes all the learning that enables a member of a family and/or community to behave appropriately within that group. This is critical to one's self-identification, and the group's approval is necessary for self-esteem (Heath, 1986a, p. 146).

Each cultural group's vernacular is characterized by unique phonological, semantic, syntactic, and pragmatic characteristics. Such a set of language variations constitutes a **dialect**. Dialects are culturally determined. Children emulate the dialect of their parents, caregivers, and educators. By the age of 3, children's language and communication styles mark them as members of a particular linguistic community.

Children from nonmainstream cultures who speak a dialect are termed **culturally-linguistically different (CLD)**. Until recently, we knew very little about how children who are CLD learned language. In fact, our knowledge of language learning was overwhelmingly derived from studies of children who were white, native English speaking, firstborn, and from the middle and upper middle classes. However, once ethnographers began to study children who are CLD and their families, the body of knowledge increased (Heath, 1983; Mertino, 1992; Stockman, Vaughn-Cooke, & Wolfram, 1982).

The cultural influences on language and language learning become clear when we contemplate the differences in communication styles of African American children in Charleston, South Carolina; Asian American children in San Francisco, California; Latin American children in Chicago, Illinois; Native American children in Tempe, Arizona; and European American children in Topeka, Kansas. Among African Americans, interruptions during conversations are tolerated and often the most aggressive speaker will get the floor (Terrell & Terrell, 1993). On the other hand, Native American children are taught to hear out a speaker before they question or comment (Harris, 1993). Asian American children are socialized to say "no" sparingly. It is considered impolite to communicate disagreement, especially if one does not know the speaker well (Cheng, 1987). Persons of Latin American ancestry are accustomed to keeping a close personal distance while talking to one another, and touching during conversation is not unusual (Kayser, 1985, 1995). Both African American and Latin American children will avoid direct eye contact with an adult who is scolding them. On the other hand, European American adults expect their children to look at them when they are being disciplined. Not to do so is considered a sign of disrespect.

Cultural Differences

Ogbu (1993) used the concepts of *primary* and *secondary* cultural differences to explain the differences in school achievement and cultural styles between mainstream and nonmainstream cultural groups in the United States. Primary cultural differences are characteristic of immigrants who have not had a subordinate relationship with European Americans. Their cultural differences, which existed prior to their immigration to the United States, are usually quite specific and easily identified. The immigrants recognize these differences as a barrier to academic and employment success and seek to overcome them in order to be more competitive. They do not hesitate to take on European American cultural behaviors in order to achieve their social and educational goals. Conversely, secondary cultural features are more likely to be exhibited by groups that have had a subordinate relationship with European Americans. Their cultural differences are more likely to develop after the two cultural groups come into contact. Ogbu referred to groups with secondary cultural features as "caste-like minorities" (p. 487), whose secondary cultural features arise from their reactions to being subordinated and exploited by the dominant group. Many African Americans, Latin Americans, and Native Americans exhibit secondary cultural features. In effect, they have not been completely woven into the European American cultural fabric. Secondary cultural features are evident after groups become subordinate to the dominant cultural group. The secondary cultural differences are more a matter of style than content (i.e., child-rearing, learning, communication, interaction, and cognitive styles); and the group with secondary cultural differences will be reluctant to relinquish these cultural behaviors in favor of those of the dominant group. Members of the group with secondary cultural features may find it emotionally painful to cross cultural barriers, and they may be penalized or socially ostracized by the group for perceived desertion of its cultural mores. For example, "talking white" and successful academic achievement ("acting white") are behaviors that may be rejected by some of the group member's peers.

Child-rearing Practices

Culturally determined child-rearing practices also influence language development and communication styles (Anderson & Battle, 1993; Heath, 1986a). For example, some parents believe that it is their responsibility to nurture their children and be their primary teacher. European American parents are likely to embrace this concept and may teach their children language by naming objects in the environment and pointing out and asking them about the objects' characteristics (e.g., color, purpose, size). Another view of child rearing is that parents are to provide basic nurturing and care giving but that children have a major role in their own development. The belief is that, if given the opportunity, children will gain from the environment and their interaction with it the information and knowledge necessary to become productive group members. For example, African American children are expected to be able to benefit from the language around them as a model for language development, and there may be very little explicit teaching. Heath (1983) and Ward (1982), in their studies of language learning and use in African American children, found that children were allowed to be present during adult conversations; however, the conversational content was not modified for them, nor were they expected to participate. Children were not expected to initiate conversations or offer topics, but rather listened and responded to the adults' questions and followed their instructions. In other cultures, communal responsibility for child rearing is the norm. Although parents are primarily responsible for the child's nurturance and well-being, the entire community participates in the upbringing and cultural teaching. Latin American and Asian American parents take such a communal perspective. Caudill (1972) noted that Japanese American mothers are less likely to talk to their infants than European American mothers. Japanese American mothers, believing that children should be allowed to continue their childhood through adolescence, are very tolerant of their children's use of baby talk and immature speech well into the school years.

These and similar research findings demonstrate that children from different sociocultural backgrounds develop language, communication, and learning styles based on their families' expectations and the cultural norms of their socializing community.

LANGUAGE ASSESSMENT WITH PRESCHOOLERS

The relationship between culture and communication style is well established. Therefore, it becomes imperative that any assessment of the language and communication of children who are CLD must account for the cultural dynamics of language. When we assess language and communication, we evaluate competence and performance, but we are also interested in understanding the child's communicative style. *Traditional assessments, which do not account for the cultural dynamics of language, provide us with data but not the insight necessary to understand them.* The lack of insight can lead to improper diagnoses and program placements, poor communication with parents and teachers, and inadequate therapeutic outcomes.

Purposes of Assessment

The purposes of communication assessment with children who are CLD is the same as with other children:

1. To determine whether the child's language is age-appropriate.

2. To determine whether the child's language will support literacy development. Reading is a language-based skill, which has its roots in oral language skills. Comprehension skills (Gerber, 1993), emergent literacy (Terrell, 1992), and metalinguistic awareness (Paul, 1995) are prerequisites for literacy development. The assessment must determine whether those

skills are present and, if not, if the child has the potential for developing them.

3. To provide information for planning language intervention. If the child is not a competent communicator, the assessment should provide information about strengths, weaknesses, and areas requiring remediation.

4. To provide guidance to family members about how to stimulate and facilitate language and literacy development. The assessment must yield information to guide families in their attempts to assist and support their child's language learning.

STANDARDIZED ASSESSMENTS: ISSUES AND CHALLENGES

One of the purposes of language assessment is to obtain an objective measure of the child's level of language development and ability. In order to accomplish this, standardized tests with proven reliability, validity, and sensitivity are often used. This assessment strategy may be appropriate for children whose cultural and linguistic characteristics are represented in the standardization population. However, the diverse languages, dialects, and cultures of children who are CLD require that alternative and/or additional assessment strategies be employed.

Cultural Issues

It is not uncommon to witness stereotypes being applied to people from nonmainstream cultures. However, there is as much diversity between various members of the African American, Latin American, Asian American, and Native American cultural groups as between those groups and European Americans. Cuban Americans, Mexican Americans, and South Americans have distinctive cultural and linguistic features, which define their ethnicity and distinguish them from other Spanish-speaking cultural groups. The same is true of other cultural minorities. However, there are also cultural characteristics and communication styles that are shared across cultural groups (Paul, 1995).

High-Context and Low-Context Communication

One paradigm for considering communication similarities across cultures was described by the anthropologist Hall (1976) in his writings about differences in communication styles between various cultures. Cultural groups vary in the amounts of information transmitted via words as opposed to situational context and physical cues, which take the place of words. Cultural groups vary along a continuum of contextualization; hence, the use of the concept of high-

and low-context cultures. Low-context cultures are more dependent on exact, precise, direct, and logical verbal communication. European Americans, including the Swiss, Germans, and Scandinavians, are low-context cultural groups. High-context cultures rely more on nonverbal and contextual cues. Less emphasis may be placed on words than on situational cues, due to established hierarchies with less emphasis on literal, precise definitions and more on the overall sense and context of the message. Describing high-context communication Hecht, Andersen, and Ribeau (1989) explain that "facial expressions, tensions, movements, speed of interaction, location of the interaction, and other subtle 'vibes' are likely to be perceived by and have more meaning for people from high-context cultures" (p. 177). African Americans, Latin Americans, Asian Americans, and Native Americans are examples of high-context cultural groups. Table 3-1 delineates some of the communication differences between high- and low-context cultures.

Lynch and Hanson (1992) explain the relationship of high- and low-context cultures to change in the following manner:

> High-context cultures tend to be more formal, more reliant on hierarchies, and more deeply rooted in the past. In contrast, low-context cultures are more informal, allow more equality of interaction, and have less knowledge about and reverence for the past. As a result, high-context cultures may change more slowly but provide a healthy stability for group members. Low-context cultures may be more responsive to and comfortable with change but lack a sense of continuity and connection with the past. (p. 45)

The differences between high- and low-context communication styles become obvious when we look at the demands that language assessment puts on a child's communication system. Language assessment is a low-context communication situation, which requires particular types of communication and precise language. The assessment usually takes place in an environment that is unfamiliar to the child, and it may be conducted by someone the child has never met. The examiner, as part of the assessment scheme, will ask the child to do things (i.e., put the block under the box) for which there may be no apparent reason. There may even be pseudoquestions (Where is your nose?) that any child should be able to answer. A child who is a high-context communicator may be penalized for lack of communicative precision and a communication style unlike that required by the assessment.

A Cultural Definition of Pathology

Acknowledgment of the cultural influences on language and communication leads us to a cultural framework in defining communication pathology. A determination of whether communication is pathological or typical must be made

Table 3-1. High- and Low-Context Communication

ETHNICITY	ORIENTATION	COMMUNICATION
High-Context Cultures		
Asian Americans Native Americans Arab Americans African Americans Latin Americans	Time: Polichronic* Kinship: Extended family Child Rearing: Authoritarian Cooperation Ethic: Cooperation Social Contracts*: Humanistic Group Orientation: Collective	Verbal: Situational cues are important; more emphasis on the overall sense and context of the message; less emphasis on literal, precise definitions Nonverbal: Physical gestures, posture, intonation are heavily relied upon
Low-Context Cultures		
European Americans Greeks Italians Scandinavians Germans Swiss	Time: Monochronic* Kinship: Nuclear family Child Rearing: Permissive Cooperation Ethic: Competition Social Contract*: Legalistic Group Orientation: Individual	Verbal: Precise, direct, logical verbal communication is valued Nonverbal: Distance is required for comfort in communication

***polichronic**—several events may be occurring simultaneously. Everything has its own schedule. Events rather than time or a schedule are important. Time is not considered money.
monochronic—events happen sequentially rather than simultaneously or on a predetermined schedule. This requires planning. Time is considered money.
social contracts—humanistic: friendship and kinship relationships are heavily relied on in making agreements and commitments. Legalistic: formal documents and institutions are heavily relied on for making agreements and commitments.

Source: Adapted from Westby, & Rouse, G. (1985). Culture in education and the instruction of language learning–disabled students. *Topics in Language Disorders, 5*(4), 15–28; Hall, E. T. (1976). *Beyond culture.* Garden City, N.Y.: Anchor Books; and Lynch, E., & Hanson, M. (1992). *Developing cross-cultural competence.* Baltimore: Brookes.

in relation to the standards and mores of the child's socializing community. To do otherwise is to run the risk of making claims and judgments about the communicative behaviors of a given group of speakers from an inappropriate or, even worse, an ethnocentric set of assumptions and norms (Taylor, 1986, p. 9). Culturally valid assessment requires the use of instruments and strategies that fairly distinguish between typical and deviant communication and do not discriminate against the child because of his or her sociocultural background (Taylor & Payne, 1983). The assessments must incorporate the standards for typical, useful communication as defined within the child's own socializing community.

Bias in Language Assessment

Taylor and Payne (1983) pointed out four types of bias inherent in standardized language assessments: situational bias, direction or format bias, value bias, and linguistic bias. Situation bias can occur when the examiner and the child are operating from different cultural expectations about the rules of communicative interaction. Cultural expectations about speakers' roles, whether to answer pseudoquestions, and styles of interaction may affect the assessment results.

Direction or format bias can become an issue if the child is unfamiliar with the structure of the assessment or the directions provided by the examiner. For example, if the child is not accustomed to telling stories to adults, then the examiner's direction to do so may not be understood or responded to appropriately. Moreover, a child's inability to respond to syntactically complex questions or requests may be interpreted as a language deficit when in fact it is a lack of experience with those syntactic structures.

Value bias can occur when a child is asked what he or she would do in a certain situation. There can be a mismatch between the child's culturally determined answer and the response the examiner is seeking. Linguistic bias occurs when the examiner alters the assessment battery to assess the child's use of dialect without considering or verifying that the child may have some facility with **Standard English vernacular (SEV)**.

Westby (1994) identified additional biases that can impact assessment results. Rudeness bias occurs when clinicians ask family members questions that are considered inappropriate or offensive. If the parent does not feel empowered to protest, the question may go unanswered or be answered incorrectly. Another danger is that the family member may be offended and form a negative opinion of the clinician.

A clinician's belief that silence implies consent can lead to courtesy bias. Family members may not agree with the clinician's perception of their child or may not trust his or her judgment and recommendations. However, rather than risk offending the clinician or creating an embarrassing situation, they appear to agree when in fact they do not and have no intention of following the clinician's recommendations (Westby, 1994, p. 48).

Norm-Referenced Versus Criterion-Referenced Tests

Traditionally, communication assessment has involved comparing a child's speech and language to a standard of developmentally appropriate communication. Speech-language pathologists have been trained to use **norm-referenced tests** as the primary means of objective determination of a communicative disorder. Norm-referenced tests provide rankings and scores (percentile ranks, *z* scores, *t* scores, scaled scores, stanines, equivalent scores) that allow the comparison of the testee's performance to that of others in the norming population. This type of test ideally possesses essential psychometric constructs that provide assurance that the test aids in the identification of a communicative disorder (McCauley & Swisher, 1984). An advantage of norm-referenced, standardized assessment tools is that they provide reliable, valid, somewhat precise measures of communication ability (Owens, 1995).

Two psychometric constructs that must be considered in the selection of a norm-referenced assessment instrument are *validity* and *reliability*. An assessment instrument is reliable if it provides precise results that remain reasonably consistent when the measurement procedure is repeated with the same individual. Validity can be defined as the extent to which the assessment instrument measures what it purports to measure (Ventry & Schiavetti, 1986).

There are some disadvantages inherent in normed tests when used with children who are CLD. The standardization populations for many norm-referenced speech and language measures do not include a diverse enough sample of children to make the norms valid for children who are CLD. Also, the tests may not accommodate the dynamic, diverse nature of the language of children who are CLD. Many standardized tests focus on the syntactic and semantic relationships that underpin SEV, with little or no consideration of the structural and pragmatic elements of the vernacular of a child who is CLD. The norm-referenced assessment allows the clinician to assess the child's knowledge of SEV but does not provide information about the child's proficiency in his or her own vernacular, nor his or her potential for learning SEV.

Procedural modifications or adaptations made during test administration to accommodate children's individual differences may jeopardize the test's validity. However, when it becomes necessary to use norm-referenced measures as part of an assessment strategy, certain adaptations may nonetheless be necessary. If done carefully and consistently, such adaptations can be justified; however, modifications should be made only on the *second* test administration (the test should be administered according to directions and without modifications the first time). After the second administration, the test-retest results can be compared. Some modifications that can be used to make norm-referenced assessments more appropriate for children who are CLD are presented in Table 3-2.

Once modifications are made, the test norms are no longer valid, so the test cannot be scored. Consequently, the examiner must give a specific description of the modifications that were made in the testing procedure and make notations about the child's responses, performance, and behaviors.

Table 3-2. Modifications for Standardized Test Administration With Children Who Are CLD

1. Select the test that has the most valid items for the skills to be assessed.
2. Examine the directions and each of the test items in order to determine whether the child who is CLD has had access to the information.
3. Develop a list of alternative directions and responses to items before administering the test.
4. The following procedural modifications may be made in order to obtain a more accurate description of the child's communication:
   A. Provide additional time for the child to respond.
   B. Continue the test even though a basal is not established.
   C. Continue the test beyond the ceiling.
   D. Ask the child to name the picture or point to actual objects for items missed on tasks that use pictures for assessing comprehension.
   E. Encourage the child to explain incorrect choices and note the explanations in the report.
5. Record all of the child's responses. When an answer is changed, give credit, especially when it is demonstrated that the correct answer was known (and was not a guess).
6. Compare the child's responses with the ones considered to be correct on the test. For responses that are the same or similar, mark them correct.
7. For those items found to be incorrect according to the test manual, compare the child's answers with reported features of the child's language or dialect and rescore when appropriate.
8. Score the test results in two ways. First, record scores as indicated in the examiner's manual, even though the directions may have been changed in your case. Next, rescore each item, allowing credit for those items that are considered correct in the child's language system and/or experience.
9. Compare both sets of scores with the norms. Most often, the adjusted scores are higher than the unadjusted scores for typically developing children. Children with communication disorders will achieve low scores no matter how the test is scored.
10. When reporting results of such testing, indicate that adjustments have been made. The evaluator should describe which items were modified, what was done to modify test procedures, and the differences in the childs responses after such modification.
11. Focus on what children can do rather than what they cannot do; look for what children know as well as what they do not know.

Source: Tolliver-Weddington, G., & Erickson, J. (1987). Guidelines for use of standardized tests with minority children. In L. Cole & V. Deal (Eds.), *Communication Disorders in multicultural populations* (pp. 21–22). Rockville, Md.: American Speech-Language-Hearing Association. Adapted by permission.

Criterion-referenced assessments are not used to compare children to an externally derived standard. They are "devised to examine a particular form of communicative behavior, not with reference to other children's achievement but only to determine if the child can attain a certain level of performance" (Paul, 1995, p. 42). The best use of these measures is to determine a baseline of functions or behaviors that can be used to assess a child's progress toward a desired goal of communication behavior. A distinct advantage of this approach is the opportunity to use a developmental sequence of the child's vernacular as the standard of comparison. Criterion-referenced procedures can be used for the assessment of both comprehension and production. Miller and Paul (1995) discussed the use of criterion-referenced procedures for the examination of both contextualized and noncontextualized comprehension performance. There is also a significant role for the criterion-referenced assessment of language performance (Paul, 1995). The obvious benefit of criterion-referenced assessment techniques is that they easily accommodate language diversity. An assessment strategy can be tailor-made for the individual child without jeopardizing the opportunity to obtain valid, reliable data for analysis and intervention planning.

An interesting approach to criterion-referenced assessment is Terrell's Parent-Child Comparative Analysis (PCCA) (Terrell, 1992). Terrell devised the strategy to assess the speech and language of a 4-year-old Nigerian girl born in the United States. The child's parents spoke only English to her and spoke their native language, Ibo, to each other. They referred their daughter for a speech and language assessment because of possible articulation and language deficits and a suspected hearing loss. The clinician wanted to determine the extent to which the child's communication was influenced by the Ibo language and culture and whether her articulation and language skills were developmentally appropriate. Since there were no standardized Ibo language assessments available to the clinician, the father (whose English was more heavily accented than the mother's and who was the child's primary caregiver) was used as the referent for assessing the child's speech and language. The father's and daughter's receptive language and articulation were assessed in English using standardized measures. The child's expressive language was assessed using three conditions: telling a story with pictures as stimuli, retelling a story after the clinician read a storybook to her, and telling a story to the clinician. The father's expressive language task was to talk about his native Nigeria. The child's and father's speech and language samples were compared to determine divergent patterns. "The child's divergent patterns that did not occur in the parent's responses were then compared to typical expectations for the child's chronological age" (Terrell, 1992, p. 35). Based on the comparison of the child's and the father's performances, the clinician was able to determine that her articulation was mildly delayed and her language moderately delayed. Her hearing was normal. Terrell offers several cautions about using the PCCA; however, it is a useful model to consider for assessing a child who is CLD.

It is difficult to justify using only standardized, norm-referenced tests for the assessment of children who are CLD. All standardized language tests are culturally based. They incorporate certain cultural assumptions about how children learn, organize, and use language. Most standardized tests are better indicators of acculturation than of language disability. Indeed, *the best use of standardized tests with children who are CLD may be to determine their familiarity with the language required for academic success* (Westby, 1994).

A Culturally Valid Assessment Strategy

The purpose of language assessment is to evaluate communicative competence. This goal is broader than the assessment of linguistic competence (Erickson & Iglesias, 1986, p. 193). Since culture influences language and communicative style in children who are CLD, a culturally valid approach to the assessment is desirable. Taylor and Payne (1983) stated that culturally valid tests do not discriminate unfairly either for or against a client, either for cultural reasons or because of cultural variations based on such factors as age, gender, socioeconomic class, or dialect (p. 11). Several authors (Dabney, Clingmon, Clark-Thoma, Coonce, & Wyatt, 1994; Erickson & Iglesias, 1986; Langdon, 1992; Taylor & Payne, 1983) have advocated culturally relevant procedures for communication assessment of children who are CLD. Incorporating ethnographic principles into the assessment strategy helps honor and preserve the cultural aspects of the child's language and communication patterns. A culturally valid assessment strategy includes: (1) extensive parent input and participation; (2) culturally valid language tests; (3) assessment of the child's potential for communication skills acquisition; (4) careful, deliberate decision making about the use of norm-referenced and criterion-referenced assessment tools; (5) careful consideration of the use of standardized and nonstandardized methods of test administration; (6) an assessment of the child's play behaviors as an indication of cognitive style and development; and (7) a comprehensive, natural context sample of the child's language. If the child's first language is not English, a culturally valid assessment strategy will also include an assessment of both the child's first and second languages to determine competence in both. If necessary, an interpreter should be used (Erickson & Iglesias, 1986).

Assessment of the child's first and second languages is important because bilingualism is a complex phenomenon. The child may be a competent communicator in the first language yet may not be proficient in the use of the second language in academic situations (Hakuta & Garcia, 1989). The assessment of both languages will also help the professional determine whether the child is **code switching** (alternating between the two languages). Code switching, which was once considered a language deficiency, is, in fact, a creative discourse strategy that allows the child the use of both languages (Hakuta & Garcia, 1989, p. 376).

Using a culturally valid assessment strategy yields the information necessary to understand a child's communication within the proper cultural context. Moreover, language is assessed under the most optimal conditions: situations in which the child feels at ease and is likely to provide the best communication behaviors. This strategy also allows for family members who are most knowledgeable about the child's communication patterns and style to provide information and help guide the clinician's impression of the child's language development and use. Finally, a culturally valid assessment ideally should be administered by a culturally competent speech-language pathologist who is familiar with the child's vernacular.

The concepts of **cultural sensitivity** and **cultural competence** are critical to the notion of culturally valid assessment. Cultural sensitivity allows the professional to view all cultures as positive, valid representations of a group's worldview. Cultural competence involves awareness of one's own cultural limitations, respect for cultural differences, and the ability to use cultural resources in interventions (Davis-McFarland, Fain, & Moss, 1995). Cultural sensitivity leads to understanding the need for a relevant assessment approach for children who are CLD. Cultural competence facilitates the implementation of the culturally valid assessment strategy.

The use of culturally valid assessment strategies helps the professional distinguish between *language difference* and *language deficiency.* A child who successfully uses the language of his or her community but has not mastered the language necessary for school success may be exhibiting a language difference. The child's communication style, as learned in the home, may be different from that of the academic environment. Here, intervention may not be necessary. Instead, explaining the concept of communication difference versus communication disorder to parents and teachers may be sufficient. If intervention is necessary to support academic achievement, it can focus on teaching the child alternative methods of expression in the classroom and formal communication situations and on adjusting the communicative demands of the classroom (Paul, 1995). If culturally valid assessment reveals that the child is not a proficient user of the language of his or her socializing community and/or that he or she experiences difficulty in communicating with family and peers, then a language deficiency exists. Culturally valid therapeutic intervention to establish the language necessary for communication and learning is warranted.

Family Participation

The Individuals with Disabilities Education Act (IDEA) Amendments (1997) mandate parent-professional partnerships. Often the families of children with CLD include extended, as well as nuclear, family members. It is not uncommon for older siblings, grandparents, aunts, uncles, or other, more distant, family relations to have caregiving responsibility for the child.

Families of children from nonmainstream cultural groups must be viewed as vehicles of change in the assessment process. Family members should be an integral part of any assessment strategy with children who are CLD. They can provide valuable information about the child's environment, behavior, preferences, lifestyle, and language. Their input also helps the clinician understand the family's perception of the child and their expectations and desires for the child's language development and performance. Their information can be used for decision making about language competence and performance, therapeutic intervention, and program placement.

There are several paradigms for including parents and families in the assessment and intervention process, including family-centered approaches (Hammer, 1994), family systems therapy (Minuchin, 1985), and ecological approaches to family intervention (Bronfenbrenner, 1985). Ethnographic techniques that use family interviews, naturalistic observations, and questionnaires can be very successful with children who are CLD and their families (Hammer, 1994).

Family participation in the assessment becomes important when considering the situation that nonmainstream parents face. They may not be familiar with the assessment process and service delivery system or understand why their child is being assessed. Their previous experiences with health or educational intervention may have been unpleasant. They may not be familiar with the assessment and intervention vernacular, and they may not think their child has a communication impairment. In fact, they may view their child as very competent or be quite accepting of the disorder. Making the family members a part of the assessment process not only allows them to share pertinent information about themselves, their lifestyle, and their child, it also allows them to become informed about the assessment and intervention process, observe the clinician's interaction with their child, and, in turn, become an advocate for the process and for their child's successful participation. According to Crais (1994), the benefits of having the family participate in the assessment include: (1) increasing the likelihood of gaining consensus on important issues, (2) getting a clearer view of the child's development, (3) saving time, (4) getting a more representative sample of the child's behaviors, and (5) arriving at assessment findings that more closely represent the family's view of the child.

There are several ways to get family input. Questionnaires can be used to identify family concerns, priorities, and resources (Crais, 1993). Interviews with a list of guide questions that cover important topics can be developed (Hammer, 1994). Some sample questions that can be used to elicit information about family members' concerns and perceptions are listed in Table 3-3.

Hammer (1994) recommended beginning the family interview with broad topics and then moving to subtopics and suggested letting the parents take the lead, asking open-ended questions, and keeping on the topic. Throughout the interview the clinician should probe and ask for clarification to ensure a thorough understanding of the parent's message and intent (1994, p. 5).

Table 3-3. Questions to Elicit Information From Family Members During Assessments

1. What activities does your child enjoy most?
2. How does your child participate in these activities?
3. When does your child communicate best?
4. When does your child have the most difficulty communicating?
5. How does your child communicate with:
   Parents (or primary caregivers)?
   Brothers/sisters?
   Extended family members?
   Playmates?
6. How does your child let you know what he or she wants?
7. Does your child start activities or conversations with other people?
8. Does your child communicate as you think he or she should at this age?
9. Does your child communicate like most children his or her age?
10. How would you compare your child's communication skills at this age with his or her brother/sister at the same age?
11. What have you been told about your child's speech?
12. What do you think about this?
13. What information do you want to get from this assessment?

Source: Adapted from Lund, N., & Duchan, J. (1988). *Assessing children's language in naturalistic contexts* (2nd ed.). Englewood Cliffs, N.J.: Prentice-Hall, Inc. Adapted by permission.

The family interview should be augmented with observations of family interactions. The clinician can observe communicative interactions and see who interacts with the child; who initiates communicative interactions, the topics of interaction, and who directs the interaction; the modes of communication used; the communicative acts used by all family members; the child's role in communicative interactions; and the parents' teaching style (Crago & Cole, 1991; Van Kleeck, 1994). The information from the questionnaire, interviews, and observations can be recorded and analyzed for themes, concepts, perceptions, and the family's desires for their child. Using the information in conjunction with other communication assessment data makes the family's concerns and information an integral part of the assessment outcomes. It also facilitates the next logical step of involving parents in making decisions about intervention.

Language Sampling

Language tests can provide useful information about a child's language competence; however, a true assessment must include examination of the child's language production. Language sampling should be a part of any assessment strategy for a child who is CLD (Damico, 1991; Iglesias, 1986; Kayser, 1995; Paul, 1995). A language sample allows for the analysis of spontaneous language without the artificial constraints of traditional assessment procedures. The sample can be analyzed for the child's use of the native vernacular *and* SEV to determine strengths in both modes of communication. Language sampling allows for the assessment in several contexts of the language performance of a child who is CLD. The child's knowledge of phonology, morphology, syntax, semantics, and pragmatics, as well as metalinguistics, can be assessed from the sample. Another advantage of language sampling is that "the examiner constructs situations in which the client can choose the topic and range of conversation" (Weiss, Tomblin, & Robin, 1994, p. 115).

A spontaneous sample of 75 to 100 utterances is adequate for an assessment of the child's production abilities. One of the best contexts for recording the language sample is in the child's own environment (home, preschool, etc.) and using interactions with a variety of people, such as a familiar adult (a family member, teacher, etc.), a peer, and an unfamiliar adult (i.e., a professional). This variety allows the professional to assess differences in the child's language production in various contexts with different conversation partners. In a clinician-child interaction, a variety of elicitation techniques may be used to stimulate various language behaviors. Lund and Duchan (1988) recommended patterning, role-playing, responding to open-ended questions, storytelling, probes, narrations, and games or problem solving. The proper techniques must be determined by the clinician based on knowledge of the child and the assessment goals. The process must be structured so that the child is comfortable and at ease, and thus capable of his or her best language performance. However, as the sampling progresses, "the clinician must challenge the child's language system to encourage the child to use higher levels of language in more communicatively demanding contexts" (Reed, 1994, p. 427).

Kayser (1985) found that speech-language pathologists used language samples with Mexican American children to successfully evaluate several areas: syntactic structures, conversational skills (topic maintenance, turn taking, and clarification abilities), questions, detailed description, and coherence in explanations. Cognitive skills were assessed through examining the children's attention to the task, auditory memory and sequencing, response time, and auditory discrimination. Elicitation methods were found to influence the child's language performance. Narratives gave more information about cognitive and organizational abilities, whereas conversational samples yielded information about the children's syntactical structures and interactional social abilities. Language sampling was judged to be a reliable procedure because "the language sample could be elicited several weeks later and the only difference would be the quantity of language, but not the quality" (Kayser, 1995, p. 267).

Kayser further noted that the language sample elicitation process can be biased by the procedures the professional uses. Two variables must be considered during the elicitation process: the child-clinician interaction and the use of conversation and narrative. In many nonmainstream cultures, children are not given the same status as adults. Therefore, a child who is CLD may not respond readily to a language task in which an unfamiliar clinician requests that he or she talk about culturally inappropriate topics or answer unfamiliar questions. Conversations and narratives are also culturally bound (Heath, 1986b; Kayser, 1990); therefore, the professional must be familiar with the child's culture and its requirements for conversation and narratives in order to appropriately evaluate the child's language sample.

Vaughn-Cooke (1986) pointed out that language sampling should be used in conjunction with other assessments to provide a global picture of language development and use and to make intervention and placement decisions. She also cautioned that language sample results must be interpreted from a developmental perspective to determine whether the child's language is developmentally appropriate. The lack of such developmental information for some nonmainstream English vernaculars is problematic. There are some developmental data for **African American English vernacular (AAEV)** (Stockman, 1996; Stockman, Vaughn-Cooke, & Wolfram, 1982), and Mexican American English Vernacular (Kvaal, Shipstead-Cox, Nevitt, Hodson, & Launer, 1988; Schnell de Acedo, 1994); however, similar data for Asian American dialects and Native American languages appears scarce.

Syntactic complexity of the language sample can be analyzed through the use of mean length of response (MLR) for younger children (up to 5 years) (Miller, 1981). Terminal units (T-units) (Hunt, 1965) should be used to analyze older children's samples. Traditionally, Developmental Sentence Scoring (Lee, 1974) has been used to assess syntactic complexity in language samples. Currently the Developmental Assessment of Spanish Grammar (DASG) (Toronto, 1976) and the Black English Sentence Scoring (BESS) test (Nelson & Hyter, 1990) are available for the assessment of syntactic complexity in Spanish- and AAEV-speaking children, respectively.

Transdisciplinary Play-Based Assessment

Transdisciplinary Play-Based Assessment (TPBA) is a comprehensive assessment approach that allows team members to assess the level and quality of a child's language and communication, cognitive, social-emotional, sensorimotor, and play behaviors (Linder, 1993). The play-based assessment takes place in an environment in which the child is surrounded by familiar toys and materials that can be used for a variety of play scenarios. One or both of the child's caregivers is present and involved in the assessment. The fact that the child is encouraged to play as he or she wishes, with minimal intrusion by the evaluator, reduces the cultural bias of the assessment situation. It also allows for extended observation of the child in a natural environment.

The TPBA is conducted by a team that can include any constellation of professions. In addition to the parents, a minimal team usually consists of a speech-language pathologist, an occupational or physical therapist, and a teacher or psychologist. Other team members may be added as needed. Team roles include the play facilitator (who interacts with the child during the assessment), the parent facilitator (who interacts with parents during the assessment), the observing team members, and a videographer (who tapes the session). The assessment room must include a variety of toys and play materials to facilitate the demonstration of an array of developmental behaviors. Gross motor equipment, manipulative toys, a sand-and-water table, an art area, blocks, and clothes and furniture for dramatic play should be available. The assessment progresses through observation of the child during unstructured play, structured play in which the child engages in cognitive and language activities, unstructured play with another child who is an age-mate, a parent-child interaction session, motor play, and snack time. These varied situations give the team an opportunity to assess the child's self-help skills, adaptive behavior, and oral motor skills. The entire assessment may take 60 to 90 minutes depending upon the child's interest and level of development. Once the videotape has been analyzed, the team can come to a consensus about the child's developmental level, in each of the aforementioned areas, based on the behaviors observed during the assessment. After a meeting with the parents to discuss the findings, recommendations for appropriate interventions can be made.

The advantages of the TPBA are several. First, parent input is an integral part of the assessment process. Second, cultural bias, which is inherent in many other standardized approaches, is minimized. Third, because the child is playing, which is a very familiar task, the issue of unfamiliarity is minimized. One caution is that the assessment of the play behavior must be made in relation to the culturally relevant play behaviors for the child. Torrefy and McCray (1996) offer strategies for facilitating play in children from various cultural backgrounds.

TPBA is a holistic approach to cognitive, language, and behavioral assessment. All the team members observe the same behaviors at the same time, which minimizes the opportunities for conflicting opinions about the child's strengths and abilities. Finally, this approach to assessment of language and communication allows for a determination of the child's level of symbolic behavior, a necessary prerequisite for assessing the appropriate level of communication function. TPBA uses the modality of play (rather than language) to determine the child's level of cognitive development.

Dynamic Assessment

Assessment of the language of children who are CLD should include a determination of their potential for language learning. **Dynamic assessment** is a term used to identify a number of distinct approaches that are characterized by guided learning for the purpose of determining a child's potential for change (Kleinman & Prizant, Chapter 2; Palincsar, Brown, & Campione, 1994; Piaget, 1952). Peña, Quinn, and Iglesias (1992) have introduced the concept of dynamic assessment to language testing with children who are CLD:

> The notion of applying dynamic methods to language assessment holds promise for the assessment of both communicative competence and language-learning potential. It is the method we propose for evaluating linguistically and culturally diverse children. Because it assesses the child's capacity to learn, given previous experiences and the opportunity to learn new skills, dynamic assessment is an inherently nonbiased process. (p. 271)

Dynamic assessment uses a test-teach-test approach. The child's language is assessed. Then a new language skill is taught using a mediated learning experience (MLE). Afterwards, the child is retested to determine whether the new skill has been learned.

Peña, Quinn, and Iglesias (1992) initially assessed Puerto Rican American and African American preschoolers' abilities to name pictures. Their subsequent mediation activities focused on teaching the children labeling strategies. Afterwards, they retested the children and found that the dynamic language assessment differentiated children who were language different from those who were language disordered. Compared to the others, children who were language disordered were less responsive to mediation, and the clinicians had to work harder in the mediation process to effect even a minimal change in their language skills (Peña et al., 1992, p. 277).

Dynamic assessment can have several advantages over traditional norm-referenced assessment strategies. One advantage is that traditional strategies assess current function without any examination of the extent to which the child's skill level can be modified through intervention. In particular, we cannot be sure that children who are CLD have been exposed to all of the skills assessed by norm-referenced tests. However, dynamic assessment includes the opportunity to teach a skill, thus enabling the assessor to determine the child's language-learning potential. A second advantage of dynamic assessment is that the child uses problem-solving strategies that are taught during the MLE. This provides an opportunity for the assessor to evaluate the child's ability to incorporate those strategies into his or her performance repertoire. Finally, dynamic assessment requires a different relationship between the assessor (teacher) and the child. With traditional assessment strategies, the assessor-child interaction is minimal and specifically related to the tasks at hand. However, with dynamic assessment, the assessor and child interact continuously and are involved in a common goal—the accomplishment of the learning objective (Bogartz, Hisama, Manni, & Wurtz, 1986). In fact, it is not uncommon for the assessor to give the child an instruction such as the following for the MLE: "I am going to teach you about word endings and we are going to work together until you have learned them all." The instruction not only tells the child what he or she will be learning, it also indicates that he or she will have help and support during the process. This approach should motivate the child to his or her best effort.

Too often children who are CLD are penalized for lacking skills that they do not exhibit during traditional language assessments, whereas dynamic assessment provides the opportunity to determine their language-learning potential. This has implications for understanding a child's current skill level and allows for the prediction of future development. All of this information is useful for intervention planning and parent counseling.

Culturally valid assessment allows the clinician to take on the child's cultural perspective. Communication ability is defined in relation to family and community standards. It yields information that allows the clinician to differentiate between the communication skills appropriate for interaction with family and friends and the language skills required for academic achievement. A culturally valid assessment strategy decreases bias and increases the validity of the assessment information. The following summarizes the principles of a culturally valid assessment strategy:

1. The clinician should be aware of the influence of personal bias. Nonbiased assessment begins with respect for the child's cultural background. The clinician's cultural sensitivity and cultural competence influence the child's test performance as well as its interpretation.

2. The clinician should conduct an **ethnographic assessment**, which begins with gaining familiarity with the family's and community's definitions of acceptable communicative skills and of communicative disorders.

3. The clinician should use the family as a resource for information about the child. The family's preferences and priorities should be honored during the assessment and intervention planning.

4. The clinician should use criterion-referenced assessment instruments where possible. Data from ethnographic studies, local norms, and other relevant data should also be used to determine whether or not the child's communicative skills are within normal limits for his or her linguistic community.

5. If norm-referenced tests are used, careful, consistent modifications in test administration may be warranted. The modifications should be documented and comparisons made between the child's achievement on the regularly administered test and the modified test.

6. The examiner should use spontaneous language sampling as one assessment of language competence and performance. Samples should be taken with different communication partners and analyzed to determine the child's facility with his or her native vernacular and with SEV.

7. A nonbiased measure of cognitive, language, and motor development can be obtained through play-based assessment. The clinician should be care-

ful to use the appropriate cultural filter to interpret and evaluate the child's play behaviors.

8. The assessment of language-learning potential is an essential part of the language assessment of a child who is CLD. The opportunity to teach the child a language-learning strategy provides insight into his or her learning style, language competence and performance, and problem-solving abilities.

Assessment is the first component of a two-part process. Once a culturally valid assessment strategy has revealed that a child has a communication disorder, intervention may be necessary. The need for cultural relevance is equally as important in intervention as in assessment.

LANGUAGE INTERVENTION WITH PRESCHOOLERS

There are two assumptions that form the foundation for planning appropriate assessment and effective service delivery with the preschooler who is CLD: First, the impetus for intervention must come from the family's desires for the child, and second, the intervention process should improve the family's communicative effectiveness, both within and outside the socializing linguistic community (Berger, 1986; Dunst, 1985). Underlying these assumptions are two basic requirements for the speech-language pathologist: conducting a culture-specific and valid assessment and developing a partnership with family members in order to plan intervention goals.

Clinical Management: An Overview

In a statement of need, members of the American Speech-Language and Hearing Association (ASHA) Committee on the Status of Racial Minorities (1985) reported that "it is firmly established that most ASHA members are aware of their limitations in language proficiency and in their competence to serve minority populations" (p. 13).

As stated earlier in this chapter, both assessment and intervention with the child who is CLD should be conducted within the framework of normative data obtained from an ethnographic study of the child's linguistic community. This is inconsistent with the mandates of PL 105-17 (IDEA, 1997) and Title VII of PL 95-561 because both require that standardized measures be used to assess language proficiency and educational achievement and determine proper educational placements. However, in order to plan and provide effective intervention with the child who is CLD, the ASHA committee recommended the following competencies for the speech-language pathologist:

Language Proficiency: Level of proficiency from familiarity to fluency in the language or dialect of the nonmainstream culture.

Typical Development:	Knowledge of normative data relative to the nonmainstream culture's language or dialect.
Cultural Sensitivity:	Knowledge of the values, mores, traditions, and beliefs of the nonmainstream culture.
Intervention:	Knowledge of, and the ability to effectively treat, communicative disorders for the nonmainstream population

It is beyond the scope of this chapter to discuss each communicative disorder that may impinge upon the communicative performance of the child who is CLD; however, the remainder will be devoted to a discussion of family-centered and curriculum-based approaches to intervention for the preschooler with a language disorder who is CLD.

The Parent-Professional Partnership

Earlier in this chapter, several models of parent-professional partnerships were presented. These partnerships included the family-centered model (Hammer, 1994), the family systems model (Minuchin, 1985), and the ecological approach (Bronfenbrenner, 1985). Relating these intervention models to the preschool population who are CLD, Terrell and Terrell (1993) advocated the inclusion and participation of family members in the intervention process. Almost 20 years ago, Adler (1979) described an intervention program for children who are CLD that also required family participation. Adler's program was a three-tiered model that incorporated home visits, group and individual parent conferences, and parental participation in intervention sessions.

During home visits, which were conducted twice a week, the professional met with a family member. Role-playing was used to demonstrate intervention techniques. During the individual and group conferences, individual therapy plans were explained, with time allocated for parents to ask questions. It was incumbent on the professional to get through to the participating family member. These conferences were held in a clinical facility. The final component involved the family member serving as a speech aide in the clinic room. The parents were taught to be paraprofessional aides.

Utilizing a three-tiered model similar to Adler's (1979) and the ecological approach to intervention recommended by Bailey and Wolery (1984), Dowell (1994) developed an early intervention program for preschoolers who are CLD. The program included individual family-child sessions, home visits, and a parent group. Titled Families and Children Interacting Together (FACIT), the program was implemented at North Carolina Central University (NCCU) Division of Speech and Hearing in collaboration with the Adaptive Physical Education Program. This transdisciplinary team-based intervention initiative included four preschoolers with language disorders between the ages of 24 and 54 months and their families; graduate students from the disciplines of speech-language pathology, nursing, and adaptive physical education; an adaptive physical educator; a special educator; and a psychologist. The four children and their families were African American speakers of AAEV.

Individual Family-Child Sessions. Sixty-minute individual sessions were held with the children at the NCCU Speech and Hearing Clinic. Immediate and extended family members were encouraged to attend as many intervention sessions with their child as their schedules allowed. These sessions were held 3 days per week. Child-oriented techniques (Fey, 1986) were utilized during the intervention sessions. These techniques were based on following the child's lead during free play. Self-talk (an adult talks aloud about objects in the immediate environment and actions as they are occurring in order to model language for the child), parallel talk (an adult talks aloud about what the child is doing or about events as they occur in the child's environment), expansions, expectations, buildups-breakdowns, and recasts were modeled during these sessions. Family members incorporated the use of these techniques while engaging their child in experiential activities such as baking cornbread, making juice pops, and popping popcorn. Interactive instruction was also utilized so that target behaviors were elicited during play-, art-, drama-, and music-based activities (Dowell, 1992, Seifert & Schwarz, 1991).

Based on the team's philosophy regarding intervention with the child who is CLD, family members became the vehicles of change throughout the course of intervention. The other team members served as intervention facilitators. Rather than using tokens or edible reinforcers, family members became the primary reinforcers by using praise, hugs, shouts of joy, physical touch, and broad smiles and laughter to reward their child's efforts to improve their communicative skills.

The Home Visit. The second author (Dowell) and the graduate student case manager visited each child's home weekly. The home visits were scheduled on a day that was convenient for the family. Family members were also consulted regarding the optimum time of day during which the child was most likely to be alert and interactive.

The communication and interaction style used during the home visits served to generate warmth and sincerity. Nonintrusive language, a pleasant tone of voice, and statements that encouraged mutual sharing of information were the specific communicative style features that were used. During these visits, family members were encouraged to share with other team members any information regarding their child that could be incorporated into the intervention program. For example, family members shared their priorities as well as information about their child's interests, favorite pastimes, and favorite toys. This information served as the basis for the development of objectives, goal selection, and the selection of intervention strategies and materials that would be most appropriate for each child. These visits served to establish optimal and effective learning situations that allowed both the child who is CLD and family member to develop active (rather than passive) roles in the intervention process.

The Parent Group. On a weekly basis, each child's family members met with each other and the team members. During the group meetings, parents were encouraged to evaluate the efforts of the team, to share information with other team members, and to obtain information from other team members regarding any needed resources. Overall, evaluative feedback ranged from positive statements about feeling respected to complaints that "one girl keeps trying to get in my business."

At the end of the program, observations from video and audiotaped sessions of each of the three program components indicated significant increases in the total number, length, and use of child-directed techniques during family-child interactions. In addition, team members established the following guidelines for developing partnerships with families.

1. Use nonintrusive language. As one parent stated, "Break it down so we all can understand what you're talking about."
2. Awareness of paralinguistic features. As one parent stated, "It's not what you said; it's how you said it. Don't tell me what to do, *ask!*"
3. Convey respect. Team members, in keeping with African-American culture, learned each family member's name and the appropriate manner to address them. For example, using Mr. Mills rather than James.
4. Understanding that major family concerns may vary. Team members learned that family survival (having a home, electricity, and water) may surpass the child's communication status as *the* family priority for a period of time.
5. Be a resource for empowerment. Team members learned to empower families to effect change in their lives and the lives of their children.

Curriculum-Based Instruction

Inclusion refers to the education of the child in the school and classroom that he or she would normally attend. It involves bringing support services to the child and requires that he or she remain in class with the other students. Ideally, inclusion involves arranging the classroom environment in such a manner that every child has an opportunity to lead and to experience success and diversity.

The concepts of high- and low-context cultures discussed earlier in this chapter are applicable to intervention as well as assessment. The professional must be sensitive to the intervention needs of the child who is CLD and provide opportunities throughout the school day and within the school curriculum to support the child's cultural and communicative learning styles.

Nelson (1994) defined **curriculum-based intervention** as the use of the local curriculum for determining a student's instructional needs and progress.

For example, using curriculum, high-context activities such as art, music, and family and consumer science, which involve group participation and less structure, may be more appropriate for the child who is CLD than using worksheets and programmed instruction.

Gilbert and Gay (1987) also reported that low-socioeconomic-status African American children prefer activities in which group sharing and nondirective intervention are utilized. The authors also stated that these children demonstrated stage-setting behaviors. These behaviors included sharpening pencils, repeatedly asking directions, and obtaining instructions from peers before beginning an assigned task. The behaviors were punished by teachers who wanted the students to begin and end the task within an allocated period of time. For the children, attempting to do the task was viewed as more important than completing it. They expected appreciation from the teacher for the effort; however, the teacher only praised them after the task was completed.

South Carolina State University Speech and Hearing Clinic developed a model program, the Extended School Year Speech Pathology and Audiology Program, which utilizes a curriculum-based format for 3- to 5-year-old preschoolers who are CLD (Gregg, personal communication, 1996). According to Gregg, the program was designed to ensure that children who are CLD who have been diagnosed as linguistically impaired, especially in cases of pragmatic impairment, would have continuous opportunities for communicative intervention beyond the preschool and home setting. The program provides intervention for preschoolers who are CLD and training for speech-language pathologists from diverse cultural backgrounds (Latinos, Anglos, and African Americans) on how to effectively interact with the child who is CLD.

This program is a 6-week summer experience that is held 4 days per week, with the daily format incorporating individual, small group, and large group sessions. Approaches to intervention combine professional- and child-oriented strategies within the context of group participation. The curriculum is context bound and includes the use of theme-based, experiential activities. Pragmatic skills are targeted within the context of a variety of routine activities such as show-and-tell and snacktime. The program incorporates the use of adolescent bridges, or partners, who serve as communicative models during these activities. Semantic skills are targeted with a set of six to eight core vocabulary words, which are introduced each week. Picture labeling, picture stories, and story retelling tasks are used to teach and elicit vocabulary words. Syntax and morphology are targeted using sequential picture cards and whole language activities. Children are engaged in experiential activities and generate stories that are audio- or videotaped and replayed for the group as the final activity of the day. Phonology is targeted using the bridge, or partner, as a communicative model as well as individuals from the child's linguistic community, who are selected based on the thematic unit. For example, a mail carrier, librarian, police officer, and firefighter might be targeted for the theme, "The Neighborhood." These individuals serve as communicative models for the children who are CLD.

A core vocabulary is selected on a weekly basis. Weekly anecdotal records provide information for communicating with family members about their child's communicative status and progress. The program is currently in its 2nd year. During summer 1995, 7 children who are CLD from one school district and 1 child from the local community participated. During summer 1996, there were 21 children who are CLD from two school districts and three surrounding communities. Currently, quantitative data from pre- and postassessment testing are being analyzed. Based on reports from school officials, classroom teachers, and parents, the benefits derived from this program were noteowrthy and its continuation was determined warranted.

CASE STUDY: CONSUELA

Four-year-old Consuela was referred to the speech-language pathologist by her Head Start teacher, who complained that Consuela was very quiet during most class activities. She often sat in class with her head down, never asked questions, and seemed hesitant to answer questions. She did not bring things to share during show and tell, nor would she participate in the show and tell discussions. The teacher reported that Consuela often used Spanish and English to communicate, and about 50 percent of her speech was intelligible. The speech-language pathologist went into the classroom to observe Consuela and noted the same things the teacher had reported.

Before doing an assessment, the speech-language pathologist spoke to Consuela's parents, who reported that Consuela was the third of four children. She had grown up in a Spanish-speaking community. Her mother spoke only Spanish, and her father spoke both Spanish and Spanish-influenced English at home. Consuela spoke mostly Spanish to her mother and younger brother, but she spoke English to her father and older siblings. Both parents reported that Consuela's development of communication skills had been similar to that of her older siblings. They said she talked a lot at home and they considered her an intelligible, competent communicator. When asked if they read to Consuela, they said they did not but that Consuela's grandmother (who lived next door) often told the children stories about their ancestors and tales from her childhood. They had no concerns about Consuela's ability to communicate and were surprised that she had been referred to a speech-language pathologist.

The speech-language pathologist observed Consuela on the playground at school. During the 30-minute observation he noted that Consuela asked the teacher to get a rope from the storage closet and then organized five other children into a game of jump rope. Once the game ended, she moved to a new group of children and began teasing one of her peers about his new haircut. She asked questions of the other children, responded to their questions, and pointed out a butterfly to another child, who had not seen it light on the swing next to her. Throughout the play period Consuela used both Spanish and Span-

ish-influenced English. Whenever she seemed unsure of a word she immediately switched to Spanish. Once back in the classroom, however, Consuela fell silent again.

The next day the speech-language pathologist invited Consuela to his office, where he asked her to tell him a story. Consuela began slowly telling him a story in English about a big brown dog who befriended a cat. When she hesitated, the speech-language pathologist told her she could use Spanish for the English words she did not know. Now her rate of speech increased and she told the story with enthusiasm and interest. The speech-language pathologist asked Consuela questions about the story and got her to offer her opinions and insights about some of the story events. He recorded the story and their conversation. Analysis of the samples revealed that Consuela's sentences were of adequate length and complexity for her age. Spanish dialectical influences included deletion of the -ed *regular-past marker, omission of the plural /s/ marker, and omission of some articles. Phonological influences included consistent devoicing of final consonants, and some substitutions:* t/θ, z/s, *and* dz/j. *Consuela used concepts of quantity and sequencing as well as nouns, pronouns, verbs, adjectives, conjunctions, and prepositions. She also used negation and possessors. Consuela was then given a vocabulary test and was found able to name 15 of 32 pictures in English and 28 of 32 in Spanish. The speech-language pathologist used a mediated learning experience to teach Consuela the English vocabulary words she did not know, and within 15 minutes, she had learned all the words. A retest 2 days later indicated an 85 percent retention rate. When the speech-language pathologist asked Consuela if she enjoyed the Head Start program, she enthusiastically said she did. When asked why she did not participate more in class, she said that she was sometimes unsure of her English and did not always understand what the teacher said to her.*

The speech-language pathologist related to the Head Start teacher that Consuela's concept development and Spanish language skills were age appropriate. Because her English language skills were less developed, she code switched. When given the opportunity Consuela was perfectly capable of increasing her English proficiency. The speech-language pathologist encouraged the teacher to assist Consuela with vocabulary learning and to encourage her to participate in show and tell and other language-oriented classroom activities. He advised her father and older siblings to continue to speak English with Consuela at home. He also recommended that she be exposed to good oral English language models such as educational television shows and English language storybooks.

Consuela had a language difference rather than a language deficit. Her age-appropriate Spanish language skills were an indication of her ability to learn and use language appropriately. Consuela's English language skills were not age-appropriate, but her assessment results indicated good language-learning potential. With good language models and vocabulary teaching Consuela's English language skills should continue to develop.

CASE STUDY: JAMAL

Jamal was one of several African American children attending the Learning Tree Child Development Center. At 4 years of age, he was the favorite of the entire staff. He had an engaging smile and was very affectionate. He was also the quietest child in his group. He spoke only when he had to. He pointed to direct teachers' attention to objects or toys he wanted. When the teacher gave directions, he usually watched the other children as if to see what they were doing before he complied. His teacher asked the speech-language pathologist what she might do to get Jamal to talk more. The teacher was also concerned because Jamal did not seem able to learn concepts as quickly as his classmates. The speech-language pathologist agreed to come into the class and observe Jamal. She noted that Jamal's attention span was limited, even for a 4-year-old. He did not join in the conversation with the teacher or other children during play and discussion times, and he was usually silent during lunch, whereas his peers chatted away. He did not respond during show and tell, even when his teacher called on him. When he did speak, he usually used two- to three-word utterances. He sometimes appeared lost in his daydreams.

When Jamal's mother came to pick him up, the speech-language pathologist asked her about Jamal's communication at home. She said Jamal had always been quiet. She remembered that he said his first words other than "mama" and "daddy" at about 16 months of age. After that, his vocabulary developed slowly, and at 30 months he was just beginning to put two words together. She said he usually played silently by himself even when his older siblings were nearby and playing together. He often expressed himself by pointing to objects or gesturing. When the speech-language pathologist asked his mother how she would compare Jamal's communication skills development with that of his two older brothers, she reported that Jamal "never talked as good as they did at his age." She said she was concerned about Jamal's communication skills and was planning to ask his teacher what she thought.

The next day the speech-language pathologist went to observe Jamal while his class was outside. Jamal played kick ball with his classmates for a while. His eye-foot coordination seemed poor as he failed several times in succession to kick the ball. When he did finally kick the ball, he ran clumsily after it. Eventually he wandered to a far corner of the play area and began kicking gravel alone. He did not talk to any of the other children. The next week the speech-language pathologist assessed Jamal's speech and language. His articulation test revealed several AAEV dialectical variations. When these were discounted, his score fell in the 25th percentile. A comprehensive language test was administered and scored according to the directions. It was then readministered with modifications to accommodate Jamal's cultural linguistic differences. With the modifications, Jamal's language was assessed to be moderately delayed. He did not identify common household objects, he did not know the primary colors, and he did not understand simple number concepts even though they had been introduced initially in his 3-year-old preschool class. Language sam-

ples were recorded in the classroom, first during a conversation between Jamal and his teacher, and then while Jamal was retelling his mother a favorite bedtime story. Analysis of the sample revealed that Jamal's vocabulary was limited to short, high-frequency words. He spoke primarily in two- and three-word phrases. He did not use irregular verbs or third-person singular tense, and articles, prepositions, and conjunctions were missing from his spontaneous speech. His pragmatic skills were age appropriate. A play assessment revealed slightly delayed gross and fine motor development, with mild oral-motor immaturity and limited, immature language skills. During a dynamic assessment, the speech-language pathologist introduced several vocabulary items with pictures as stimuli. After considerable teaching, Jamal mastered only 10 percent of the new words. A retest the next day revealed only 5 percent retention. The speech-language pathologist explained her assessment findings to Jamal's teacher and mother.

Upon receiving consent to enroll Jamal in speech-language therapy, the speech-language pathologist began the intervention process by conducting another home visit. The speech-language pathologist observed that Jamal's siblings and parents quickly responded to his nonverbal communicative behaviors. For example, when he pointed to the box of cookies on the kitchen table, his mother handed him the entire box. When Jamal wanted to play with a puzzle that his older sister and brother had been putting together, he grabbed as many pieces as he could and covered them with his body, looking at his brother and sister the entire time. Jamal's siblings looked back at him and, without a word, pushed the remaining puzzle pieces to him and found a different puzzle to play with. Following this attempt to engage his siblings, Jamal sat quietly and played alone. As the speech-language pathologist prepared to leave their home, she asked the parents to share their goals for Jamal. Both parents expressed their wish for Jamal to "use the words he does say more" and to "talk more." The speech-language pathologist also asked them to spend some time thinking about goals that would include all members of the family. Jamal's father responded quickly, saying, "We want to know what we can do here at home with Jamal to help you and his other teacher." During their conversations, the speech-language pathologist determined that Jamal's parents were African American English Vernacular speakers who would be good language models for Jamal.

Jamal's parents and the speech-language pathologist decided on a 4-day-a-week intervention program in which she would visit both the home and the preschool classroom twice a week for 60-minute sessions. Initial goals included increasing receptive and expressive vocabulary, increasing mean length of utterance, increasing opportunities to develop and engage in conversational exchanges and dialogue, and improved oral motor skills.

During the home visits, the speech-language pathologist used role-playing to demonstrate three techniques: self-talk, parallel talk, and expansion. She also talked to the family about following Jamal's lead and observing him to identify and use his attempts to engage them in play and or conversations.

The speech-language pathologist used her observations from her first home visit to provide examples. She pointed out that when Jamal pointed to objects or people, he was requesting an action or an answer. She also told them that by pausing and not immediately responding to Jamal's gestural or nonverbal behaviors, they gave him the opportunity and motivation to use words to communicate, especially if they modeled the correct word for him. She instructed them that using the self-talk technique would provide Jamal with opportunities to hear the label for the desired item without pressuring him to respond at that moment. "You might say, 'Jamal wants cookies. Jamal is pointing to cookies,' to provide him with an opportunity to make the request again and to have the model verbal behavior repeated." In order to strengthen Jamal's oral motor skills, she instructed his parents to teach Jamal to blow bubbles from a bubble wand and chew and blow bubbles with sugarless bubble gum. The speech-language pathologist ended the visit by asking them to keep a diary of all the words and phrases Jamal used, and their contexts, for a period of 1 week. This diary, along with the journal entries made each week by Jamal's teacher, identified vocabulary strengths to be shared with each member of Jamal's intervention team.

During her preschool classroom sessions, the speech-language pathologist collaborated with Jamal's preschool teacher to determine the vocabulary words that would be targeted each week within the classroom. A set of six words was introduced to Jamal each week based on the teacher's weekly theme or unit (i.e., food, clothing, community helpers). Picture labeling, story retelling, and language experience activities were used as a means of eliciting and reinforcing linguistic targets. Gross motor skills were observed and monitored on the playground by the teacher during outside physical activities.

Jamal had a language disorder. Although he was a dialect speaker, he was not able use the vernacular for self-expression or to interact with family, teachers, or peers. Therefore, it was necessary to teach Jamal vocabulary and to model proper language use so that he could learn how to communicate effectively. Jamal's parents and teachers were instructed on how to teach Jamal the language he needed. Through intervention at home and in the classroom, Jamal was exposed to the good language models and his opportunities to learn and enhance his communication skills were increased.

The preceding two case studies represent models for intervention with the preschooler who is CLD. As Bunce (1990) reported, not much has been written regarding specific instructional or intervention techniques for bicultural children with language disorders (p. 493). Bunce provided the following suggestions for intervention:

1. Begin intervention where the child can be successful.
2. Base intervention on culturally valid assessment and observations.
3. Plan for generalization from the beginning.

4. Take advantage of teachable moments or follow the child's lead.

5. Train receptive skills first and generalization to productive skills may occur.

6. Make assessment and observation a component of the intervention process.

Awareness of both the linguistic and cultural influences on learning serves to increase the effectiveness of intervention for the child who is CLD with a language disorder. Appropriate communicative intervention relies on an integration of cultural values and normative data to facilitate the acquisition of linguistic skills. Even though achieving this integration is challenging, it must be accomplished if the communicative needs of the child who is CLD with a language disorder are to be met.

SUMMARY

Assessment and intervention with the preschoolers who are CLD presents challenges that must be addressed from a cultural perspective. Some children who are CLD are not exposed to SEV in their immediate, socializing environment. Therefore, a comprehensive assessment is necessary to determine the child's level of language function in their native vernacular and SEV. The clinician must also find nonculturally biased methods of assessing the child's cognitive level and language-learning potential. There must also be an assessment of emergent literacy skills. This approach requires a careful selection of appropriate tests to assure valid, nonbiased results. Culturally valid methods, which include ethnographic techniques and family participation, enable the clinician to distinguish between culturally determined language differences and language pathology. The choice of intervention strategies is dependent on valid assessment outcomes. Here, too, close attention must be given to cultural variables. Parent involvement in the choice of intervention strategies and in the intervention program itself has been shown to be particularly successful with children who are CLD.

REFERENCES

Adler, S. (1979). *Poverty, children and their language.* New York: Grune and Stratton.

American Speech-Language-Hearing Association Committee on the Status of Racial Minorities, (1985). *Clinical management of communicatively handicapped minority language populations* (pp. 13–17). June 6. Rockville, Md.: American Speech-Language-Hearing Association.

Anderson, N., & Battle, D. (1993). Cultural diversity in the development of language. In D. Battle (Ed.), *Communication disorders in multicultural populations* (pp. 158–186). Boston: Andover Medical Publishers.

Bailey, D. (1989). Assessment and its importance in early intervention. *Assessing infants and preschoolers with handicaps* (pp. 1–21). Columbus, Ohio: Merrill.

Bailey, D. B., & Wolery, M. (1984). *Teaching infants and preschoolers with handicaps.* Columbus, Ohio: Merrill.

Berger, M. (1986). Contributions of family therapy to the development of early childhood special education services that enhance individual and family development. *Training professional to interact with families.* (Monograph 2). Moscow, Ida.: University of Idaho.

Bogartz, B. E., Hisama, T., Manni, J. L., & Wurtz, R. G. (1986). Cognitive assessment of nonwhite children. In O. L. Taylor (Ed.), *Treatment of communication disorders in culturally and linguistically diverse populations* (pp. 67–114). San Diego: College Hill Press.

Bronfenbrenner, U. (1985). *Ecology of human development.* Cambridge, Mass.: Harvard University Press.

Bunce, B. (1990). Bilingual/bicultural children and their education. In L. McCormick & R. Schielfelbusch (Eds.), *Early language intervention: An introduction* (pp. 473–498). Columbus, Ohio: Merrill.

Cheng, L. (1987). Cross-cultural and linguistic considerations in working with Asian populations. *Asha, 29*(6), 33–41.

Crago, M., & Cole, E. (1991). Using ethnography to bring children's communicative and cultural world into focus. In T. Gallagher (Ed.), *Pragmatics of language: Clinical practice issues* (pp. 99–131). San Diego: Singular Publishing.

Crais, E. (1993). Families and professionals as collaborators in assessment. *Topics in Language Disorders, 14*(1), 29–40.

Crais, E. (1994). *Increasing family participation in the assessment of children birth to five.* Inservice manual and tapes. Chicago: Applied Symbolix.

Dabney, M., Clingmon, I., Clark-Thoma, E., Coonce G., & Wyatt, T. (1994). *ASHA position paper on assessment of the African-American child.* Sacramento: California Speech-Language-Hearing Association.

Damico, J. S. (1991). Descriptive assessment of communicative ability in LEP students. In E. V. Hamayan & J. S. Damico (Eds.), *Limiting bias in the assessment of bilingual students* (pp. 157–218). Austin, Tex.: Pro-Ed.

Davis-McFarland, E., Fain, M. R., & Moss, S. E. (1995). *Developing culturally valid research paradigms for African-Americans with Alzheimer's disease.* Paper presented at the American Speech-Language-Hearing Association Convention, Orlando, Fla.

Dowell, B. (1992, November). *An Ethno-Social Study of Mother-Child Interaction.* Paper presented at the American Speech-Language Hearing Association Convention, San Antonio.

Dowell, B. (1994, spring). Do you hear what I hear? In *ACCESS: Newsletter of the North Carolina Health Careers Access Program.* Chapel Hill: University of North Carolina.

Dunst, C. J. (1985). Rethinking early intervention. *Analysis and Intervention in Developmental Disabilities, 5,* 165–201.

Erickson, J., & Iglesias, A. (1986). Assessment of communication in non-English proficient children. In O. Taylor (Ed.), *Nature of communication disorders in culturally and linguistically diverse populations* (pp. 181–217). Austin, Tex.: Pro-Ed.

Fey, M. (1986). *Language intervention with young children.* San Diego: College Hill Press.

Gerber, A. (1993). *Language-related learning disabilities: Their nature and treatment.* Baltimore: Brookes.

Gilbert, S., & Gay, G. (1987). Improving the success in school of poor black children. *Phi Delta Kappa, 67,* 133–137.

Gudykunst, W., & Ting-Toomey, S. (1988). *Culture and interpersonal communication.* Newbury Park, Calif.: Sage.

Hakuta, K., & Garcia, E. (1989). Bilingualism and education. *American Psychologist, 44*(2), 374–379.

Hall, E. T. (1976). *Beyond culture.* Garden City, N.Y.: Anchor Books.

Hammer, C. (1994). *An ethnographic approach to providing family centered early intervention services.* Paper presented to the American Speech-Language-Hearing Association meeting, New Orleans.

Harris, G. (1993). American Indian cultures. In D. Battle (Ed.). *Communication disorders in multicultural populations* (pp. 78–113). Boston: Andover Medical Publishers.

Heath, S. (1983). *Ways with words: Language, life and work in communities and classrooms.* New York: Cambridge University Press.

Heath, S. (1986a). Sociocultural contexts of language development. In *Beyond language: Social and cultural factors in schooling language minority students* (pp. 132–156). Developed by the Bilingual Education Office, California State Department of Education. Los Angeles: California State University.

Heath, S. (1986b). Taking a cross-cultural look at narratives. *Topics in Language Disorders, 7*(1), 84–94.

Hecht, M., Andersen, P., & Ribeau, S. (1989). The cultural dimensions of nonverbal communication. In M. Asante & W. Gudykunst (Eds.), *Handbook of international and intercultural communication* (pp. 163–178). Newbury Park, Calif.: Sage.

Hilliard, A. (1983). Psychological factors associated with language in the education of the African-American child. *Journal of Negro Education, 52*(1), 24–34.

Hunt, K. (1965). *Grammatical structures written at three grade levels* (Research Report No. 3). Champaign, Ill.: National Council of Teachers of English.

Iglesias, A. (1986). *The cultural-linguistic minority student in the classroom: Management decisions.* Workshop presented at the State University of New York at Buffalo.

Individuals with Disabilities Education Act Amendments, Public Law 105-17. (1997). Washington, D.C.: Federal Register, June 4.

Kayser, H. (1985). *A study of speech language pathologists and their Mexican American language disordered caseloads.* Unpublished doctoral dissertation. Las Cruces, N.M.: New Mexico State University.

Kayser, H. (1990). Social communicative behaviors of language-disordered Mexican-American students. *Child Language Teaching Therapy,* 6(3), 255–269.

Kayser, H. (1995). *Bilingual speech-language pathology: A Latino focus.* San Diego: Singular Publishing.

Kvaal, J. T., Shipstead-Cox, S. G., Nevitt, S. G., Hodson, B. W., & Launer, P. B. (1988). The acquisition of 10 Spanish morphemes by Spanish-speaking children. *Language, Speech and Hearing Services in the Schools, 19,* 384–394.

Langdon, H. W. (1992). Speech and language assessment of LEP/bilingual Latino students. In H. W. Langdon & L. L. Cheng (Eds.), *Latino children and adults with communication disorders* (pp. 201–271). Gaithersburg, Md.: Aspen.

Lee, L. (1974). *Development sentence analysis.* Evanston, Ill.: Northwestern University Press.

Linder, T. (1993). *Transdisciplinary play-based assessment: A functional approach to working with young children.* Baltimore: Brookes.

Lund, N., & Duchan, J. (1988). *Assessing children's language in naturalistic contexts* (2nd ed.). Englewood Cliffs, N.J.: Prentice-Hall.

Lynch, E., & Hanson, M. (1992). *Developing cross-cultural competence.* Baltimore: Brookes.

McCauley, R. J., & Swisher, L. (1984). Psychometric review of language and articulation tests for preschool children. *Journal of Speech and Hearing Disorders, 49,* 34–42.

Mertino, G. (1992). Acquisition of syntactic and phonological features in Spanish. In H. W. Langdon & L. Cheng (Eds.), *Latino children and adults with communication disorders* (pp. 57–98). Gaithersburg, Md.: Aspen.

Miller, J. (1981). *Assessing language production in children: Experimental procedures.* Baltimore: University Park Press.

Miller, J., & Paul, R. (1995). *The clinical assessment of language comprehension.* Baltimore: Brookes.

Minuchin, P. (1985). Families and individual development: Provocations from the field of family therapy. *Child Development, 56,* 289–302.

Nelson, N. (1994). Curriculum based language assessment and intervention across the grades. In G. Wallach & K. Butler (Eds.), *Language learning disabilities in school-age children and adolescents* (pp. 111–121). New York: Maxwell Macmillan.

Nelson, N. W., & Hyter, Y. D. (1990). *Black English Sentence Scoring (BESS): Development and use of a tool for non-biased assessment.* Unpublished manuscript.

Ogbu, J. (1993). Differences in cultural frames of reference. *International Journal of Behavioral Development, 16*(3), 483–506.

Owens, R. (1995). *Language disorders: A functional approach to assessment and intervention.* Needham Heights, Mass.: Allyn & Bacon.

Palincsar, A., Brown, A., & Campione, J. (1994). Models and practices of dynamic assessment. In G. Wallach & K. Butler (Eds.), *Language disabilities in school age children* (pp. 24–53). New York: Maxwell MacMillan.

Paul, R. (1995). *Language disorders from infancy through adolescence: Assessment and intervention.* St. Louis: Mosby.

Peña, E., Quinn, R., & Iglesias, A. (1992). The application of dynamic methods to language assessment: A non-biased procedure. *Journal of Special Education, 26*(3), 269–280.

Piaget, J. (1952). (M. Cook translator). *The origins of intelligence in children.* New York: International Universities Press.

Reed, V. A. (1994). *An introduction to children with language disorders* (2nd ed.). New York: Merrill/Macmillan.

Schnell de Acedo, B. (1994). Early morphological development: The acquisition of articles in Spanish. In J. L. Sokolov & C. Snow (Eds.), *Handbook of research in language development using CHILDES* (pp. 210–253). Hillsdale, N.J.: Erlbaum.

Seifert, H., & Schwarz, I. (1991). Treatment effectiveness of large group basic concept instruction with Head Start students. *Language, Speech, and Hearing Services in Schools, 22*(4), 60–64.

Stockman, I. (1996). *Demographics are changing: Improving skills to better serve culturally and linguistically diverse preschoolers, their families, and communities.* American Speech-Language-Hearing Association Tele-Seminar.

Stockman, I., Vaughn-Cooke, F., & Wolfram, W. (1982). *Development of Black English: The first phase* (Final Research Report, National Institute of Education, NIE-G-80-0135). (ERIC Clearinghouse on Language and Linguistics, microfiche no. N2455556).

Taylor, O. (Ed.). (1986). *Nature of communication disorders in culturally and linguistically diverse populations.* Austin, Tex.: Pro-Ed.

Taylor, O., & Payne, K. (1983). Culturally valid testing: A proactive approach. *Topics in Language Disorders, 3*(3), 8–20.

Terrell, B. (1992). Emergent literacy: In the beginning there was reading and writing. In D. Ripich & N. Creaghead (Eds.), *School discourse problems* (pp. 9–28). San Diego: Singular Publishing.

Terrell, S. (1992). Parent-child comparative analysis: A criterion-referenced method for the nondiscriminatory assessment of a child who spoke a relatively uncommon dialect of English. *Language, Speech and Hearing Services in Schools, 23,* 34–42.

Terrell, S., & Terrell, F. (1993). African-American cultures. In D. Battle (Ed.), *Communication disorders in multicultural populations* (pp. 3–37). Boston: Andover Medical Publishers.

Tolliver-Weddington, G., & Erickson, J. (1987). Guidelines for use of standardized tests with minority children. In L. Cole & V. Deal (Eds.), *Communication disorders in multicultural populations* (pp. 21–22). Rockville, Md.: American Speech-Language-Hearing Association.

Toronto, A. S. (1976). Developmental assessment of Spanish grammar. *Journal of Speech and Hearing Disorders, 41,* 150–171.

Torrefy, C., & McCray, A. (1996). *Ready, set, PLAY: Promoting integration of children from diverse cultures.* Southern Louisiana University, Department of Special Education.

Van Kleeck, A. (1994). Potential cultural bias in training parents as conversational partners with their children who have delays in language development. *American Journal of Speech-Language Pathology, 3,* 67–78.

Vaughn-Cooke, F. B. (1986). The challenge of assessing the language of nonmainstream speakers. In O. Taylor (Ed.), *Treatment of communication disorders in linguistically diverse populations* (pp. 23–48). San Diego: College Hill Press.

Ventry, I., & Schiavetti, N. (1986). *Evaluating research in speech pathology and audiology.* Englewood Cliffs, N.J.: Prentice-Hall.

Ward, M. (1982). *Them children: A study in language learning.* New York: Irving Press.

Weiss, A. L., Tomblin, J. B., & Robin, D. A. (1994). Language disorders. In J. B. Tomblin, H. Morris, & D. C. Spriestersbach (Eds.), *Diagnosis in speech-language pathology* (pp. 99–131). San Diego: Singular Publishing.

Westby, C. (1994). Multicultural issues. In J. B. Tomblin, H. L. Morris, & D. C. Spriestersbach (Eds.), *Diagnosis in speech-language pathology* (pp. 29–52). San Diego: Singular Publishing.

Westby, C., & Rouse, G. (1985). Culture in education and the instruction of language learning-disabled students. *Topics in Language Disorders,* 5(4), 15–28.

CHAPTER 4

A Model for Linking Assessment and Intervention for Children With Developmental Disorders

Diane Bricker, Ph.D.
Professor, Early Intervention Program
University of Oregon
Eugene
Angela Losardo, Ph.D., CCC-SLP
Associate Professor
Department of Language, Reading, and Exceptionalities
Appalachian State University
Boone, North Carolina

Key Terms

curriculum-based assessment (CBA)
developmental disabilities (DD)
diagnosis
evaluation
linked system approach
measurement processes
program-relevant assessment
screening

Overview

The quality of language intervention services provided to infants and young children with **developmental disabilities (DD)** has improved steadily over the past two decades (Bricker, 1993). However, many children and their families still are offered communication programs that are inappropriate and fail to produce successful outcomes. Significant barriers to the delivery of quality intervention services arise, in part, from the limitations of traditional approaches to early communicative assessment, as well as the tools and procedures often chosen by communication specialists and other interventionists. The purpose of this chapter is to provide a rationale, conceptual model, and set of practical procedures for linking assessment and intervention. We begin with a brief historical review of early communicative assessment and intervention with young children from birth to 5 years who have developmental disabilities. Following that, we differentiate between the different types and purposes of assessment and identify major measurement concerns with traditional approaches, which, we believe frustrate efforts to improve intervention services. Next, we propose and discuss an alternative to the traditional approach to early communicative assessment and intervention that directly and functionally links assessment and intervention to each other and to evaluation. Finally, we provide an overview of the model and use a case study to illustrate its application.

HISTORICAL PERSPECTIVE ON EARLY COMMUNICATIVE ASSESSMENT AND INTERVENTION

Over the years, changing views on language acquisition have influenced the procedures used in both the identification and treatment of communication deficits in infants and young children with moderate to severe developmental disabilities. Focuses of assessment have tended to reflect the predominant theory of language acquisition and communicative competence, moving from the assessment of isolated components of language (e.g., syntax, semantics, and pragmatics) to a more interactive approach, which appears to recognize the multifaceted aspects of communication, the rich interplay between cognitive and linguistic processes, the importance of dialogic exchanges, and the context in which communicative exchanges occur.

The interactive approach to language assessment has emerged as a synthesis of previous syntactic, semantic, and pragmatic theory and research on the social reciprocity of the child-caregiver exchange. The social reciprocity research has shown that infants communicate through facial and body signals, gestures, and vocal expressions long before more formal language processes develop. Communication is viewed as a dyadic and contingent process in which the child both affects, and is affected by, the social environment (Carlson & Bricker, 1982). Early reciprocal transactions between the child and the caregiver are assumed to lay a foundation for the development of more formal linguistic processes (Stark, 1981; Stern, 1981). Reciprocal transactions are dependent, in part, on the ability of caregivers to "read" the early communicative signals of children. When a mismatch occurs between prelinguistic interaction patterns of children and the input of caregivers, a serious possibility exists for delays in linguistic development (Guralnick & Bennett, 1987).

Delays in the development of prelinguistic communication skills have been reported consistently for infants and young children with different etiologies of developmental disability (Yoder & Warren, 1993). Despite the wide variation in etiologies of developmental disability (e.g., autism, mental retardation, fragile X syndrome, Down syndrome) and developmental patterns of young children in this highly heterogeneous group, the importance of early language assessment and intervention cannot be overemphasized. Information gleaned from early communicative assessment can be used to develop functional communication intervention programs for young children with developmental disabilities and their families. For example, if we determine that an infant does not provide signals of communicative readiness, strategies can be developed to enhance her or his general attentiveness or readiness for communicative exchanges.

However, many of the assessment tools used by communication specialists and other interventionists who have adopted the interactive perspective do not offer information that is relevant to the formulation of intervention goals and content. The authors often find diagnostic tests being used as program assessments to determine Individual Education Plan (IEP)/Individual Family Service Plan (IFSP) goals and objectives. This practice is inappropriate because items on diagnostic instruments are selected to discriminate between groups of children at different ages, and not because they are educationally relevant. For example, a common item on a diagnostic test might be to determine whether a child can fit a shape into a form board. Although this item may be appropriately used to establish developmental norms, a program assessment is needed to help practitioners develop meaningful intervention content. Using this example, a correlate item on a program assessment might be to determine whether a child can fit objects into defined spaces. The selection of this, more functional and generative, skill as an IEP/IFSP objective would involve teaching children that food belongs on a plate, soap belongs in a soap dish, and a sock belongs on a foot. A major challenge exists for the development and adoption of instruments and procedures that directly link assessment, IEP/IFSP development, intervention plans and activities, and evaluation.

CONCERNS WITH TRADITIONAL APPROACHES TO EARLY COMMUNICATIVE ASSESSMENT AND INTERVENTION

We have identified three measurement concerns with traditional approaches to assessment, which, we believe, are major barriers to improving intervention services for children with moderate to severe developmental disabilities.

The first measurement concern is that few instruments exist that are suitable for assessing and evaluating the progress of infants and young children with developmental disabilities. Traditionally, two types of assessment—norm referenced and criterion referenced—have been used to assess the communication abilities of young children. Norm-referenced assessments compare a child's development to a normative group similar in age and relevant demographic variables (Meisels, 1996). Criterion-referenced assessments compare a child's performance to a standard of mastery or a criterion set of behaviors in a particular domain (Hamilton & Swan, 1981).

Norm-referenced instruments are generally not appropriate to assess the baseline or to chart the progress of infants and young children with developmental disabilities for several reasons: (a) most of these tests have no norms for children with special needs (Bricker, 1989); (b) the items were selected for their ability to differentiate between children of varying age or skill levels, thus making questionable their use as educational targets; (c) the intervals between items are often sizable, which makes it difficult to track the progress of or accurately assess behavior in children who learn and change slowly; (d) these tests generally require administration by trained specialists and do not permit procedural modifications or adaptations, which means that children with developmental disabilities may be penalized for an inability to respond in the expected fashion to a test item; and (e) these tests are generally administered in unfamiliar settings, often resulting in a depression of the child's performance.

The use of criterion-referenced assessments avoids many of the problems associated with norm-referenced instruments; however, many of these instruments also have drawbacks. Many criterion-referenced tests have been developed by selecting items from norm-referenced instruments, which may cause problems (Cohen & Spenciner, 1994; Johnson, 1982; Sheehan, 1982). For example, selected items may not assess functional behaviors and are therefore of no more assistance in developing intervention targets than norm-referenced tests (e.g., putting pegs in a pegboard). Picking items from other tests to create a new test may result in a tool that lacks conceptual integrity, internal consistency, and hierarchical arrangements. In addition, many criterion-referenced measures lack adequate psychometric data. In a review of 10 criterion-referenced measures commonly used with young children with special needs, Notari, Slentz, and Bricker (1990) concluded that none of these tests had adequate validity, reliability, or utility data.

The second measurement concern is that many service delivery personnel appear to have received little training and information about the necessary criteria to employ when selecting assessment and evaluation tools. Measures developed for one purpose are often used for other, inappropriate purposes. **Measurement processes** can involve at least four processes with uniquely different purposes: **screening**, **diagnosis**, **program-relevant assessment**, and **evaluation**. Screening involves a quick, economical look at a child's repertoire. If used, it should occur prior to the other measurement processes. The purpose of screening is to decide whether or not a child's performance is sufficiently different from that of other children of the same chronological age to warrant more comprehensive testing. Diagnosis is the process used to determine the nature of the problem and whether a child is eligible for services. After the child enters a program, a program-relevant assessment can be used to gather baseline information and to establish specific intervention goals and objectives. Evaluation provides a comparison of the child's performance before and after intervention. Communication specialists and interventionists should understand the purposes for which they are measuring a child's performance before choosing an assessment instrument.

The third, and most troubling, measurement concern is that often there appears to be little or no relationship between assessment, intervention, and evaluation activities. That is, often initial assessment information is not used to develop intervention goals and content, and subsequent evaluation is unrelated to assessment or intervention efforts. The dysjunction found between assessment, intervention, and evaluation program components likely occurs because of the nature of the assessment and evaluation tools used or the procedures used to conduct the assessment and evaluation. Attempting to use outcomes from norm-referenced tests or trying to implement an IFSP developed by a diagnostic and evaluation team unfamiliar with the child or the receiving program does little to promote a direct link between assessment, intervention, and evaluation. Systems that rely on assessment tools and procedures to yield intervention-relevant findings do much to promote a strong and reciprocal relationship between assessment, intervention, and evaluation program components.

A conceptual appreciation for systems that directly relate assessment outcomes to functional IEP/IFSPs and intervention plan development needs to be accompanied by the necessary tools and procedures that permit efficient and effective application of the approach. The remainder of this chapter describes one such approach with an emphasis on its application. A clinical case study will be used to illustrate how a **linked system approach** to early communicative assessment, intervention, and evaluation can be used with young children with developmental disabilities and their families.

AN ALTERNATIVE MODEL: NECESSARY COMPONENTS

An effective intervention program requires the development of functional IEP/IFSPs and intervention plans that serve to keep program staff and caregivers focused on appropriate and meaningful intervention activities. Development is based on a system that employs assessment procedures designed to yield the necessary information on children and families to develop these documents. Such systems require a direct link between program components, such as assessment, and IEP/IFSP goals and outcomes, as shown in Figure 4-1. Variations of this simple model have been described elsewhere by a number of authors (Bagnato, Neisworth, & Munson, 1989; Bricker, 1989, 1993; Hutinger, 1988).

The present model is composed of five components: (1) assessment, (2) IEP/IFSP goals and outcomes, (3) intervention planning, (4) intervention activities, and (5) evaluation. Each component is linked to the next in a linear fashion, and all five components are regulated, or influenced, by the program's philosophy. *Program philosophy* refers to the pervasive climate and guiding principles that drive the program; for example, a commitment by staff to family involvement in assessment and intervention activities, professional team collaboration to develop and implement intervention plans, or a developmental perspective of children's growth might all be guiding principles for a state-of-the-art program. The model shown in Figure 4-1 illustrates the direct relationship between assessment and IEP/IFSP development, which, in turn, drives the formulation of intervention plans. Then, the plans provide the structure for intervention activities.

The evaluation component provides ongoing and direct feedback as to the success of the intervention activities, intervention planning, and progress toward IEP/IFSP goals and outcomes.

CURRICULUM-BASED ASSESSMENT: THE NECESSARY TOOL

A linked system in which assessment outcomes are used directly to develop functional IEP/IFSP goals and intervention plans requires the use of assessment tools and procedures that yield relevant information. The general category of assessment most useful for developing functional IEP/IFSPs and intervention plans is a type of criterion-referenced test referred to as **curriculum-based assessment** (CBA) or, preferably, a curriculum-based assessment/evaluation test. CBAs have been defined as "a direct application of criterion-referenced assessment strategy to instructional content. Assessment and curricular content are coordinated to address the same skills and abilities" (Notari et al., 1990, pp. 162-163).

The explicit design of CBAs provides a direct and ongoing link between an assessment and intervention (curriculum). A number of CBAs have been developed for use with infants and young children who are at risk and have de-

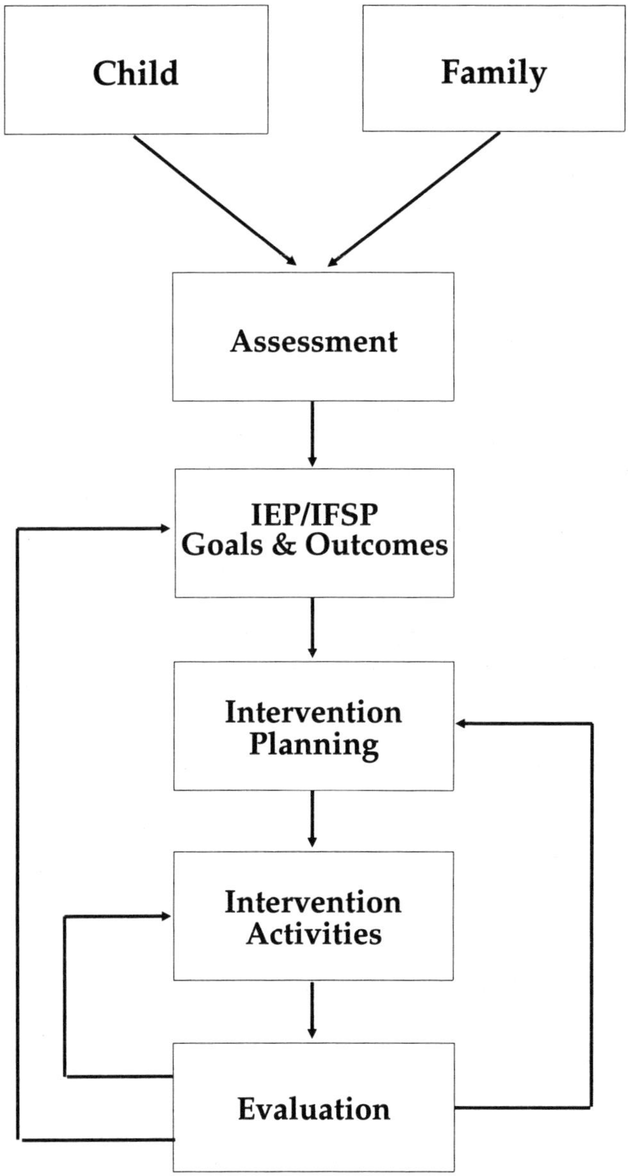

Figure 4-1. Model directly linking program components.

velopmental disabilities. Notari et al. (1990) reviewed 10 such CBAs, examining features such as number of items, test organization, adaptations, administration time, data collection method, scoring options, type of outcome, standardization and psychometric data. Although these CBAs varied across the features, each was judged to provide interventionists and caregivers with more information that is directly applicable to the development of functional intervention plans and intervention activities than could screening tests, norm-referenced tests, or even other criterion-referenced tests that lack accompanying curricular materials.

When selecting a CBA, communication specialists and interventionists should consider the following features to promote the links between assessment, intervention, and evaluation. First, CBAs should target functional skills—that is, skills thought to be essential for infants and young children to manage themselves independently and to cope with environmental demands. Each item on this type of an assessment should potentially be an appropriate intervention target. Second, CBAs should be comprehensive, covering the major areas of development (e.g., fine motor, gross motor, cognition, adaptive, social-communication, and social).

Although a communication specialist may be primarily focused on a child's social communication behavior, there are many reasons why it is essential for this person to have an appreciation for the child's total repertoire. First, it is often difficult when working with infants and young children, to separate the intimately related domains of early development (e.g., Is a smile a communicative or social behavior, or both?). Second, the communication specialist can do a more effective job, whether working with a caregiver or professional team, if assessment and intervention activities are coordinated rather than offered in isolation. This coordination of effort requires a thorough and comprehensive knowledge of the child's entire repertoire.

Third, the recommended method of obtaining information should involve observations of children's skills while they participate in daily activities. The scoring system should be sensitive enough to reflect how each child performed the skill and if the skill was performed independently, with different people, or in different settings (Bricker, 1989). A range of scoring options should be provided to reflect those skills that are emerging. Fourth, because these assessments are generally not standardized, CBAs should provide the user with suggestions on how to adapt or modify item presentation and/or item criterion to accommodate children with developmental disabilities. Fifth, CBAs should include procedures for the formal inclusion of input from parents or primary caregivers to help ensure involvement in developing functional intervention plans. Sixth, CBAs should provide activities that can be used to assist children in acquiring each targeted goal or objective. For example, if an item on the social-communication domain requires using action words appropriately—and that item is chosen as an IFSP goal—the interventionist should be able to refer to an associated curriculum to find suggested teaching activities and strategies that may be useful when working on this target with the child. Finally, although few CBAs report reliability and validity data, preference should be given to those that do (Notari et al., 1990).

One of the CBAs available for use with infants and young children, the Assessment, Evaluation and Programming System (AEPS) particularly emphasizes the use of its test outcomes to develop functional IEP/IFSPs and intervention plans (Bricker, 1993). The AEPS system is composed of four separate volumes: *AEPS Measurement for Birth to Three Years* (Bricker, 1993), which contains the AEPS Test; *AEPS Curriculum for Birth to Three Years* (Cripe, Slentz, & Bricker, 1993); *AEPS Measurement for Three to Six Years* (Bricker & Pretti-Frontczak, 1996); and *AEPS Curriculum for Three to Six Years* (Bricker, 1996). As Bricker, Pretti-Frontczak, and McComas (1998) point out, the AEPS Test has several of the preferred features that promote the link between assessment and intervention. In addition, the AEPS test has been studied extensively (Bailey & Bricker, 1986; Bricker, Bailey, & Slentz, 1990; Cripe, 1990; Hsia, 1993; Notari & Bricker, 1990). Congruent validity, test stability, interrater agreement, and test-retest reliability have all been examined and found to be acceptable to good (Bricker et al., 1990; Hsia, 1993). In addition, the utility of the AEPS Test has been addressed by asking a series of questions of test users in the field. These data indicate that the respondents generally found the content of the test appropriate and useful for developing IEP/IFSPs and intervention plans.

In a well-controlled study, Notari and Bricker (1990) examined the usefulness of the AEPS Test for developing IEP/IFSPs. Forty-eight interventionists developed IEP/IFSPs; those who used the AEPS Test wrote significantly better goals and objectives than did the control subjects, who did not use the test.

A study conducted by Cripe (1990) examined the effectiveness of the AEPS associated family measures when developing IFSPs for children aged 6 months to 3 years. Following treatment, which included training on the AEPS materials, interventionists (N=30) wrote significantly better IFSPs and included significantly more family outcomes on their IFSPs than before the training.

The data collected on the AEPS Test, and particularly the Notari and Bricker (1990) and Cripe (1990) studies, suggest that the AEPS Test and associated family measures do enhance an interventionist's capacity to write more functional IEP/IFSPs, which should, in turn, assist in the development of functional intervention plans.

Application of the model shown in Figure 4-1, which links assessment, IFSP/IEP goals and outcomes, intervention planning, intervention activities, and evaluation, is dependent on the use of a measurement tool or system that yields comprehensive, accurate, and meaningful data for IEP/IFSP development and intervention planning. In the following sections, an overview of the model is provided and a clinical case study is used to illustrate how these vital processes can be linked.

AN OVERVIEW OF THE MODEL

As indicated earlier, the use of a model that directly links program components is dependent on the availability of an assessment tool and procedures that provide the necessary and relevant information to develop functional

IEP/IFSPs and intervention plans. The AEPS Test is one such tool. Three features of the AEPS Test make the link between assessment, intervention, and evaluation direct and relevant. First, the AEPS Test is comprehensive and covers all developmental areas for which one is likely to program (i.e., fine motor, gross motor, adaptive, cognitive, social-communication, and social). Second, to the extent possible, each domain is composed of items that are hierarchically arranged from simple to increasingly complex, which is helpful in determining the sequence of skills to be taught. Third, items on the AEPS Test measure functional skills and are thus all potentially relevant intervention targets.

The importance of family participation in a child's intervention program, particularly for the infant or young child with a developmental disability, cannot be overemphasized; therefore, it is important to use a linked assessment, intervention, and evaluation process that generates meaningful caregiver participation. One strategy for enhancing active family participation in this process is to provide information to help the family select relevant goals and objectives for their child and outcomes for their family. Two associated AEPS family measures, included in the *AEPS Measurement for Birth to Three Years* (Bricker, 1993), can be used, in conjunction with the AEPS Test, for this purpose. The first measure, the AEPS Family Report, is designed to obtain information from the family about the child's skills and abilities across multiple domains of development. The items on this tool correspond directly to the items on the AEPS Test. The second measure, the AEPS Family Interest Survey, is designed to assist caregivers and interventionists in identifying the family's interests and priorities that are child focused (e.g., ordering adaptive equipment), family focused (e.g., accessing family recreational programs), and community focused (e.g., locating day-care or respite care services). The items on the Family Interest Survey are designed to reflect a family's interest in accessing information, resources, and services, rather than identifying problems associated with parenting a child with a developmental disorder.

The first step in developing an IEP/IFSP from the AEPS Test and associated AEPS family measures is summarization of the results. Caregivers and interventionists can review the results from each developmental domain and collaboratively select goals and objectives for inclusion on the child's IEP/IFSP. This procedure provides a direct tie with assessment and a common base for the selection of IEP/IFSP goals by caregivers and interventionists.

Once the goals and their associated objectives have been selected, the next step is for program staff and caregivers to prioritize the goals. Caregivers and interventionists should select only the highest priorities as intervention targets. Our experience suggests that interventionists often select more goals and/or outcomes than they and caregivers can comfortably address. Two to four well-selected goals that target important response classes or skills or relevant family outcomes are sufficient and generally manageable by program staff and caregivers.

The next step is to develop intervention plans for the selected priority goals or outcomes. An intervention plan can follow a number of formats but should always contain the following information: (1) identification information, such as child's name and that of the interventionist; (2) dates for the initiation of training and the expected completion; (3) intervention domain; (4) types of settings where intervention may occur; (5) specification of the goal or outcomes and associated objectives, if appropriate; (6) specification of more discrete intervention targets if necessary (particularly appropriate for children with severe disabilities); (7) specification of child or family progress evaluation procedures; and (8) decision rules to be used. Decision rules are used to decide whether change to the intervention plan or activities is in order. For example, if the child progress data indicate no movement toward a specific goal after 2 weeks of intervention, different intervention activities may be in order.

Once intervention plans have been designed, intervention activities can be initiated. This process is greatly facilitated when using a CBA tool such as the AEPS. The intervention activities described in the *AEPS Curriculum* (Cripe et al., 1993) correspond directly to the AEPS test items, making it simple to relate intervention activities directly to selected goals and objectives. For each AEPS test item (goal and objective), the *AEPS Curriculum* has an associated section that describes the importance of the targeted skills, lists preceding and concurrent objectives, and provides a series of suggested intervention activities.

The final step is to conduct systematic evaluation procedures to determine progress toward priority IEP/IFSP goals and family outcomes. As shown in Figure 4-1, evaluation results are used to provide systematic feedback on the success of the intervention activities and intervention plans as well as to monitor progress toward IEP/IFSP goals and outcomes and to offer guidance for modification, as necessary. Once the criterion has been met, training should begin on the next goal or outcome. If progress is nonexistent, extremely slow, or variable, some form of change (e.g., to specified decision rules) is likely in order. Without a systematic documentation of change, interventionists and caregivers cannot determine the effects of their intervention efforts.

CASE STUDY: CASIE

The director of an inclusive early intervention program received a call from the mother of Casie, a 24-month-old child with Down syndrome. Casie's mother expressed concern that her daughter was not talking. She wanted to enroll Casie in the early intervention program and learn ways she could help Casie to talk at home. At the initial intake meeting, the program director provided an overview of an approach to early intervention in which all assessment and intervention activities are conducted in collaboration with families. The director offered several options for Casie's mother to be involved in her daughter's program. For example, she provided a copy of the AEPS Family Interest Survey, and they discussed its relevance for planning Casie's program. The director explained that for the first few weeks of school, classroom activities would be arranged to allow the classroom teacher and other interventionists, such as the communication specialist, physical therapist, and occupational therapist, to observe and assess Casie's performance in typical play activities using the AEPS test. She invited Casie's mother to participate in assessment of her daughter and provided her with the AEPS Family Report. She encouraged her to read it through and, over the next few weeks, to fill out any items she could answer from home or through observations in the classroom.

Assessment

Casie arrived at the preschool on Monday morning with her mother and her grandmother. Both adults decided to stay for the first day to ease Casie's transition into the classroom. Casie's mother observed that the classroom had large open spaces, with some areas of the room partitioned off and used as small activity centers. She glanced at a large schedule posted on the door and noticed that assessment activities were planned during the first 2 to 4 weeks of school. Each morning began with an opening circle activity, followed by three different small-center activities. The children had an outdoor playtime and snack, and the morning ended with a closing circle activity. Just then, music for circle time began and the adults and children were asked to find a carpet square and sit in a circle. Casie's mother and grandmother were invited to participate in the activity with Casie. Throughout the morning, they observed that while one interventionist conducted an activity, another interventionist was recording observations on the AEPS test protocol. At home that evening, Casie's mother read over the items on the AEPS Family Report and completed much of it based on her knowledge of what Casie could and could not do. For some of the items, she consulted with Casie's grandmother, and they made a note of those items that they were unable to score immediately and would need to observe further.

Within a period of 2 weeks, the classroom staff completed the AEPS test on Casie. Figure 4-2 (pp. 123, 124, 125) contains a scored AEPS data recording form for Casie from the social-communication domain. For the purposes of this case study, only the social-communication domain was used to identify a target goal and objective to include on Casie's IFSP. (For more information on the AEPS Measurement for Birth to Three Years *or the AEPS Family Report, see Bricker, 1993.) The AEPS test permits scoring items (goals and objectives) with a 2, 1, or 0, indicating respectively that the child met the stated criterion for the item, inconsistently performed the item, or did not meet the item criterion. As shown in Figure 4-2, Casie met the criteria (i.e., scored a 2) for Goals 1, 2, and 3 in Strand A. Her performance on Goals 1 and 2 in Strand*

Social-Communication Domain

S = Scoring Key	Q = Qualifying Notes
2 = Pass consistently	A = Assistance provided
1 = Inconsistent performance	B = Behavior interfered
0 = Does not pass	R = Reported assessment
	M = Modification/adaptation
	D = Direct test

Name: Casie

	IEP	S	Q	S	Q	S	Q	S	Q
Test Period:		First							
Test Date:		6/95		/		/		/	
Examiner:		Jones							
A. Prelinguistic communicative interactions									
1. Turns and looks toward person speaking		2							
1.1 Turns and looks toward object and person speaking		2							
1.2 Turns and looks toward noise-producing object		2							
2. Follows gaze to establish joint attention		2							
2.1 Follows pointing gesture to establish joint attention		2							
2.2 Looks toward object		2							
3. Engages in vocal exchanges by babbling		2							
3.1. Engages in vocal exchanges by cooing		2							
B. Transition to words									
1. Gains person's attention and refers to object, person, or event		0							
1.1 Responds with vocalization and gesture to simple questions		1							
1.2 Points to object, person, or event		1							
1.3 Gestures and/or vocalizes to greet others		1							
1.4 Uses gestures and/or vocalizations to protest actions or reject objects/people		1							
2. Uses consistent word approximations		0							
2.1 Uses consistent consonant–vowel combinations		0							
2.2 Uses nonspecific consonant–vowel combination and/or jargon		1							
C. Comprehension of words and sentences									
1. Locates objects, people, or events *without* contextual cues		0							

Figure 4-2. AEPS Data Recording Form for Casie, Social-Communication Domain. (From Bricker, D. [Ed.]. [1993]. *Assessment, evaluation and programming system for infants and children: Vol. 1. AEPS measurement for birth to three years.* Reprinted by permission of Paul Brookes, Baltimore).(continues)

AEPS **Social-Communication Domain**

Name: Casie

	Test Period: First		Test Period:		Test Period:		Test Period:	
	Test Date: 6/95		Test Date: /		Test Date: /		Test Date: /	
	Examiner: Jones		Examiner:		Examiner:		Examiner:	

	IEP	S	Q	S	Q	S	Q	S	Q
1.1 Locates common objects, people, or events in unfamiliar pictures		0							
1.2 Locates common objects, people, or events in familiar pictures		0							
1.3 Locates common objects, people, or events with contextual cues		0							
2. Carries out two-step directions without cues		0							
2.1 Carries out two-step directions with cues		0							
2.2 Carries out one-step directions without cues		0							
2.3 Carries out one-step directions with cues		0							
D. Production of social-communicative signals words, or sentences									
1. Uses 50 single words		0							
1.1 Uses five descriptive words		0							
1.2 Uses five action words		0							
1.3 Uses two pronouns		0							
1.4 Uses 15 object or event labels		0							
1.5 Uses three proper names		0							
2. Uses two-word utterances		0							
2.1 Uses two-word utterances to express agent–action, action–object, and agent–object		0							
2.2 Uses two-word utterances to express possession		0							
2.3 Uses two-word utterances to express location		0							
2.4 Uses two-word utterances to describe objects, people, and/or events		0							
2.5 Uses two-word utterances to express recurrence		0							
2.6 Uses two-word utterances to express negation		0							
3. Uses three-word utterances		0							
3.1 Uses three-word negative utterances		0							

Figure 4-2. (continued)

AEPS — Social-Communication Domain

Name: Casie

Test Period:		First							
Test Date:		6/95		/		/		/	
Examiner:		Jones							
	IEP	S	Q	S	Q	S	Q	S	Q
3.2 Asks questions		0							
3.3 Uses action–object–location		0							
3.4 Uses agent–action–object		0							

A raw score can be computed for the domain by adding all the 2 and 1 scores entered in the S column for a specific test period. To determine the total percent score divide the total score by the total score possible.

RESULTS

Test Date	6-95			
Total Score Possible	84	84	84	84
Total Score	21			
Total Percent Score	25			

Figure 4-2. (continued)

B was scored as inconsistent (i.e., 1), and all goals in Strand C were scored with 0.

Figure 4-3 contains an AEPS Family Report data recording form for the social-communication domain completed by Casie's mother. She was told to score each item with a Y indicating that Casie met the criterion, an S indicating that Casie met the criterion inconsistently ("sometimes"), or an N indicating that Casie did not meet the criterion.

IEP/IFSP Development

Two weeks after Casie began attending the program, her mother received a call from the program director, who was responsible for scheduling IEP/IFSP meetings. The director explained the purpose of the meeting and asked Casie's mother to bring along her completed copy of the AEPS Family Report. At the meeting, the director introduced Casie's mother to other team members and asked her to share her observations of Casie at home using the AEPS Family Report as a guide. Casie's mother confidently shared information about her child's development across six domains of development: gross motor, fine motor, cognitive, social, social-communication, and adaptive. Other team members joined in the discussion, citing instances in the classroom where the same behaviors were observed. Table 4-1 shows a summary of the results of the AEPS Test and Family Report.

Social-Communication Domain

	6-95			Date
1. Does your child turn to look at someone who is talking nearby? For example, when playing near you, your child looks at you when you speak. (A1)	Y			
2. Does your child turn to look in the same direction that you are looking? For example, when playing together, you turn and look out the window and your child turns and looks out the window. (A2)	Y			
3. Does your child make at least two vocal exchanges with others by babbling? For example, you say, "Hi baby," and your child says, "ba-ba." You then say, "What?" and your child says, "ba-ba-ba." (A3)	Y			
4. Does your child get your attention and then point to an object, person, or event? For example, he or she pulls on your arm and then points to a ball, or looks at you and then looks at a cat. (B1)	S			
5. Does your child use *at least 10* consistent word approximations to name objects, people, or events. (A word approximation is a sound that resembles the word or is part of the word.) For example, your child sees a dog and says, "gog," or says, "ju" when asking for juice. (B2)	N			
6. Without help, does your child locate *at least 20* familiar objects, people, or events after you have named them? The people, objects, or events should not be immediately present, but they should be familiar to your child and easy to find. For example, you say, "Where's Spot?" and the child goes to the window and points to the doghouse. (C1)	N			
7. Does your child carry out two-step directions that do not relate to the immediate situation? For example, when your child's doll is not in the same room, you tell the child to "Go get your doll and put it on the chair." Your child gets the doll and puts it on the chair. (C2)	N			
8. a. Does your child use at least five descriptive words (e.g., red, big, hot) correctly? For example, your child sees a red ball and says, "red," or looks at the stove and says, "hot."	N			

Figure 4-3. AEPS Family Report Data Recording Form. (From Bricker, D. [Ed.]. [1993]. *Assessment, evaluation and programming system for infants and children: Vol. 1. AEPS measurement for birth to three years.* Baltimore: Paul H. Brookes. Reprinted with permission.) (continues)

AEPS **Social-Communication Domain**

Item	6-95			Date
b. Does your child use at least five action words (e.g., go, want, run, eat, sit) correctly? For example, your child hands you a box and says, "open," or walks to the door and says, "go."	N			
c. Does your child use at least two pronouns (e.g., me, my, it, I, he, you) correctly? For example, your child looks in a mirror and says, "me," or takes a toy and says, "mine."	N			
d. Does your child use at least 15 words to label objects or events correctly? For example, your child looks at a cat and says, "kitty," or points to a ball and says, "ball."	N			
e. Does your child use at least three proper names (e.g., Mommy, Daddy, Anita, Spot) correctly? For example, your child looks at his or her mother and says, "Mama." (D1)	N			
9. a. Does your child use two words together to talk about a person and an action, an action and an object, and a person and an object? For example, your child says, "Mama go" (person and action), "Roll ball" (action and object), and "Daddy truck" (person and object).	N			
b. Does your child use two words together to talk about who has an object or who owns an object? For example, the child points to a car and says, "Mama's car," or takes a book from a friend and says, "My book."	N			
c. Does your child use two words together to talk about where an object, person, or event is located? For example, the child points to his or her mother and says, "Mama there," or holds up a cup and says, "In cup."	N			
d. Does your child use two words together to describe people, events, or objects? For example, your child points to a pan and says, "Pan hot," or picks up a ball and says, "Red ball."	N			

Figure 4-3. (continued)

AEPS **Social-Communication Domain**

	6.95				Date
e. Does your child use two words together to tell you when he or she wants more of something or when he or she wants something to happen again? For example, your child holds up a cup and says, "More juice." When being pushed in a swing, your child says, "Go again."	N				
f. Does your child use two words together to tell you when he or she does not want something, has not done something, or that something is gone? For example, your child finishes some juice and says, "All gone," or gives a wind-up toy to an adult and says, "Not go." (D2)	N				
10. a. Does your child use three words together that include a negative word (e.g., no, not, don't, can't). For example, your child says, "No do that," or "Not baby's ball."	N				
b. Does your child ask three-word questions using "Wh"-words (e.g., what, who, where) or a rising voice? For example, your child asks, "Where my coat?" or "We get lunch?"	N				
c. Does your child use three words together to tell you where to place an object or where to find an object? For example, your child says, "Put baby in," or "Roll ball here."	N				
d. Does your child use three words together to tell you about a person, an action, and an object? For example, your child says, "He throw ball," "Baby drink bottle," or "Mama drive car." (D3)	N				

Priority Goals: ______________________

Figure 4-3. (continued)

Casie's mother commented to the director and other team members that the AEPS Family Report prepared her to come to the meeting with a comprehensive picture of Casie's present status (i.e., what she can currently do) and what the next developmental targets should likely be (i.e., IEP/IFSP goals). For example, on the social-communication domain, she noted that Casie was

Table 4-1. Summary of the AEPS Test and Family Report

Fine Motor	Gross Motor	Adaptive
Casie is able to grasp and release handheld objects. She is beginning to stack objects (e.g., large blocks) with some spilling. Casie is beginning to use a turning motion with either wrist when she tries to turn door knobs.	Casie can walk around large toys or furniture that are in her way. She is beginning to bend over to reach objects on the floor without sitting or falling down. She is also beginning to walk up stairs provided an adult holds her hand.	Casie bites and chews hard and chewy foods and drinks from a sipper cup, with some spilling. She cooperates during hand washing and teeth brushing. She will raise her arms, with some prompting, to allow an adult to dress or undress her.
Cognitive	**Social-Communication**	**Social**
Casie is beginning to locate objects that are partially covered. She participates in familiar interactive games such as patty-cake and is beginning to imitate large motor movements such as clapping.	Casie turns and looks toward a person speaking or a noise-producing object. She is beginning to play with sounds, especially during circle time. Casie follows a person's pointing gesture used to establish joint attention.	Casie is beginning to play near other children in the sand box and observes their play. She is beginning to entertain herself for short periods of time by playing with pop-up toys and toy pianos.

inconsistent in getting her attention and pointing to desired objects, persons, or events. The team referred to the AEPS Curriculum for Birth to Three *(Cripe et al., 1993) and Casie's mother selected a goal: "Gains person's attention and refers to an object, person and/or event," and its associated objective: "Points to an object, person, and/or event" (p. 356).*

Intervention Plans

Next, the team developed and wrote an intervention plan focused on the selected social-communication goal and its associated objective. This intervention plan provided Casie's mother and the other team members with a framework and guidance for choosing and directing intervention activities. The intervention plan addressing Casie's social-communication goal and its associated objective is shown in Figure 4-4. As shown in Figure 4-4, intervention plans contain more detail and specification than the IEP/IFSP document.

Child: Casie Interventionist: Martha Jones

Initiated: 09/01/95 Expected Completion: 12/02/95 Completed: / /

Domain: Fine Motor Gross Motor Adaptive Cognitive (Social-Communication) Social

Type of Setting: Free Play & Small Group Group ______ Individual ______ Home

Goal 1: Gains person's attention and refers to an object, person, and/or event

Objective 1.2: Points (10–12 times per day) to objects, persons, and/or events across settings for 10 consecutive days

Developmental Programming Steps:

Confirmation function: The adult says, "There's the ball." The child points to the ball.

Comment/reply function: The adult asks, "What happened?" The child points to the spilled milk.

Information function: The adult asks, "Where's your teddy?" The child points to the teddy bear.

Request function: The child points to the bottle. The adult models, "Want bottle?"

Attention function: The child points to a sibling jumping in a swimming pool. The adult says, "There's Billy."

Question function: The child points to a new stuffed animal. The adult asks, "What's that?"

Comment/describe function: The child points to a truck. The adult says, "That's a truck."

Child Progress Procedures: During free play activities, three times a week, frequency of pointing will be monitored.

Decision Rule: If frequency of pointing does not double within 3 weeks, review teaching procedures and the number of opportunities provided to practice the skill.

Figure 4-4. Functional Intervention Plan for Casie's Priority Social-Communication Goal. (From Bricker, D., [Ed.]. [1993]. *Assessment, evaluation and programming system for infants and children: Vol. 1. AEPS measurement for birth to three years.* Baltimore: Paul H. Brookes. Reprinted with permission).

Intervention Activities

Using the intervention plan as a guide, Casie's mother and other team members discussed an array of daily activities that could be used to address the targeted social-communication goal and objective for Casie. The professional staff also consulted the AEPS Curriculum for Birth to Three *(Cripe et al., 1993) for intervention suggestions and activities. The director asked Casie's mother to describe some typical routines at home, and the team suggested specific strategies to use within those routines to provide opportunities for Casie to practice*

Goal: Gains person's attention and refers to an object, person, and/or event

Home Routines:		**Classroom Routines:**	
Getting Dressed	Pretend not to notice the phone ringing, giving the child an opportunity to direct your attention.	Circle Time	Activate a noise-producing toy. Wait for the child to use a gesture or vocalization before activating the toy a second time.
Taking a Bath	Use gestures with your words. Ask the child, "Do you want up?" while modeling holding up your arms.	Activity Center Time	Model gaining a person's attention to refer to objects, people, and/or events using the child's peers in different activities.
Mealtime	When the child consistently focuses on an object, person and/or event of interest, refrain from offering the desired material until the child uses a gesture.	Snack Time	Arrange the snack table so that desirable foods are in view, but slightly out of reach. If the child looks at the food and gestures, pass the desired food.
Trips in the Car	Watch for the child to indicate interest in objects, persons and/or events. Respond to any gesture or vocalization consistently.	Outdoor Play	Help child to get on swing. Pause before pushing or make sure you are within an optimal distance for the child to attempt to gain your attention.

Objective: Points to objects, persons, and/or events across settings

Home Routines:		**Classroom Routines:**	
Getting Dressed	Put one shoe on the child's foot and put the other shoe just out of reach. Ask the child, "Where's the shoe?"	Circle Time	Use songs and finger plays that incorporate the use of pointing.
Taking a Bath	When the child touches a body part, say, "That's your foot." Repeat with different body parts and model pointing.	Activity Center Time	While looking at books, name the pictures and take turns pointing to them.
Mealtime	When pouring drinks for dinner, ask the child questions containing choices, "Do you want milk or juice?" Wait for the child to gesture or point.	Snack Time	Give the child a small piece of cracker or any favorite food. Hold the next piece within view and ask, "What do you want?" Wait for the child to gesture or point.
Trips in the Car	During trips to new places, watch the child's gaze, name the objects and events the child looks at, and model pointing.	Outdoor Play	As the child is reaching for or pointing to a favorite toy, label it, talk about it, and give it to the child to play with.

Figure 4-5. Examples of Home and Classroom Activity Plans. (From Bricker, D. & Pretti-Frontczak, K. [1996]. *Assessment, evaluation and programming system for infants and children: Vol. 3. AEPS measurement for three to six years.* Baltimore: Paul H. Brookes. Reprinted with permission).

her social-communication goal and objective. As shown in Figure 4-5, activity plans were developed that can be used both at home and in the classroom.

As shown in Figure 4-5, Casie's mother and the interventionists planned to provide opportunities for Casie to practice her social-communication goal and objective in several different familiar routines throughout the day, as opposed to creating artificial teaching environments.

Evaluation

Finally, the team discussed several options for monitoring Casie's progress toward the selected social-communication goal and objective, both at school and at home. At school, interventionists decided to conduct brief, frequent probes of the targeted goal and objective, observe and note Casie's response, and prompt her if necessary. The resulting data can be plotted on a simple graph, as shown in Figure 4-6.

At home, Casie's mother decided it would be easiest for her to record the data as anecdotal progress notes. An example of an anecdotal progress monitoring form is shown in Figure 4-7. Finally, the director explained that readministration of the AEPS Test and Family Report could provide the team

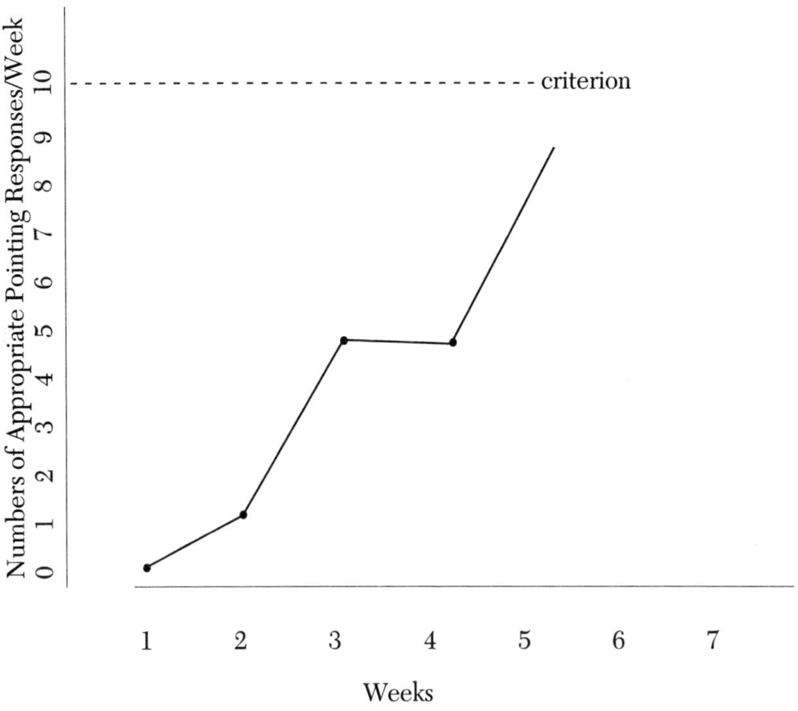

Figure 4-6. Number of Appropriate Pointing Responses by Casie Collected During Weekly Probes.

Goal: Gains person's attention and refers to an object, person, and/or event

Describe Casie's Behavior: Describe Context:

Objective: Points to objects, persons, and/or events across settings

Describe Casie's Behavior: Describe Context:

Figure 4-7. Example of Anecdotal Progress Monitoring Form. (From Bricker, D., & Petti-Frontczak, K. [1996]. *Assessment, evaluation and programming system for infants and children: Vol. 3. AEPS measurement for three to six years.* Baltimore: Paul H. Brookes. Reprinted with permission.)

with an important record of Casie's progress toward targeted goals and objectives. The team decided to readminister both measures at 3- to 4-month intervals. Results from such quarterly evaluations can be displayed on the summary graphs included with the AEPS Test protocols.

SUMMARY

Observations of the assessment and evaluation of infants and young children with developmental disabilities lead to the inescapable conclusion that many approaches currently being used could benefit from serious revision. In particular, in our observation of programs we found little attempt to relate assessment and intervention to each other, or to evaluation activities. We believe this occurs largely because communication specialists and other interventionists select assessment and evaluation measures that do not lend themselves to the development of a direct and logical linkage between program components. When norm-referenced tools developed to discriminate between groups of children are used to generate intervention content, it is predictable that the relationship between initial assessment, intervention, and evaluation will be unconnected and remote.

If early communicative assessment and intervention practices are to improve, two important factors should be at work. First, there must be clear vision, or visions, on the part of leaders and experts as to what constitutes improvement for the field. Without such vision (even if time should show it to be flawed), it seems unlikely that there can, or will, be concerted efforts to move in a new direction or change current policy or practice. Second, specification, often at a concrete level, of how to actualize a desired change is necessary. For many individuals, a conceptual model or framework is of limited use unless accompanied by a set of clear practices that clarify how the approach can be applied.

This chapter described our vision for the improvement of intervention services to infants and young children with developmental disabilities. Accompanying this vision is a set of relatively specific procedures for its application. The use of this approach, in which the assessment/evaluation tool is pivotal to the development of functional IEP/IFSPs and intervention plans, has much to recommend it over alternative approaches; however, the collection of future data will, without doubt, show us its flaws and suggest new, and even better, alternatives. The future will offer many challenges, which we can best meet by using our current state-of-the-art knowledge and practice as the foundation for formulating new and better visions.

REFERENCES

Bagnato, S. J., Neisworth, J. T., & Munson, S. M. (1989). *Linking developmental assessment and early intervention: Curriculum-based prescriptions*. Rockville, Md.: Aspen.

Bailey, E., & Bricker, D. (1986). A psychometric study of a criterion-referenced assessment instrument designed for infants and young children. *Journal of the Division for Early Childhood, 10*(2), 124-134.

Bricker, D. (1989). *Early intervention for at-risk and handicapped infants*. Palo Alto: VORT Corp.

Bricker, D. (Ed.). (1993). *Assessment, Evaluation and Programming System for Infants and Children: Vol. 1. AEPS measurement for birth to three years*. Baltimore: Brookes.

Bricker, D. (Ed.). (1996). *Assessment, Evaluation and Programming System for Infants and Children: Vol. 4. AEPS curriculum for three to six years*. Baltimore: Brookes.

Bricker, D., Bailey, E., & Slentz, K. (1990). Reliability, validity and utility of the Evaluation and Programming System: For Infants and Young Children (EPS-I). *Journal of Early Intervention, 14*(2), 147-160.

Bricker, D., & Pretti-Frontczak, K. (Eds.). (1996). *Assessment, Evaluation and Programming System for Infants and Children. Vol. 3: AEPS measurement for three to six years*. Baltimore: Brookes.

Bricker, D., Pretti-Fontczak, K., and McComas, N. (1998). *An activity based approach to early intervention* (2nd ed.). Baltimore: Brookes.

Carlson, L., & Bricker, D. D. (1982). Dyadic and contingent aspects of early communicative intervention. In D. D. Bricker (Ed.), *Intervention with at-risk and handicapped infants* (pp. 291-308). Baltimore: University Park Press.

Cohen, L., & Spenciner, L. (1994). *Assessment of young children*. New York: Longman.

Cripe, J. (1990). *Evaluating the effectiveness of training procedures in a linked system approach to individual family service plan development*. Unpublished doctoral dissertation. University of Oregon, Center on Human Development, Eugene.

Cripe, J., Slentz, K., & Bricker, D. (Eds.). (1993). *Assessment, Evaluation, and Programming System. Vol. 2: AEPS curriculum for birth to three years*. Baltimore: Brookes.

Dunst, C. J., & Rheingrover, M. A. (1981). Discontinuity and instability in early development: Implications for assessment. *Topics in Early Childhood Special Education, 1*(2), 49-60.

Guralnick, M. J., & Bennett, F. C. (1987). *The effects of early intervention for at-risk and handicapped children*. New York: Academic.

Hamilton, J., & Swan, W. (1981). Measurement references in the assessment of preschool handicapped children. *Topics in Early Childhood Special Education, 1*(2), 42-48.

Hsia, T. (1993). *The evaluation of the psychometric properties of the Assessment, Evaluation, and Programming System*. Unpublished doctoral dissertation, University of Oregon, Eugene.

Hutinger, P. L. (1988). Linking screening, identification, and assessment with curriculum. In J. B. Jordan, J. J. Gallagher, P. L. Hutinger, & M. B. Karnes (Eds.), *Early childhood special education: Birth to three* (pp. 29-66). Reston, Va.: Council for Exceptional Children and Its Division for Early Childhood.

Johnson, N. M. (1982). Assessment paradigms and atypical infants: An interventionist's perspective. In D. Bricker (Ed.), *Intervention with at-risk and handicapped infants: From research to application* (pp. 63-76). Baltimore: University Park Press.

Meisels, S. J. (1996). Charting the continuum of assessment and intervention. In S. J. Meisels & E. Fenichel (Eds.), *New visions for the developmental assessment of infants and young children* (pp. 27-52). Washington, D.C.: Zero to Three, National Center for Infants, Toddlers, and Families.

Notari, A., & Bricker, D. (1990). The utility of a curriculum-based assessment instrument in the development of individualized education plans for infants and young children. *Journal of Early Intervention, 14*(2), 117-132.

Notari, A., Slentz, K., & Bricker, D. (1990). Assessment-curriculum systems of early childhood special education. In R. Brown & D. Mitchell (Eds.), *Early intervention for disabled and at-risk infants* (pp. 117-132). London: Croom-Helm.

Sheehan, R. (1982). Infant assessment: A review and identification of emergent trends. In D. Bricker (Ed.), *Intervention with at-risk and handicapped infants* (pp. 47-61). Baltimore: University Park Press.

Stark, R. (Ed.). (1981). *Language behavior in infancy and early childhood.* New York: Elsevier North-Holland.

Stern, D. N. (1981). The development of biologically determined signals of readiness to communicate which are language "resistant." In R. Stark (Ed.), *Language behavior in infancy and early childhood* (pp. 45-62). New York: Elsevier North-Holland.

Yoder, P. J., & Warren, S. F. (1993). Can developmentally delayed children's language development be enhanced through prelinguistic intervention? In A. P. Kaiser & D. B. Gray (Eds.), *Enhancing children's communication: Research foundations for intervention* (pp. 35-62). Baltimore: Brookes.

CHAPTER 5

Collaboration With Families in Communication Intervention

Yvonne Gillette, Ph. D., CCC-SLP
Associate Professor
School of Speech-Language Pathology and Audiology
University of Akron
Akron, Ohio

Key Terms

assessment
consultant
ecological communication program (ECO)
family
intervention
partners
routines

Overview

Professionals function most effectively when they empower the **family**. In fact, family empowerment is the central theme of the Individuals with Disabilities Education Act Amendments (IDEA) 1997, which mandates that services enhance the family's capacity to meet the needs of their children in the areas of communicative, cognitive, social, emotional, and motoric development. These mandates can serve to foster an effective role relationship for families and professionals as collaborators in facilitating the child's development. In this context, *family* refers to the parent-child unit that meets the child's needs, whether met by one or more parents (Bailey & Simeonsson, 1988), as well as siblings and extended family.

Assessment and **intervention** in the area of communication are particularly adaptable to a collaborative effort between families and professionals because children can only use their communication skills within exchanges with others. In the case of this chapter, *assessment* will refer to the process of conducting activities used to plan intervention (Crais, 1995). *Intervention* will refer to those activities and strategies used to nurture the child's development, particularly, but not exclusively, in the area of communication.

In many cases, family-child exchange may provide the most effective context for assessment and/or intervention due to the intimacy of the communicating partners. In fact, theorists have long argued that the development of child communication skills can be viewed as a function of interaction strategies employed by partners, that is, those who regularly interact with the child (Bronfenbrenner, 1979; Bruner, 1978; Greenspan, 1985; Watzlawick, Beavin, & Jackson, 1967). In this light, it is important to explore the expectations that families have for assessment or intervention. It is also important to support their capacity to participate in assessments and to provide effective interventions to meet their own expectations. A contextual approach to assessment sets the stage for families to begin to view themselves as a primary consumer of communication intervention services, rather than the child alone.

When early intervention (EI) professionals successfully support families in their role as primary change agents in the lives of their children, they can benefit the family as well as society at large. The family may find benefit in an improved relationship with the child, and society may find reduced demand for more costly services as these children mature. To effectively empower families, professionals must develop skills to promote child development within a consultative model. The guidelines in this chapter will assist professionals as they develop a systematic communication assessment/intervention model to employ with the families of children from birth through age 5, which has implications across the lifespan.

THE PROFESSIONAL AS A CONSULTANT

Although a **consultant** could be viewed as an expert who gives advice, Weinberg (1985) suggests that with successful consulting, this is rarely the case. Instead, the consumer takes the lead and the consultant shapes a path toward consumer-selected goals with ongoing input from the consumer.

EI professionals working as consultants to families are more successful when they realize that the families themselves are the experts in relation to their own child and family. Intervention plans must arise from both the family's dreams and their realities. A family with the primary dream of having a child walk cannot, and should not, be convinced to adopt a primary dream of improved communication. Instead, activities that promote skill in walking can become a context for communication enhancement. A family that wishes to keep a child at home during the preschool years should not be convinced to enter center-based EI programming. Instead, the home can become the location of intervention, allowing the family to continue their preferred role as the primary agent of change in the life of the child and the family as a whole. As these examples illustrate, consultants negotiate with families to develop plans that match the latter's view of the desired services to enhance the child's development.

AN ECOLOGICAL MODEL OF COMMUNICATION INTERVENTION

During the 1980s, the **ecological communication program (ECO)** evolved from a series of research and development projects (MacDonald & Gillette, 1984, 1985, 1986, 1988, 1989). The projects were motivated by the realization that traditional models of one-to-one, behaviorally oriented speech-language intervention were not effective with children who had not yet developed consistent communication with their families. In addition, traditional approaches are not compatible with the mandates of IDEA (1997) to empower families to promote the development of their children. The close, and almost exclusive, ties between families and their young children demand a communication assessment/intervention model to guide the families as they develop increasingly more sophisticated communicating partnerships with their children. The ECO model can best be defined as a system for intervention that proposes to guide the development of interactions between children and their partners from play through conversation. ECO has been successfully applied to children from birth through age 5 as well as other individuals functioning at this level of development.

The model that evolved continues to assess skills and then project outcomes for the child's communication skills, as is traditional in communication intervention planning. The ECO model, however, operates within a collaborative context of communication between the family and a professional. Consequently, the program guides consultants to develop assessment and intervention plans with families that include (1) communication contexts, (2) current child skills and projected outcomes within these contexts, and (3) partner communication strategies that support current skills and can facilitate the desired outcomes. This context-rich plan is the essence of the consultation process.

ECO ASSESSMENTS

Using the collaborative context described in the previous section, ECO assessments address three primary questions:

- What does the family expect to gain from the assessment?
- How does the child interact and communicate across daily routines and communication partners?
- How can communication partners promote the child's communication development within these daily routines?

Family Expectations

The first question guides the remainder of the assessment. Here, the family identifies any particular concerns regarding their child's communication skills, their desire to facilitate development of communication skills, and the priority they ascribe to communication skill development in relationship to other child and/or family concerns. When consultants proceed from the family's agenda, they will find clear direction for any further work with that family. Families are inevitably diverse in their attitudes and desires, and it is the job of the professionals to match their priorities and needs. For example, one family may be eager to obtain advice on getting their child to use words instead of gestures, whereas another may be so concerned about their child's health that they have little time to consider the need for communication intervention. While both of these examples may result in an ECO assessment, the family in the first example has already identified a desired outcome, whereas the family in the second example may need more time to consider whether improving communication skills is a priority for them at this time.

Child's Interaction and Communication

Once a family has identified communication as a developmental skill that they wish to facilitate, the professional and the family can address the second assessment question by identifying how the child interacts and communicates across daily routines and partners. **Routines** are predictably occurring contexts in which children find themselves engaged in the same activity with a partner or partners. Assessment should address both the range of the child's daily life experiences and the child's behavior within typical routines.

As consultants develop a view of children in their daily life routines, they come to realize the diversity in the range of opportunities available for children to practice communication or other developmental skills. Opportunities differ for children who are physically impaired and whose care may occupy a major portion of shared time with others (Light & McNaughton, 1993); children in adverse social circumstances, which may limit their range of experiences; and children in two-parent families, which afford children many opportunities for diverse interactions. Differences between a child's actual life experience and an "ideal" childhood experience must be considered in assessment and addressed in intervention. As the ECO assessment proceeds, it often becomes clear to the consultant as well as the family that communication partners are essential keys to developing a child's communication skill.

Role of Communication Partners

The third question addresses the key role of the partner in developing communication. Ideally, observations include the child interacting with a range of partners, including the consultant, in order to determine the communication strategies that foster the most productive interaction and communication. Using interactions as a source of discussion assists in discovering effective communication strategies. When silent waiting prompts the child to initiate a message, families and their consultants should note it. If questions yield head shakes instead of words, partners can try commenting and then discuss the difference between questions and comments. Consultants who model the act of noticing effective communication strategies will generally find that families will be more likely to share their observations. In addition, families, drawing on a much wider range of experience with the child, can provide many more insights from daily life with the child.

DETERMINING THE NEED FOR A COMMUNICATION INTERVENTION PLAN

Under IDEA (1997) mandates, young children and their families participate in communication assessment as part of multifaceted assessments. In addition to their traditional role of informant regarding the child's health, social life, and past experiences, families can contribute to these assessments in a variety of unique ways. These may include (1) their expectation for the assessment, (2) their observations of the child in his or her typical environments, (3) their interpretation of the child's behavior in typical, as well as other, environments, (4) their participation in an assessment to elicit child behaviors, and (5) their validation of the assessment findings (Crais, 1993). Consultants also contribute to these assessments in a variety of ways, but particularly by informing families why certain information is requested and by summarizing results as a source of information for developing a plan of service. Professionals who can facilitate a shared view of assessment as a two-way process between families and consultants often gain more useful communication assessment information. Discovering the varied reasons behind communication exchange may help families look at communication as a process between the child and significant others, rather than as a product produced by the child alone.

Initially, consultants can use the four ECO Outcomes (described in more detail in a later section) as issues to guide an interview with the family.

- Establishing a partnership between partner and child (Participation)
- Developing routines together (Balance)
- Acting and communicating in progressively matched ways (Match)
- Sharing enjoyment

Addressing these issues highlights the centrality of the family to the communication intervention process. The first outcome addresses, as the core of the communication development process, shared experiences, which typically evolve during family life. The remaining outcomes characterize communication as depending on two partners who are balanced, matched, and emotionally in tune. When families and their consultants mutually consider these aspects of communication, the team becomes better able to determine the need for communication intervention and to contribute to the design of the intervention plan.

GATHERING INFORMATION FOR A COMMUNICATION INTERVENTION PLAN

To demonstrate how information might be gathered for an ECO assessment, two new tools derived from the original ECO materials are described in this section (Gillette, 1989; Gillette & MacDonald, 1989; MacDonald, 1989; MacDonald, Gillette, & Hutchinson, 1989). The ECO Environmental Scan and the ECO Partnership Guidelines shape interviews and observations toward a contextual perspective as consultants gather information with families for planning communication interventions.

The ECO Environmental Scan

Consultants can use the ECO Environmental Scan to discover with the family the richness of the child's participation in daily life (Figure 5-1). Measures relevant to an environmental scan include determining: (1) where the child spends time (situations), (2) the frequency and variety of social and functional routines in which the child participates, (3) the range of partners across routines, (4) the length of time for which the child participates in routines, and (5) the range of reasons for participating. Through using an environmental scan, consultants will avoid making assumptions about the circumstances of the child's life and be in a better position to individualize plans to the family's and child's unique experience. Families live in diverse circumstances, and few assumptions can be made about the life of any family.

While a complete environmental scan does take time, the process creates an excellent context for building a relationship with the family. In addition, the complete scan need only be performed once, with updates as circum-

Partners / Situations/ Routines	MOM	DAD	MIKE	MITCHELL	SARAH (PT)						
Home											
taking a bath	O	S									
eating	O	S									
getting dressed	O	S									
doing PT exercises	O										
bedtime (2 times)	O	S									
Physical Therapy											
session	O				O						
Home (play)											
smile at faces		R									
bang for attention	R										
smile at dog play				R	R						

1. Review child's daily life noting where the child spends time and typical routines that occur in each situation (Column 1).
2. Note the child's typical partners in these routines across the top.
3. In the squares that show the intersection of partners with the child, rate each square as O = Often, S = Sometimes (R= rare, if including infrequent routines).
4. Determine key routines with the family. Enhance these with other descriptors such as range of reasons for participating, and typical length of time.

Figure 5-1. ECO Environmental Scan. (From Gillette, Y. [1996]. Early intervention in communication development: A collaborative model for professionals consulting with families. In M. Smith & J. Damico [Eds.], *Childhood language disorders* [pp. 300–324]. New York: Theime Medical Publishers. Reprinted with permission.)

stances change. The scan can also include situations such as day care, home, the bus or car, and more novel locations, such as a frequently visited park. The professional should probe for functional routines such as bathtime, getting the groceries, or cleaning house. The scan also should explore for social routines, including going for walks, playing with toys, or watching television.

Identified partners can include parents, grandparents, neighbors, cousins, and sitters, to name a few. Once the scan's visual display becomes available, families and their consultants can negotiate to select a few key intersections of routines and partners to focus toward the goal of enriching the child's communication experience. The display also assists in pinpointing more routine-partner combinations as communication intervention expands.

An environmental scan can also provide concrete measures relevant to the child's communication status and change. The measures are ecological and contextual in nature, recognizing that more regular routines and partners, as well as longer contacts for more varied reasons, can have a strong impact on overall communication development. While these measures may not seem immediately relevant to communication itself, consider the following example. A young child spends most of his days in a day-care setting with 12 other children in his age group. Content to play quietly on his own and being well-behaved, he receives little attention. When an older sister is scheduled to work at night, she cares for the child during the day, taking him with her on errands and to the park. Here he learns about the community and finds one or two peers to play with at the park. An ecological component of this child's communication plan may be to determine if the sister could provide more regular day care by rearranging her work schedule. This change alone could have significant impact on the child's communication. If such a change is combined with professional consultation with all the child's caregivers, the communication plan could be even more effective.

The ECO Partnership Guidelines

No individual can communicate in isolation. Consequently, logic dictates that communicating partnerships provide the context for assessment, intervention, and change monitoring rather than isolating the child. Families and their consultants can use the ECO Partnership Guidelines to provide a systematic view of child skills and partner strategies that contribute to any communicating partnership across the four ECO Outcomes. Families and their consultants can participate with, and observe, the child in typical functional (mealtime, bedtime) and social (play, watching television) routines, and then plan for communication outcomes based on the results of their participation and observation.

The theoretical and empirical bases for the outcomes that comprise the ECO Partnership Guidelines follow. This background can assist in developing a complete rationale for a partnership approach to intervention. In addition, specific child skills, partner strategies, and measures suggested for each of the four outcomes can provide guidance in developing individualized plans for partnership interventions.

Outcome 1: Participate—Establish a Partnership. Table 5-1 presents the child skills, partner strategies, and measures of participation that contribute

Table 5-1. ECO Partnership Guidelines

Outcome 1: Participate—Establish a partnership

Child Skills

- participates in a range of settings
- participates in a range of routines and conversations
- participates with a range of partners
- interacts/converses for social and functional reasons
- continues interacting for varying lengths of time

Partner Strategies

- contact the child frequently
- follow the child's lead
- keep the child interacting

Measures of Participation

- where the child spends time (situations)
- frequency and variety of social and functional routines
- range of partners across routines
- length of time spent in routines
- range of reasons for participating

Source: Gillette, Y. (1996). Early intervention in communication development: A collaborative model for professionals consulting with families. In M. Smith & J. Damico (Eds.), *Childhood language disorders* (pp. 300–324). New York: Theime Medical Publishers. Reprinted with permission.

to developing Outcome 1. Routines result when partners contribute turns (Kaye & Charney, 1980) in the form of actions and messages. They have been described as formats (Bruner, 1983), joint activity (Bronfenbrenner, 1979), and social interactions (Stern, 1977). Children who are successful communicators contact others, respond to contacts from others, and stay in the interactions. In addition, they use these skills in functionally and socially motivated routines. Partners who promote this behavior follow the child's lead; they also contact the child frequently and do so in a variety of extended routines.

Why are routines considered so essential to communication? Bruner (1983) likened the development of the routine to Chomsky's (1973) concept of the deep structure and surface structure of language. Bruner used a game of peekaboo as his exemplar. To be recognized as peekaboo, the game must follow certain rules (the deep structure); however, no two games of peekaboo are exactly alike (the surface structure). This analysis can apply to any routine. Attempting to enhance a child's communicative experience must logically address the frequency and variety of routines and partners to ensure that the child experiences how communication works.

Unfortunately, children who are disabled or at risk may not have the variation in experience that produces a robust, generative communication system (Mahoney, 1988; Merighi, Edison, & Zigler, 1990). Their limited experience can result not only from the child's personal microsystem (his or her daily life) but also his or her society (Bronfenbrenner, 1979). When assessing communication or planning and monitoring communication intervention programs, consultants should consider how personal, community, state, and federal funding priorities can affect a child's communication development when an ecological approach is used. If a family lacks the resources to purchase a wheelchair for a child who cannot walk, his or her community experiences will be limited. When public funds for transportation are limited, the child who is at risk may be confined to the immediate environment. With these concepts in mind, consultants can make a strong case for including frequent, repeated experience with familiar and motivating routines in plans designed to develop a wide variety of integrated skills, including communication (Goodman, 1992).

When planning with families, consultants should keep in mind that family priorities, culturally based preferences, and opinions on raising children will all influence their choices in planning. ECO provides a wide range of outcomes, skills, strategies, and measures, so it is usually possible to identify some options that families and their consultants will both find valuable. Consultants must be sensitive to family values as they work to facilitate a child's communication development.

Outcome 2: Balance—Develop Routines Together. Table 5-2 presents the child skills, partner strategies, and measures of match related to Outcome 2. Many researchers have noted less balance in interactions that include a child with special needs than in pairs where the child is not disabled (Buckhalt, Rutherford & Goldberg, 1978; Cunningham, Reuler, Blackwell, & Deck, 1981; Jones, 1980; Mahoney, Finger, & Powell, 1985). Moreover, Merighi et al. (1990) found that when children experienced mostly relationships dominated by partners, they became less effective adults. Scholars of parent-child interaction appear to agree that children learn to communicate by gradually contributing to the routines of daily life in ways similar to their partners. Bronfenbrenner (1979) suggested that development occurs within relationships in which the balance of power gradually shifts toward the developing persons, and that more learning occurs when the developing person participates rather than simply observes. Bruner (1983) struck a similar note in his "handover principle," which recommends that "where before there was a spectator let there now be a participant" (p. 60). Stern (1986) looked for "attunement"; Kaye and Charney (1980) for "turnarounds"; and Als, Tronick, and Brazelton (1979) for "mutual feedback systems."

While families and their consultants may understand the need for balance, achieving it may be hampered by interaction habits the family has developed with a child who may be slow to react due to sensory, motor, social, or cognitive needs. These habits may develop from daily pressures, incorporating work outside the home, demands of other children, and similar influences. Atten-

Table 5-2. ECO Partnership Guidelines

Outcome 2: Balance—Develop routines together

Child Skills

- initiates routines and conversations and responds to initiations from others
- shows a back-and-forth interaction style
- imitates others

Partner Strategies

- maintain balance in play, then conversation
- wait, signal, and expect
- respond to the child with actions and messages
- imitate the child at times

Measures of Balance

- frequency of initiations as well as responses to initiations of others
- ratio of actions that each partner contributes to the routine
- ratio of messages that each member contributes to the routine

Source: Gillette, Y. (1996). Early intervention in communication development: A collaborative model for professionals consulting with families. In M. Smith & J. Damico (Eds.), *Chidhood language disorders* (pp. 300–324). New York: Theime Medical Publishers. Reprinted with permission.

tion to subtle factors such as timing and structure (Stern, 1977) can easily be obscured by the rush of life.

Timing and structure also influence the relationship between the consultant and partner, a point that the former should recognize in conducting intervention. Consultants may provide more effective services if they respond to the family's concerns as they present them. Consultants who are skilled in timing provide the pauses needed to elicit these family concerns. While a consultant's question will generally draw an answer from the family, a pause may elicit a family concern that provides the consultant with new information. Consultants may find it useful to observe the structure of their family interviews and planning sessions to make sure that they balance their own interaction with the family, much as they strive to balance the partner's interactions with the child.

A few highlights from clinical experience may be helpful in designing programs to achieve balance. A frequent profile of partner-child interaction consists of partners who talk and children who act. Consider a child playing while the partner comments on the play. Balance may be achieved by creating an interaction in which the partner performs a play action accompanied by a message about the play, then waits for the child to take a turn.

When partners can observe the change in the child's participation in response to these strategies, they are often motivated to try such an approach themselves. When a child would benefit from imitating the actions and messages of others, partners often need to practice with the consultant in order to change their interaction style, even when they are already motivated to do so. It is a big change for a partner to modify his or her participation by, for example, performing one action (place a block on a table) and saying one message ("block" or "on") rather than building a block tower and saying to the child, "Can you make a block tower like I did?" When families repeatedly experience the effectiveness of these simpler models, they may begin to appreciate their role as a primary agent of change in their child's life.

The measures suggested in Table 5-2 accent the strong emphasis that the ECO program places on balance. A one-to-one relationship in terms of actions as well as messages is ideal and can be achieved when partners provide the child with communication opportunities by modeling actions and messages, then waiting for the child to contribute to the routine.

Outcome 3: Match—Act and Communicate in Progressively Matched Ways. Progressive matching (MacDonald & Gillette, 1985, 1986, 1988) is closely related to balance. Progressive matching fine-tunes the partner's contribution to a routine so that it provides a model within the "zone of proximal development" (Vygotsky, 1962). Vygotsky found that children became bored with models that were below their own level of behavior or too redundant with it, while models that were too advanced also discouraged the child's behavior. Recently, Mahoney and Neville-Smith (1996) found similar results when measuring the effects of directive communication on children's interactive engagement. Ideally, progressively matched models are actions and messages that match the child's level and occasionally are a challenging step above. Additionally, models provide examples of actions and/or messages the child can try, but without a question or command that elicits a specific behavior.

Many scholars across the second half of the twentieth century have acknowledged the importance of this notion to development. For example, Piaget (1951) noted that children form schemas based on experiences that are moderately incongruent with their existing mental models but cannot incorporate schemas that are highly novel. The notion is central to Van Dijk's sequence of interpersonal methods (see Stillman & Battle [1984], Hunt's [1965] minimal discrepancy, and Bruner's [1983] fine-tuning). Bandura (1977) developed his social learning theory largely from the notion that learning occurs through observation and practice. His theory postulates that children learn much of what they know by observing adult models and repeating their behavior. Once learned, the behavior becomes a part of the child's repertoire without the necessity of the model's presence.

Experimental work also supports the notion of progressively matched models to foster communication development, as well as the fact that matching may not be the strategy that some adults use naturally with some children. As early as 1930, Valentine showed that infants imitate their mother more than they imitate other individuals, and that while they may have failed to respond to initial demonstrations, they did respond after the action was repeated a number of times. Bandura (1977) concluded that the infants appeared to vary in their performance based on who the models were, what they selected to model, and how they did it. Kaye (1976) showed that mothers modeled tasks that children came close to performing on pretests. However, they were directive, using commands and questions, if the child did not exhibit a similar performance. Cheseldine and McConkey (1979) instructed parents of children with Down syndrome to teach 20 target words to their children. The children who learned the most words had parents who modeled the words as their teaching strategy. Other, less successful parents used a question and command approach.

All the evidence suggesting the importance of modeling within the range of the child's performance implies that partners must fully understand the child's current performance in terms of action and messages in order to provide an appropriate match (Goodman, 1992). Here, consultation can provide the insight to assist the partner in identifying effective strategies for interacting with the child. A review of the list of child skills and partner strategies in Table 5-3 shows the flexibility of the notion of match across various children and partners over time. Early on, a child may be able to imitate simple actions (clapping hands together, touching or holding an object) and simple messages (reaching for a desired object, squealing in delight). Later, the same child may need more complex actions and messages in order to learn from the interaction and stay interested in it.

The pragmatic impact of a message is another subtle point of intervention that often requires attention. Messages presented as statements ("flower," "The fish is swimming") provide models, not only of the words and messages themselves, but also of the act of commenting on what is observed in the environment. On the other hand, questions ("What is that?", "What is the fish doing?") do not give the child information, but rather test for it. Questions also set the stage for a limited exchange, which often must be reinitiated by the partner to be sustained. Commands may also limit communication development in that the expected response to the command is rarely a message (consider, "Show me the flower," or "Look at the fish."). When the command does require a message, the exchange that occurs is not typical of free-flowing communication between partners but rather emphasizes the subordination of the developing person to the more advanced partner.

Outcome 4: Share Enjoyment. Many scholars postulate the importance of emotional attachment to the development of effective communication (Bruner, 1983; Greenspan, 1985; Stern, 1986). Bronfenbrenner (1979) hypothesized that one learns more from a teacher with whom one has a close relationship. Experimental evidence also supports the idea that emotion-based outcomes are essential to the development of a rich communicative experi-

Table 5-3. ECO Partnership Guidelines

Outcome 3: Match—Act and communicate in progressively matched ways

Child skills

- imitates actions and messages partners use
- uses actions and messages in functional and meaningful ways
- uses varied actions and messages (gestures, sounds, signs, words, phrases)
- uses increasingly novel and sophisticated messages
- makes self understood

Partner strategies

- observe, then build on the child's action-message repertoire
- model actions and messages the child may be able to imitate
- match the child's behavior, play in childlike ways
- communicate in ways close to the child
- comment more than question or command

Measures

- frequency of actions and messages sent
- balance between actions/messages imitated vs. spontaneous
- appropriateness of action/messages
- variety of messages
- complexity of messages (MLU)
- similarity between these measures for each partner

Note: MLU = mean length of utterance

Source: Gillette, Y. (1996). Early intervention in communication development. A collaborative model for professionals consulting with families. In M. Smith & J. Damico (Eds.), *Childhood language disorders* (pp. 300–324). New York: Theime Medical Publishers. Reprinted with permission.

ence between a child and his or her significant partners. Tronick, Als, & Adamson (1979) had mothers interrupt a happy play routine by showing the infant a passive face. At first, infants reacted by vocalizing and turning or waving their hands to attract the mother's attention. They became distressed and gave up when their efforts were not successful. Clearly, these infants expected to have an effect on the behavior of their partners. Murray and Trevarthen (1986) devised an ingenious experiment to show that a mother's behavior is affected by her child's actions. Three- and four-month-old infants were shown to their mothers over video in a real time versus a lagged time condition. In the real time condition, mother and child reactions were transmitted to each other immediately. In the lagged time condition, the mother was shown a replay of the child that was not related to her actions and reactions. In both cases, the mother presumed the real time condition. When the presentation was real time, the mother worked from the infant behavior, commenting positively and responding to the infant's behavior. In the delayed presentation, the mothers called for attention, made negative comments, and frequently corrected the child. This finding showed that the same mothers performed in either a responsive or directive manner, depending on the responsiveness of the infant.

In order to be effective, communication programs must address the issue of social-emotional attachment in order to foster the positive exchanges that benefit the child as well as the partner. Consultants who have dealt with communication development using traditional methods, however, may be uncomfortable with including an emotion-based outcome in an intervention plan. One means to facilitate an awareness of the tie between emotion and communication, for both professionals and families, is to observe the child, or other children, under both stressful and pleasant conditions. It soon becomes clear how emotional environment contributes to communication skill development.

The ECO partnership guidelines related to sharing enjoyment present child skills and partner strategies using language that is nonthreatening and can provide valuable guidance to families and their consultants as they incorporate shared enjoyment into their communication plan (Table 5-4).

DYNAMIC ASSESSMENT AND MONITORING

The partnership guidelines have value for families and their consultants as they assess, intervene, and monitor child communication in relationship to a

Table 5-4. ECO Partnership Guidelines

Outcome 4 : Share Enjoyment

Child skills

- shows enjoyment through face and voice
- contacts others for fun

Partner strategies

- be animated
- use positive comments

Measures of enjoyment

- for each partner, use a range scale such as 1 = little enjoyment to 5 = considerable enjoyment

Source: Gillette, Y. (1996). Early intervention in communication development. A collaborative model for professionals consulting with families. In M. Smith & J. Damico (Eds.), *Childhood language disorders* (pp. 300–324). New York: Theime Medical Publishers. Reprinted with permission.

partner or partners. In addition, the guidelines can direct dynamic assessment and monitoring (Feuerstein, Rand, & Hoffman, 1979; Olswang, Bain, & Johnson, 1992). Dynamic assessment and monitoring is analogous to a clinical probe in which the consultant or family member varies interaction methods with the child to determine how his or her communication may change when alternative partner strategies are employed. For example, the consultant may notice that the partner is quick to fill the silence if the child does not offer an action or message turn immediately. During dynamic assessment, the consultant suggests that the partner incorporate a wait of 10 seconds following any turn. If the child's communication increases, waiting may prove to be an ideal strategy. Another example involves family program monitoring. In this case, the family may have successfully employed waiting and matching and the child may communicate frequently during the interaction. However, the family may express concern that the child's messages are somewhat repetitive and primarily consist of object names. Through a process of dynamic monitoring, the consultant fine-tunes the plan with the family by demonstrating with a "truck and sand" routine. For example, the family is encouraged to incorporate action words and names of people into the sand routine as well as other daily routines with the child. Soon, the family will report that the child has begun to use these new words and even combines them in phrases, saying "dig in sand," rather than "sand," or "make a tunnel," rather than, simply, "truck." Through dynamic monitoring, the family will discover how progressive matching can facilitate their child's communication skills.

The results of dynamic assessment and monitoring become the fuel to energize the plan for intervention; this is particularly true when the partner actually participates with the child and notes promising responses to an intervention strategy or set of strategies. Both the consultant and the partner will witness the child achieve new outcomes; intervention is designed to transform these fragile behaviors into habits.

ECO INTERVENTION PLANNING

The *ECO Communication Intervention Planning Guide* (Gillette, 1996) provides a systematic guide to developing the communication component of an Individualized Family Service Plan (IFSP) or Individualized Educational Plan (IEP). Figure 5-2 shows a completed plan. The *ECO Communication Intervention Planning Guide* summarizes information gained from the ECO Environmental Scan and observations analyzed by the ECO Partnership Guidelines. Using the guide can assist the consultant in developing the ECO Model of communication intervention with the team. It pinpoints the ecological components of ECO intervention such as situation, routines, communication outcomes, child skills, and partner strategies. When a more in-depth presentation seems desirable, other educational materials may be useful. One example is the video program, *An Introduction to the Ecological Communi-*

SITUATION: Home School Other *Home*

ROUTINES/CONVERSATIONS:
(social) *dog play, funny face game, ignoring game*
(functional)

PARTNERS: *Mom Dad Mitchell Mike*

MESSAGES: *All messages in all routines will be simple sounds*
Routine/Conversation 1: Dog play
"hey" "ooo" "papa"

Routine/Conversation 2: Funny Face Game
"eee" "hi" "baba"

Routine/Conversation 3: Scarf Game
"ah" "mmm" "hi"

COMMUNICATION OUTCOMES/CHILD SKILLS/MEASURES
1. *Outcome: Balance*

   Matthew's Skill: show a back-and-forth interaction style

2. *Outcome: Match*

   Matthew's Skill: imitate others

COMMUNICATION STRATEGIES (Partner):
1. *Wait, signal, and expect*
2. *Model sounds Matthew may be able to imitate*

PRACTICE SCHEDULE: *avoid practicing all day long*
Routine: _______ Times of Day: _______ Length of Time: ______
Routine: _______ Times of Day: _______ Length of Time: ______
Routine: _______ Times of Day: _______ Length of Time: ______

Figure 5-2. ECO Communication Intervention Plan. (From Gillette, Y. [1996]. Early intervention in communication development: A collaborative model for professionals consulting with families. In M. Smith & J. Damico [Eds.], *Childhood language disorders* [pp. 300–324]. New York: Theime Medical Publishers. Reprinted with permission.)

cation Program (MacDonald & Gillette, 1989). The goal of these presentations is to ensure that families and other team members participate fully in the development of the communication intervention plan.

The *ECO Communication Intervention Planning Guide* provides a template that families and their consultants can use together over time to guide a systematic discussion of communication intervention and gain commitment from all members of the team to an ecological plan of intervention. The following steps may provide guidance for such interactive and systematic planning.

1. Select situations, routines, and partners for the sites of intervention: Doing this in the forum of the team provides opportunities for team input regarding optimal selection—one consultant cannot know all the implications of selecting a particular routine or partner, but the team may. Team participation facilitates a greater possibility of success when using an ecological approach.

2. Select communication outcomes: Using the ECO outcomes—participation, balance, match, and enjoyment—increases the likelihood that all team members will be able to contribute to the selection of outcomes because these kinds of outcomes arise from direct experiences with the child. The consultant may gain alternative perspectives on the child's performance that may not be available in a clinical assessment.

3. Select child skills to develop as well as partner strategies to facilitate that development: Use the ECO Partnership Guidelines to select child skills and partner strategies related to the outcomes selected by the team. Partners and consultants who have observed and participated in a dynamic assessment can effectively contribute to the selective process based on their actual experience with the child.

4. Select progress measures: The team must decide how to measure progress, how frequently the measures should be performed, and who is responsible. The ECO Partnership Guide recommends measures for each ECO Outcome, such as the numbers of routines in which the child participates (participation outcome), or the ratio of actions each partner contributes to the interaction (balance outcome). The team also needs to be aware that the source of the measures will differ depending on the direction of the outcome. The family may provide the best report of participation in daily life, whereas the consultant may more objectively measure the balance of actions between participating partners. When a measure is selected, discussion must include the team member responsible for collecting the data and a method designed to fit the individual's available time and motivation (Schwartz & Olswang, 1996).

It often proves to be an optimal balance of responsibility if the consultant monitors the partnership program in terms of the written summary of data collected. The summary content will be guided by the data source. For example, a documented interview with the family may be the most valid record of participation data whereas balance data may be collected during partner-child routines that the consultant charts on an interval basis, such as weekly, biweekly, or monthly. Another potential source of data is a partnership calendar (Figure 5-3). While many partners may be reluctant to collect frequency data due to time constraints, they may be happy to summarize one highlight daily or, perhaps, three times a week. This responsibility may also keep them focused on the importance of their role in the program.

WEEK:____________________

CHILD: ____________________

PARTNER: ____________________

1. List in column one the routines that you have agreed to practice this week.

2. Write a note or record data about each routine you practiced each day.

Routine	Monday	Tuesday	Wed.	Thurs.	Friday	Sat.	Sunday

WEEK:____________________

CHILD: ____________________

PARTNER: ____________________

1. List in column one the routines that you have agreed to practice this week.

2. Write a note or record data about each routine you practiced each day.

Routine	Monday	Tuesday	Wed.	Thurs.	Friday	Sat.	Sunday

Figure 5-3. ECO Communication Partnership Calendar.

5. Select an intervention schedule that fits the family. At first, families may benefit from regularly scheduled practice sessions on specific routines. In this respect, ecological communication programming shares some features with weight loss clinics. While ECO families and weight loss clients both know what to do, it is often difficult to establish a new habit without specific commitments and schedules. Securing a commitment to direct, scheduled intervention in terms of days of the week, times of the day, and length of time for each selected routine may help some partners establish habits while they give thought as to how they will incorporate these new habits into their daily routines. Once habits are established, more creative implementation of the plan generally evolves. As habits strengthen and more potential contexts emerge, the intervention can begin to occur naturally in spontaneously occurring contexts.

In this way, communication intervention can be woven into the pattern of the child's life. The ECO Environmental Scan provides a way for all team members to see how this is possible as they contribute to an evolving plan. Once families and their consultants have collaborated on the ECO Communication Plan, a regularly scheduled consultation with involved partners can form the basis for implementing the details of the plan. The next section will review the components of a consultation session directed toward implementing an ECO Plan.

CONSULTING WITH PARTNERS TO IMPLEMENT AN ECO COMMUNICATION INTERVENTION PLAN

Once an initial plan has been developed, the team continues to work together to achieve the plan's outcomes and implement the plan as the family-child communication partnership develops. Effective consultants hone their skills through analyzing their interactions with consultees, in a manner analogous to the intervention they are recommending to a communicating partnership. They follow the partner's lead, present models of interaction progressively matched to the partner's skill level, and foster a spirit of enjoyment. These ongoing consultation sessions should not be viewed as the child's "therapy" but rather as opportunities to share observations and modify the plan along a course of positive communication growth between the two communicating partners—the child and the family. With these principles in mind, the format presented next may serve as an ongoing consultation strategy.

Monitor

Consultants monitor partnership programs with families by sampling data from the sources they have jointly selected. The source of the data may be interview or observation. A sample could be a videotaped interaction between the partner and child, a partnership calendar, or a directed interview related to specific communicative interactions between the partner and child. In any case, the family and their consultant should know from the plan the kind of data that will be used to monitor progress and how it will be collected.

Monitoring also involves an interpretation of the data. The family and their consultant consider together what a summary of the data reveals. For example, they consider what strategies to implement if, for example, data reveal that the child has begun to communicate with more people and that vocabulary in play routines has increased more than in functional routines, but that message length has not increased since the last session. When collaborating with the partner to interpret the data, the consultant should probe for additional insights. For instance, in the previous example, it may be that the child's number of immediate contacts has increased but the new partners use fewer effective communication strategies than the family uses, making these new contacts less effective than they could be. Monitoring and interpreting data and sharing insights with partners are essential ingredients for implementing the intervention plan over time.

Plan and Educate

Discussion during the monitoring portion of the session will lead to modification of the plan's implementation. Perhaps new routines need to be added to the plan, or, as in the previous example, additional partners need to learn some specific strategies. In other cases, routines may need to be adjusted to promote growth—adding new vocabulary, longer messages, or increased participation in the routine. Partners could be having trouble implementing a specific strategy. During the planning/educating portion of the session, begin to revise the details of the plan implementation on paper. These details may be altered as the session progresses, but the rough draft will provide an initial outline.

While developing the draft of the revised plan, topics related to the plan's components will arise. The discussion provides a forum in which partner education can take place. The success of partnership programs depends on the understanding of the program's components that is shared by the partner and consultant. The reasoning behind each new outcome, child skill, and partner strategy chosen for the plan is essential to its success. Consultants should be prepared to illustrate each program component with a variety of techniques besides direct discussion. Varied teaching tools provide more avenues for learning for all partners, and some allow for sharing with partners who cannot directly participate due to family work schedules and other complications. Written materials and video programs can help to fill the need for education. If video samples of routines are collected during the training sessions, sharing the tapes with a range of partners can provide a useful educational tool when used as a basis for discussion led by the partner in the program. Prepared video programs, or portions of them, can also be useful (Cripe, 1995; Gillette, 1993; MacDonald & Gillette, 1989; Manolson, Ward, & Dodington, 1995; McConkey, 1988). Some partners may wish to review written materials after they leave the session or provide them as guidance for other partners. Materials such as the *ECO Resources* (Gillette & MacDonald, 1989) and the *CATCH Guide to Planning Services with Families* (Gillette, 1992) have been designed to clarify new points or give further examples of implementation.

Practice

Once the plan's implementation details have been revised, the family and their consultant practice with any new components to see if they make sense and can actually be implemented. The family or consultant may wish to take the lead and practice a routine and selected strategies with the child. Providing feedback to each other helps to determine what seems to work well, what could work if slightly altered, and what does not work at all. Actually performing with the child often shows most effectively what can be done and how rather than depending on words alone. This is another application of the ECO principles of participation, balance, match, and enjoyment to partner education.

The following three-step approach often works effectively: (1) practice a routine with the child while another person (family or consultant) observes; (2) share observations on performance that are related to outcomes, child skills, and partner strategies in the plan, (3) practice another routine with the child, but switch observer and participant roles and share observations on the second routine. In this practice session, timing is important. The consultant and partner should take turns practicing brief (1-minute or less) interactions with the child. Share perspectives on the routines and provide positive comments before suggesting an avenue for change. Often the most effective feedback is provided in the form of another model or suggesting what a partner could do through positive comments, rather than a directive approach that involves pointing out errors.

Integrate Into Daily Life

While the session with a consultant provides direction for implementing the program, daily intervention works to promote the child's total life experience toward promoting effective communication partnerships. As the child and the family develop a partnership together, daily life can become a series of frequent, spontaneous, and enjoyable routines.

Some partners may easily incorporate new communication skills into their daily life with the child, whereas other partners may need a bridge to practice these communication behaviors with the child. When a family expresses frustration with their skill development, they can be encouraged to schedule brief, but regular, practice sessions with the child. The scheduled practices provide opportunities to consciously practice the strategies recommended in the plan. Once they are more confident in their skills, partners should gradually begin to incorporate the strategies into their spontaneous contacts with the child. The consultant and partner should also develop a method for monitoring the program. Charts, calendars, and interviews at consultation sessions are possible examples. Partners who keep a record may be more likely to remember the components of the plan and to practice them regularly. They also come prepared to discuss the program at consultation sessions. However, the method must suit the value and lifestyle of the partner, or it may become a dreaded task (Gillette & MacDonald, 1989).

Consultants familiar with the ECO model have found the following guidelines to be essential in working with families to develop communicating partnerships with the child (adapted from Gillette, 1989, p. 13):

1. Start small and build. Work for a small, but noticeable, change. Avoid constructing an elaborate plan, which the partner may find cumbersome and discouraging. Partners will be encouraged to build on small, but successful, plans. Too much planning and not enough action early on can be discouraging.

2. Use strong points as well as problems to implement plans: Consider the entire profile to build the plan logically. A partner may be skillful at consciously practicing, but less successful in implementing certain strategies. Here, spontaneous use of strategies may be recommended. For example, place a "WAIT" reminder or two around the house. Whenever the partner notices it, the reminder will prompt longer waiting before communicating with the child. The partner's report on the effectiveness of this approach could show that conscientiousness provided the fuel for change. Be flexible and point out the strong points before discussing concerns.

3. Trust your partners. Consultants may inadvertently assume the attitude that "we know best." In the ECO model, partners contribute to, and execute, the plan; they are essential to its success. Use their input to guide the plan. Strategies they think work best may be the most motivating to use. Routines they enjoy are most likely to be successful. Practice schedules must be reasonable to their daily life, whatever the consultant feels are the child's needs. Negotiating the plan with the partner develops a realistic plan—a plan partners will follow because it includes their work and ideas. See Table 5-5 for contrasting productive and nonproductive consultant behaviors (Bailey, Buysse, Edmondson, & Smith, 1992; Bailey, Palsha, & Simeonsson, 1991; Crais, 1993, 1999).

APPLYING THE ECO MODEL

A case study, related from the point of view of the mother, illustrates the details of ECO assessment and intervention with one family. The case study fol-

Table 5-5. Productive and Nonproductive Consultant Behaviors and Attitudes

Productive Consultant Behaviors and Attitudes
1. Support the family in their efforts to communicate effectively with their child.
2. Collaborate with the family in developing intervention plans.
3. Reflect the family's stated concern in the information you provide.
4. Present alternative levels of involvement to families and encourage them to choose the level that best meets their unique situation.
5. Obtain the family's perspective to assist in determining a program's success.

Nonproductive Consultant Behaviors and Attitudes
1. Involve families in *your* treatment program for their child.
2. Explain the treatment plan *you* have developed to remediate the problem.
3. Provide the family with information *you think* they need to understand their child's problem.
4. Present the required level of family involvement and encourage the family to adapt to it.
5. Use standardized tests to verify a program's success.

lows the format advocated here to: (1) determine the family's priority for communication intervention for their child; (2) determine the situations in which the child participates as well as regular partners and routines using the ECO Environmental Scan; (3) complete a focused observation and interaction—to share observations of the child's communication across routines and persons based on the ECO Partnership Guidelines; (4) derive a plan of intervention with the family from the information collected using the *ECO Intervention Planning Guide*; and (5) implement the plan and provide ongoing fine-tuning of the plan as the partnership develops.

CASE STUDY: MATTHEW

My husband and I love our son very much, and we had learned to adjust to his cerebral palsy and hydrocephaly. However, we weren't prepared for the frustration we experienced every time we tried to communicate with him. Doctors and other professionals had suggested early intervention programs that included speech, physical, and occupational therapy as well as family training on a variety of issues. But we wanted to focus on Matthew's physical problems, so we opted to take him to physical therapy three times a week.

Communication Intervention Becomes a Priority

The therapy was helpful, but over time, we began to realize that it was hard to communicate with Matthew and things weren't getting any better on their own. Matthew was 16 months old now. I took out the baby books of my other children. They said words at 12 months, not very many, but a few. I remember how they worked so hard to get their message across using their gestures, eyes, and sounds even when they didn't have words. I didn't see this much effort with Matthew—maybe because movement for him is such a chore. Since he doesn't seem to try to imitate our words, it is difficult to tell if he even can move his mouth in all the ways he would need to for talking.

I discussed this with my husband and we decided we needed to contact someone to find some systematic approach to getting Matthew communicating with us. Our physical therapist recommended a few schools and clinics. We called around to find out what was offered. We decided to attend a family training program that lasted 8 weeks and met in the evening, so my husband and other children could attend at least occasionally.

At our first meeting I ended up pouring out my frustrations to our speech-language pathologist, Jill, "He does cry softly to get our attention if he needs us, but it's not as easy as it used to be to figure out what he wants. He really frustrates us during play times. He is content to watch while we play and talk, but doesn't do much vocally. Sometimes he will smile, but laughing seems like a big effort, so we rarely see that. I guess I should be glad that he does observe us—he must be learning from that! But we can't really know what he's learning or thinking or feeling without more reaction from him."

"You seem to have a good handle on communication," she told us, "it definitely does involve all of those behaviors you mentioned, as well as words and phrases."

"I know, but I'm tired of waiting, I want Matthew to say some words. I've thought about it, he really only needs a few, at least to start with. It would be so nice to hear him say, 'Hi, mom.'" I whispered, fighting back the tears.

"It sounds like you are more than ready for communication intervention," Jill whispered back.

Taking a Look at Matthew's Communication Environment

Matthew hadn't been invited for this first communication intervention session. I was surprised, because he always attended physical therapy sessions, right from the first. Jill explained to us that communication intervention would probably function differently from physical therapy in a lot of ways. She wanted to see us alone today to take an objective look at Matthew's communication environments and partners in particular—an "environmental scan," she called it. I didn't see what this had to do with talking, but I decided to see what happened (see Figure 5-1).

What we found was that Matthew's life was pretty utilitarian. He mainly stayed at home with us, other than his physical therapy appointment. We did take him other places, like the store, or to a school event, but we realized these were actually pretty rare. Jill helped us to see that Matthew participated in many functional routines, like diapering, eating, or taking a bath, but not many social ones. Each of these functional routines can take a very long time, however. His major feedings happen three times a day and can take up to an hour because of his various motor difficulties. Because of his physical needs, he just takes a lot more time than other kids.

Seeing the scan, I worried out loud. "I think Matthew really frustrates me when I try to be social with him, so I give up. So do my other kids. They stop by and tickle him or kiss him on the head, but he's just not very responsive to us. I did try reading to him every night, but he would just fall asleep. So, there really isn't much we do with him regularly that I would call social. Now that I see this in black and white, I feel terrible. Am I neglecting him?"

"You are hardly neglecting him," my husband piped in. "Our little guy takes a lot of work and he's not getting any lighter. You do most of the work—I wish I could pitch in more."

"Nobody is really at fault here, " Jill reminded us. "What you have been doing is responding to Matthew's messages, which seem to indicate that he's okay on his own. By coming here, you are showing him that you would like a variety of messages. You want more going on with him. He's lucky to have you two as parents!"

"So, what do we do now—start playing with him more?" I asked.

Jill asked us to slow down a bit and share any memories of positive play activities we may have had with Matthew. We came up with three: Matthew smiling when we make silly faces, Matthew banging on his high chair when we ignore him on purpose, and Matthew smiling and vocalizing when our other kids play with the dog.

"None of these really happen too often, however. The other kids are so involved in school activities that by the time they actually play with the dog, Matthew is usually asleep. I personally don't take the time to play with the dog," I shared.

"I do the funny face thing," offered my husband, "but it really only lasts a second. I wouldn't call it play, really."

"Perhaps not," said Jill, "but it is a place to start. I think we'll add these three routines to our environmental scan, even though they are rare. For our next meeting, I'll come to your home, so I can meet your dog, Matthew, and your other children, and see what you are talking about. In the meantime, look for other tiny examples of play or social interactions at home and share them with me. I also want you to look over these partnership guidelines. Next time, all of us will be looking at how Matthew interacts and communicates with each of us during different activities. You also might want to look at this video program, Communicating Effectively with Young Children [Gillette, 1993]. This should give us more to discuss next time."

On the way home we talked about our session. It seemed to us that Matthew needed more varied experiences than he was getting. The environmental scan helped us see that. He also could use more fun in his life. No wonder he was bored—if that's what he is. Jill helped us see that it wasn't our fault that this had happened—it was probably inevitable, as we were just reacting to the messages Matthew sent us. Best of all, we did have a place to start. We just hoped the dog would behave at the next session.

We spent the week looking at our life with Matthew in a more playful way. He did seem to light up more now that we were focused on it. And the video program we watched suggested a few topics to discuss with Jill. Like matching—it seemed they wanted us to talk down to Matthew by using sounds and single words, and which seemed like a bad idea to us.

Playing with Matthew and Observing Him Play with Others

"So, how did your week go?" Jill asked after we introduced her to two of our sons, Matthew and Mitchell, and Sammy, the dog.

"We looked for play and we found a little more. Matthew likes scarves that are jiggled in his face, especially silk ones. He does respond if we point out things on television. We showed him some computer games that our other kids like and he responded for awhile. They are really beyond him, though," I shared.

"But, he's still not talking!" my husband offered, a little out of frustration.

"Well. I'm not expecting things to happen that fast," said Jill, "and neither should you. Let's just start with play as our first objective."

That sounded fair enough to all of us. We shared our concern about the video program. Jill explained to us that children will imitate sounds or single words more easily if they are used in place of complete sentences, at least sometimes. It's something we agreed to experiment with while we played with Matthew, and it seemed to make sense. Our oldest son, Mike, learned Spanish last year and he started out with single words. We discussed the partnership guidelines, too. It seemed like a lot of lists to me. I needed Jill to make sense of it for us.

"Just think of the four big goals—Participation, Balance, Match, and Enjoyment. Each outcome contributes to more effective communication. Your family may want to focus on all of them to get more communication going with Matthew," Jill told us.

"Yes, I did figure that out. But where to start? He doesn't participate much—we found that out last week. He doesn't play much and I do most of the work during functional routines like eating and dressing—so that's not balance. And enjoyment—he does have his little, tiny smiles, but not a lot of fun. I guess we have work to do!"

"Actually, it can be quite fun," Jill encouraged us. "In fact, I think we should all play with Matthew for a while and see what happens."

Playing with the Dog. *"Me first," said Mitchell, dying to get into the center stage. "I can show you the dog thing! I run around like a maniac, Sammy chases me, and Matthew smiles and even sometimes laughs."*

And that was exactly what happened. Mitchell and Sammy nearly knocked themselves out, and Matthew smiled slightly. Jill suggested that we take Matthew off the couch and put him on the floor. The dog came to Matthew—something that doesn't happen very often. But, then, Matthew is usually not on the floor. Here's what happened:

Sammy brushed up against Matthew's cheek.
Matthew moved his cheek slightly toward Sammy.
Sammy snuggled back a little harder.
Matthew snuggled back.
Sammy pushed at Matthew with his nose.
Matthew: fell over.

"Oh no!" Jill exclaimed.

"Don't worry, Matthew falls over a lot in chairs. This floor looks pretty soft with carpet on it, and he's not crying—he's actually smiling and making sounds. Matthew doesn't use many sounds," I noted as I reached for him.

"Let's just leave him there a second," Jill whispered to me. "Let's see what happens." It was odd, but Matthew seemed to be waiting quietly for someone to pick him up. He eventually began to make some sounds when nothing happened—then Jill gestured to me to pick him up. This little episode made me realize something about waiting which had been a topic in the video program. I had thought I did wait for Matthew to communicate, but it was obvious that sometimes I hadn't waited long enough.

"He can make some pretty cute sounds, Mom," commented Mitchell.

"Yes, and I think if we give him more time, he might make more," I winked at Jill and my husband. They obviously agreeed.

Funny Faces. *Now it was my husband's turn to communicate with Matthew. I could tell he was more than ready to try out his funny face routine—he had really gotten Matthew going a few times with it last week.*

Dad: *"Let's get up here in this high chair, my man—I'm gonna make you giggle" (Dad hoists Matthew up in the chair)*

Matthew: *(Looks straight at Dad, then around the room)*

Dad: *"Here we go, you know what daddy wants. A big smile—you can do it, I know you can!" (Makes his faces)*

Matthew: *(Looks at Dad's silly face and smiles—gets a little bit stiff in his limbs as a reaction)*

"But, how do I get some sounds with that?" Dad asks Jill.

"Maybe slow down your mouth and slow down your body?" I offered.

"It's worth a try," said Jill.

"Your turn," my husband turned the stage over to me.

Mom: *(Slowly moves her head up to Matthew's tray)*

Matthew: *(appears to examine her carefully)*

Mom: *"Hi" (very softly)*

Matthew: *(Purses his lips slightly)*

Mom: *(Imitates his action, but adds the sound that comes out naturally from this position) "Ooo"*

Matthew: *"Ooo" (very softly, while pursing his lips)*

Dad applauded. So did Mitchell. It looked so easy, but it was hard—I felt as if I was moving in slow motion. Mitchell tried for the same reaction, but didn't get it. He talked too much, moved too fast, and made his sound very explosively. Matthew didn't even try to imitate. Slow motion seemed to be the key. I told Jill and she agreed, as did my husband.

"So, is that our program—slow motion?" I asked.

"For now, it is," said Jill.

Communication Intervention Planning

Jill showed us what she had been checking off on the ECO Partnership Guidelines (Tables 5-1 through 5-4) while we had been playing. It made sense to me and my husband—after just 2 weeks, we knew we needed more balance and more match with our son if he was ever to start communicating with us. Jill explained it to Mitchell.

"It takes Matthew a long time to move, even in tiny ways," said Jill. "That means we need to give him more time to make sounds or other movements. We also have to watch him very carefully, because some of his movements are really tiny. But if we want him to do more, we have to do a whole lot less. Make one sound, then wait—let your face tell him that you expect him to make a sound, too. If you flip a scarf toward him—just do it once and then see how he reacts. It's different than playing with other little kids, but it's what Matthew needs right now. He's already showed us that," Jill explained.

In the meantime, I had been looking over the ECO Partnership Guidelines. The child skill we were clearly looking for right now was imitation. We seemed to get what we wanted by using sounds and tiny movements and by waiting, signaling, and expecting—both were partner strategies in the ECO Guidelines. Little did I know I had already completed part of our communication intervention plan.

Jill pulled out a form titled "ECO Communication Intervention Plan." She told us that the work we had done this week and last were major contributions to the plan. We had already identified some routines to practice last week, and we all agreed that this would be a good place to begin for now. As far as choosing partners, we wanted everyone in the family to be involved, at least in a small way. As far as messages, we thought we would just use very simple sounds right now and see if Matthew would start to imitate more often before we did anything fancy. Jill suggested that Matthew would benefit from a back-and-forth interaction style.

"You take a turn, I take a turn": she illustrated the back-and-forth movement with a hand. Think of it as a conversation without words. Start by imitating his behavior first in order to keep the interaction going. Do one thing at a time, something you know he can do, and expect Matthew to take his turn. Don't always expect a sound—an eye blink, a finger flick, any kind of movement counts for now. Just take turns with actions and sounds and don't use words in between. Keep things flowing and see how long they flow," she suggested.

"Don't use words?" Mitchell asked. "How is Matthew supposed to know what to do if we don't tell him it's his turn?"

Jill explained that this turn taking was like a conversation in which everyone takes a turn when they encounter an opportunity to do so. Turn taking is actually an important rule for Matthew to learn since the rest of us do it naturally. He isn't taking his turn very often yet, but perhaps with practice and lots of opportunity, he'll start. Jill told us that next time she would be looking to see if Matthew stayed in an interaction for more than one turn and how often he repeated the initial behavior. We would be looking for the same thing at home. I told Jill that I thought the best strategies for getting Matthew communicating were waiting, signaling, and expecting and modeling messages he could imitate.

Last, we wondered how often we should practice. Jill told us that we seemed to be highly motivated, so she wouldn't recommend a schedule for now. Instead, she suggested that we "salt and pepper" the day with tiny interactions. Keep it fun and keep working away no matter what happens. She objected when I told her I would do it all day long.

"We don't usually communicate with each other all day long," she told me. "Be sure to give Matthew some free time, and yourself as well."

I would try, but I was really too excited to make any promises.

Implementing the Plan

Two weeks later, it was time for another session with Jill. I was accompanying Matthew this time. I was excited about what happened between Matthew and me. But I was disappointed in everyone else. They didn't practice like I had. When they failed to get results after one or two tries, they just gave up. Matthew can't have only one communication partner—I want this to be a family program. I hoped Jill could help, because I was getting nowhere on my own. I poured out my problem to Jill as I entered the session.

"Let me think about this for awhile," she told me. "In the meantime, tell me about the progress you are making with Matthew."

"Well, we have really gotten into these sound-making games. We do them all the time when we are together—taking a bath, getting dressed, as well as the

playtimes we decided on earlier. I have to say that Matthew's sounds are still pretty soft, and he mainly does one, the "ooo," but that's exciting to me. His movements are so limited that he really can't do much with the objects I try to use—like the scarf we told you about. He bats his hand around, but that doesn't get him much. No wonder he mainly watches what the rest of us do," I told her.

"So you think the men in the family would be more excited if there was some movement involved?" asked Jill.

"Yes, I really do. But, we've never really found any toys that were very effective with Matthew. Our physical therapist has suggested some single-switch toys and maybe a computer. What do you think? Would that be helpful for Matthew?" I asked.

"We can't know until we try," said Jill. "We are lucky because we can borrow some single-switch toys from the Toy Lending Library. And they also have an in-house computer you could try him out on. That might be a place to start."

"But, what can I do in the meantime about these lazy guys I'm dealing with?" I nagged.

"Do you think they'd be willing to develop a practice schedule for themselves? Maybe you could all set up a chart. Are you chart people?" Jill asked.

"Not usually, but I think this is important enough for us to try. Once they get in the habit of reaching out to Matthew more regularly, I think they will come around." I told her.

"So do I," said Jill. She gave me a copy of the ECO Partnership Calendar (Figure 5-3) and suggested that we use one for each of Matthew's potential partners.

"How often should we schedule them?" I asked.

"If I were you, I'd let them decide," suggested Jill.

These seemed like pretty good directions for the communication program to take. I would have to see if I could get more communication partners for Matthew. I think the schedule might really work. And who knows, maybe it is time for a little bit of technology. We were resisting it, but it does seem like an opportunity for providing action in Matthew's life. We could get a lot more routines going then.

SUMMARY

The ECO Program is designed to provide a framework that assists professionals as they help families develop communicating relationships with their children. The components of the plan consider the ecology of the child as essential. These include identifying situations, routines/conversations and associated messages, partners and partner strategies, and the outcomes anticipated from manipulating these components. A systematic consultation strategy provides the framework for developing the plan with families over time by (1) monitoring programs through varied data samples; (2) planning with them, and teaching them as needed; (3) practicing routines with them before they return home; and (4) integrating the plan into their daily life.

Matthew's story illustrates the importance of recognizing uniqueness in the family as well as in the child. Within the ECO system, professionals will find that they can thoroughly exercise their creative abilities when working with families.

REFERENCES

Als, H., Tronick, E., & Brazelton, T. (1979). Affective reciprocity and the development of autonomy. *Journal of the American Academy of Child Psychiatry, 19,* 22–40.

Bailey, D. B., Buysse, V., Edmondson, R., & Smith, T. M. (1992). Creating family-centered services in early intervention: Perceptions of professionals in four states. *Exceptional Children, 58,* 298–309.

Bailey, D. B., Palsha, S., & Simeonsson, R. (1991). Professional skills, concerns, and perceived importance of work with families in early intervention. *Exceptional Children, 58*(2), 156–165.

Bailey, D. B., & Simeonsson, R. J. (1988). *Family assessment in early intervention*. Columbus, O.: Merrill.

Bandura, A. (1977). *Social learning theory*. Englewood Cliffs, N.J.: Prentice-Hall.

Bronfenbrenner, U. (1979). *The ecology of human development.* Cambridge, Mass.: Harvard University Press.

Bruner, J. S. (1978). Learning the mother tongue. *Human Nature, 1,* 42–48.

Bruner, J. S. (1983). *Child's talk: Learning to use language*. New York: W.W. Norton.

Buckhalt, J. A., Rutherford, R. B., & Goldberg, K. E. (1978). Verbal and non-verbal interaction of mothers with their Down syndrome and nonretarded infants. *American Journal of Mental Deficiency, 82,* 337–343.

Cheseldine, S., & McConkey, R. (1979). Parental speech to young Down's syndrome children: An intervention study. *American Journal of Mental Deficiency, 83,* 612–620.

Chomsky, N. (1973). *Aspects of a theory of syntax*. Cambridge, Mass.: M.I.T. Press.

Crais, E. (1993). Families and professionals as collaborators in assessment. *Topics in Language Disorders, 14*(1), 29–40.

Crais, E. (1995). Expanding the repertoire of tools and techniques for assessing the communication skills of infants and toddlers. *American Journal of Speech-Language Pathology, 4,* 47–59.

Crais, E. (1999). Detecting communication difficulties in infants and toddlers with feeding difficulties. In D. B. Kessler & P. Dawson (Eds.), *Failure to thrive in infants and children: A transdisciplinary approach to nutritional adequacy in childhood* (pp. 319–333). Baltimore: Brookes.

Cripe, J. (1995). *Family-guided activity-based intervention for infants and toddlers*. Baltimore: Brookes.

Cunningham, C., Blackwell, J., Reuler, E., & Deck, J. (1981). Behavioral and linguistic development in the interactions of normal and retarded children with their mothers. *Child Development, 52,* 62–70.

Feuerstein, R., Rand, Y., & Hoffman, M. (1979). *The dynamic assessment of retarded performers.* Baltimore: University Park Press.

Gillette, Y. (1989). *Ecological programs for communicating partnerships: Models and cases.* Chicago: Riverside.

Gillette, Y. (1992). *CATCH guide to planning services with families*. Tucson: Communication Skill Builders.

Gillette, Y. (1993). *Communicating effectively with young children: A video-assisted training program.* Tucson: Communication Skill Builders.

Gillette, Y. (1996). Early intervention in communication development: A collaborative model for professionals consulting with families. In M. Smith & J. Damico (eds.), *Childhood language disorders* (pp. 300–324). New York: Theime Medical Publishers.

Gilette, Y. (1996). *ECO Communication Intervention Planning Guide*. Unpublished manuscript, University of Akron.

Gillette, Y., & MacDonald, J. D. (1989). *ECO resources: Using the ECO model for communicating partnerships.* Chicago: Riverside.

Goodman, J. F. (1992). *When slow is fast enough: Educating the delayed preschool child.* New York: Guilford.

Greenspan, S. (1985). *First feelings: Milestones in the emotional development of your baby and child.* New York: Viking Press.

Hunt, J. (1965). *Intelligence and experience*. New York: Ronald Press.

Individuals with Disabilities Education Act Amendments (Pub.L.No. 105–17) (1997). Washington, D.C.: Federal Register, June 4.

Jones, O. H. M. (1980). Prelinguistic communication skills in Down syndrome and normal infants. In T. M. Field, S. Goldberg, D. Stern, & A. Sostek (Eds.), *High risk infants and children* (pp. 205–225). New York: Academic.

Kaye, K. (1976). Infant's effects on their mother's teaching strategies. In J. C. Glidewell (Ed.), *The social context of learning and development* (pp. 173–206). New York: Gardner Press.

Kaye, K., & Charney, R. (1980). How mothers maintain dialogue with two-year-olds. In D. Olsen (Ed.), *The social foundations of language and thought: Essays in honor of Jerome Bruner* (pp. 211–229). New York: Norton.

Light, J., & McNaughton, D. (1993). Literacy and augmentative and alternative communication (AAC): The expectations and priorities of parents and teachers. *Topics in Language Disorders, 13,* 33–46.

MacDonald, J. D. (1989). *Becoming partners: From play to conversation.* Chicago: Riverside.

MacDonald, J. D., & Gillette, Y. (1984). Conversational engineering: A pragmatic approach to early social competence. *Seminars in Speech and Language, 5,* 171–183.

MacDonald, J. D., & Gillette, Y. (1985). Taking turns: Teaching communication to your child. *The Exceptional Parent, 15,* 49–52.

MacDonald, J. D., & Gillette, Y. (1986). Communicating with handicapped persons: roles of parents and professionals. *Journal of the Association for the Severely Handicapped, 11,* 255–264.

MacDonald, J. D., & Gillette, Y. (1988). Communicating partners: A conversational model for building relationships with handicapped children. In K. Marfo (Ed.), *Parent-child interaction and developmental disabilities: Theory, research, and intervention* (pp. 220–241). New York: Praeger.

MacDonald, J. D., & Gillette, Y. (1989). *An introduction to the Ecological Communication program.* Chicago: Riverside.

MacDonald, J., Gillette, Y., & Hutchinson, T. (1989). *ECO Scales.* Chicago: Riverside.

Mahoney, G. (1988). Enhancing the developmental competence of handicapped infants. In K. Marfo (Ed.), *Parent-child interaction and developmental disabilities: Theory, research, and intervention* (pp. 203–219). New York: Praeger.

Mahoney, G., Finger, I., & Powell, A. (1985). The relationship of maternal behavior style to the development of organically impaired mentally retarded infants. *American Journal of Mental Deficiency, 90,* 292–302.

Mahoney, G., & Neville-Smith, A. (1996). The effects of directive communications on children's interactive engagement: Implications for language intervention. *Topics in Early Childhood Special Education, 16*(2), 236–250.

Manolson, A., Ward, B., & Dodington, N. (1995). *You make the difference in helping your child learn.* Toronto, Canada: Hanen Early Language Resource Centre.

McConkey, R. (1988). Educating all parents: An approach based on video. In K. Marfo (Ed.), *Parent-child interaction and developmental disabilities: Theory, research, and intervention* (pp. 253–272). New York: Praeger.

Merighi, J., Edison, M., & Zigler, E. (1990). The role of motivational factors in the functioning of mentally retarded individuals. In R. Hoddap, J. Burack, & E. Zigler (Eds.), *Issues in the developmental approach to mental retardation* (pp. 114–130). Cambridge, U.K.: Cambridge University Press.

Murray, L., & Trevarthen, C. (1986). The infant's role in mother-infant communications. *Journal of Child Language, 13,* 15–29.

Olswang, L. B., Bain, B. A., & Johnson, G. A. (1992). Using dynamic assessment with children with language disorders. In S. Warren, & J. Reichle (Eds.), *Causes and effects in communication and language intervention* (pp. 187–216). Baltimore: Brookes.

Piaget, J. (1951). *Play, dreams, and imitation in childhood.* New York: Norton.

Schwartz, I., & Olswang, L. (1996). Evaluating child behavior change in natural settings: Exploring alternative strategies for data collection. *Topics in Early Childhood Special Education, 16*(1), 82–101.

Stern, D. (1977). *A first relationship.* Cambridge, Mass.: Harvard University Press.

Stern, D. (1986). *The interpersonal world of the infant: A view from psychoanalysis and developmental psychology.* New York: Basic Books.

Stillman, R., & Battle, C. (1984). Developing prelanguage communication in the severely handicapped: An interpretation of the Van Dijk method. *Seminars in Speech and Language, 5,* 159–169.

Tronick, E., Als, H., & Adamson, L. (1979). Structure of early face-to-face communicative interactions. In M. Bullowa (Ed.), *Before speech: The beginning of interpersonal communication* (pp. 349–372). Cambridge, U.K.: Cambridge University Press.

Valentine, C. W. (1930). The psychology of imitation with special reference to early childhood. *British Journal of Psychology, 21,* 105–132.

Vygotsky, L. S. (1962). *Thought and language.* Cambridge, Mass.: MIT Press. (Originally published in 1934).

Watzlawick, P., Beavin, J. & Jackson, D. (1967). *Pragmatics of human communication.* New York: Norton.

Weinberg, G. (1985). *The secrets of consulting: A guide to giving and getting advice successfully.* New York: Dorset.

CHAPTER 6

Language Intervention for Young Children With Language Impairments

Susan Ellis Weismer, Ph.D., CCC-SLP
Associate Professor
University of Wisconsin at Madison

Key Terms

child-centered approaches
clinician-based intervention
clinician-directed approaches
developmental disabilities (DD)
late talking toddlers
milieu teaching
parent-based intervention
specific expressive language delay
specific language impairment (SLI)

Overview

For a young child who is discovered to have a problem with language development, there are a number of treatment options available. The children who are the focus of this chapter are **late talking toddlers** (i.e., toddlers producing less than a 50-word vocabulary or not producing multiword combinations by age 2), preschoolers with **specific language impairment (SLI)** (i.e., with a language disorder not associated with general cognitive, sensorimotor, or emotional deficits), and those with language disorders associated with mild **developmental disabilities (DD)**. A variety of **clinician-based intervention** approaches where the clinician serves as the primary agent of intervention may be employed, including those that incorporate typical language peer models, as well as various **parent-based intervention** approaches, where the parent is the primary agent. The intervention approach and treatment options selected for a particular child depend on a number of factors, including the child's linguistic and cultural background. These issues are discussed in this chapter, which also reviews the evidence for the effectiveness of various intervention approaches. Finally, the role of early language intervention for these populations is considered and exemplar case studies are provided.

CLINICIAN-BASED LANGUAGE INTERVENTION APPROACHES

Language intervention models stem from differing theoretical frameworks and vary along a number of dimensions, including the extent to which the approach is clinician versus child directed, whether specific linguistic targets are selected or the goal is general communication enhancement, the degree to which the treatment context is naturalistic, and the particular teaching techniques that are employed. Focusing on the dimension of clinician directiveness, Fey (1986) designated three categories of intervention approaches, which were subsequently elaborated by Paul (1995). The categories were identified as trainer-oriented approaches (referred to by Paul [1995] as **clinician-directed approaches**), **child-centered approaches**, and hybrids. The discussion of intervention approaches in this chapter will be organized, for the most part, along a continuum of clinician versus child directiveness, though the role of the other defining characteristics mentioned here is clearly acknowledged. Although intervention approaches are distinguishable on the basis of their particular combination of features, it is also important to keep in mind that there is a good deal of overlap within certain dimensions (e.g., a number of the approaches employ elicited imitation or modeling teaching procedures).

Direct Instruction

Intervention approaches that follow a direct instruction model are highly clinician-directed (cf. Cole, 1995). They involve explicit and systematic instruction conducted within discrete time periods of massed practice and often focus on a predetermined sequence of skills. All aspects of the intervention are controlled by the clinician, and structured tasks that minimize distracting stimuli are used in an effort to elicit a high number of target responses in a short amount of time. Extrinsic reinforcement (such as tokens or verbal praise) is typically provided for responses that the clinician deems acceptable. A premium is placed on the efficiency of treatment rather than on naturalistic contexts or contingencies for communication. Examples of programs following the direct instruction model include the Distar Language Program (Englemann & Osborn, 1976) and the Communication Training Program (CTP) (Waryas & Stremel-Campbell, 1983). In the Distar program the clinician models a particular linguistic form, elicits an imitation using cuing, and then either provides a corrective imitation sequence (if the child's response was not correct) or gives verbal praise and token reinforcement (for appropriate responses). CTP entails a set sequence of lexical and syntactic goals, as well as prerequisite nonverbal goals, using stimulus pictures to elicit responses. Investigations of highly clinician-directed approaches comprised of imitation-based drill procedures have reported successful results for phonological, syntactic, and semantic targets (Connell, 1986, 1987; Hegde, 1980; Shriberg & Kwiatkowski, 1982). With the shift away from viewing language learning within a behavioral perspective, direct instruction/drill-type approaches are not as widely used as they once were (Bricker, 1993; Cole, 1995). However, Cole (1995) has pointed out that when direct instruction approaches have been compared to more child-centered approaches, there is no clear difference in overall effectiveness, as assessed by mean length of utterance (MLU) or by performance on standardized measures of language comprehension and production (Cole, Dale, & Mills, 1991; Yoder, Kaiser, & Alpert, 1991).

Milieu Teaching

Milieu teaching approaches are conducted within a naturalistic setting, such as a preschool classroom, yet employ among their methods various operant-teaching techniques. In milieu approaches, treatment occurs within the context of typical conversational exchanges, with the goal of addressing language function as well as form. Naturally occurring reinforcement is utilized in these approaches (e.g., obtaining the object that was requested). Although an attempt is made to capitalize on child-initiated interactions, primary teaching techniques within these approaches can be viewed as including both adult- and child-directed procedures (cf. Schwartz, 1987). The mand-model technique involves the use of a prompt ("Tell me what to get") or a request for response to a direct question ("What's this?"), followed by a corrective imitation sequence or reinforcement (Rogers-Warren & Warren, 1980; Warren, McQuarter, & Rogers-Warren, 1984). Time delay is another technique used in milieu approaches; it consists of withholding help for 5 to 15 seconds while nonverbal prompts (e.g., an expectant look) are given (Halle, Marshall, & Spradlin, 1979). Incidental teaching is primarily a child-centered procedure in which more elaborated language is required in situations such as those where a child requests assistance (Hart & Risley, 1980). Other teaching techniques that have recently been employed within milieu approaches consist of systematic commenting (Warren, 1992) and child-cued modeling (cf. Kaiser, Yoder, & Keetz, 1992). A number of studies have demonstrated the effectiveness of milieu approaches in increasing the frequency of language use, particularly requesting behavior (see reviews by Kaiser et al., 1992; Schwartz, 1987; Warren & Kaiser, 1986). More recent investigations have further documented the benefits of milieu approaches in facilitating the acquisition of early semantic relations (Warren & Bambara, 1989; Warren & Gazdag, 1990) and vocabulary (Warren, 1992; Yoder et al., 1991) in young children with mild to moderate cognitive and language delays.

Structured Discourse and Conversational Recasting

Vertical discourse structuring strategies and conversational recasting treatment utilize types of exchanges that are observed in naturally occurring adult-child interactions. The structured discourse approaches entail an adaptation of expansion procedures in which the framework of the dialogue is designed to help the child establish semantic and syntactic links across utterances or conversational turns. The following is an example of a vertical structure:

> Clinician: "Who's this?"
> Child: "Girl."
> Clinician: "What's the girl eating?"
> Child: "Cookie."
> Clinician: "Right. The girl is eating the cookie."

Schwartz, Chapman, Terrell, Prelock, and Rowan (1985) first used this type of structured discourse strategy to successfully facilitate multiword productions in young children (2- and 3-year-olds) with specific language impairment (SLI) who were functioning at the one-word stage. Picture stimuli and verbal prompts (as in the example given here) were used in the Schwartz et al. study, such that the clinician initiated the communicative exchanges. Scherer and Olswang (1989) also demonstrated the effectiveness of structured discourse techniques in increasing the use of two-term semantic relations by 5 children with autism. In their version of the approach, structured discourse sequences were initiated by the child as well as the clinician. Conversational recasts consist of replies to child utterances that maintain the child's basic meaning but incorporate elements that are slightly above her or his current language level. For example, if the child comments, "Look, the cup fell down," the adult might recast the child's utterance by responding, "Yes, the cup that was on the table fell down." Investigations by Nelson and colleagues (Baker & Nelson, 1984; Nelson, 1991) have shown that children with typical language development can learn advanced grammatical forms with conversational recast training. Similarly, studies by Camarata, Nelson, and Camarata (1994) and Nelson, Camarata, Welsh, Butkovsky, and Camarata (1996) have demonstrated the effectiveness of this approach for facilitating grammatical skills in 4- to 6-year-old children with specific language impairment.

Focused Stimulation

In focused stimulation approaches, concentrated exposure to models of specific linguistic targets are provided within meaningful contexts. Following exposure to the models, opportunities to respond are usually provided in an attempt to elicit spontaneous productions of the target from the child as in the following exchange (targeting the verb "bounce"):

> Clinician: "I'm *bouncing* the ball. It *bounces* up and down. You try it. Can you make it *bounce*?"(Calls to another child.)
> "Sonya, come here a minute. Ricky, tell her what we're doing."
> Child: "Bounce ball."
> Clinician: "That's right, we're *bouncing* the ball. You try it, Sonya."

In some versions of this approach, certain modifications of the linguistic stimuli, such as exaggerated stress on the target (Culatta & Horn, 1982; Ellis Weismer, 1997), are employed to increase the saliency of the linguistic form being modeled. Leonard (1981, 1993) has used the term *focused stimulation* to refer to intervention approaches that share these basic characteristics but may employ a variety of teaching methods, including an interactive storytelling format (Lee, Koenigsknecht, & Mulhern, 1975), structured role-playing based on a story (Brooks & Benjamin, 1989), and naturalistic pretend play settings such as grocery store interactions (Culatta & Horn, 1982). This intervention approach has been used to address semantic and syntactic aspects of language development and is useful for both comprehension and production goals. Other investigations that have demonstrated the effectiveness of some version of focused stimulation approaches include those by Olswang, Bain, Rosendahl, Oblak, and Smith (1986); Schwartz (1988); Leonard, Camarata, Rowan, and Chapman (1982); and Ellis Weismer, Murray-Branch, and Miller (1993).

Script Therapy

The underlying assumption of script-based approaches is that intervention conducted within the context of a familiar routine will reduce children's cognitive load such that they can better focus on new language forms being presented. Scripts have been proposed as one model of event representation in human memory (Schank & Abelson, 1977) and are thought to be learned as a product of the child's experiences (cf. Nelson, 1986). For example, most young children have scripts for common events or routines such as birthday parties, bedtime, and so forth. In language training the clinician can make use of scripts the child has already developed, or new scripts can be developed by establishing certain routines within the preschool setting. Once a script has been firmly established, violations of that script can be used to prompt commenting or to demonstrate how variations in routines can be achieved (cf. Paul, 1995). For example, a snacktime script might be established in a preschool class in which the children first wash their hands, set the table, sit down, and then pass around the snack. After this routine has become firmly established, the clinician might intentionally violate the typical sequence of events by giving out the snack before the table has been set in order to elicit the use of negative forms such as "not ready" or "don't have plates." Constable (1986) has reported successful use of a script-based intervention approach to address a variety of semantic, syntactic, and pragmatic language goals in a group of preschoolers with language impairment. Similarly, Kim and Lombardino (1991) found that script treatment was effective in improving comprehension of agent-action-object and action-object-location semantic relations in three of four preschoolers with DD whom they studied.

Whole Language/Language Stimulation

There are various child-centered, functional approaches to language intervention, which usually occur in preschool classroom settings, where treatment is embedded in naturalistic social interactions. The clinician engineers the environment to allow opportunities for language use but then follows the child's lead rather than directing the activities and does not make demands for particular responses. Activities are often organized around themes or common routines, making them similar in certain respects to script-based approaches. These child-centered approaches typically target language and communication goals in a broad sense rather than addressing a limited number of specific linguistic forms (as is the case for the approaches described previously). Examples of child-centered language intervention approaches include facilitative play techniques (cf. Hubbell, 1981) and language stimulation approaches centered around the cognitively oriented High/Scope program (cf. Cole, 1995). Whole language approaches represent another type of functional, child-centered intervention, though they are generally used with children above the preschool level (Norris & Damico, 1990; Norris & Hoffman, 1990, 1993). A basic assumption of the whole language approach is that oral and written language are best learned in meaningful discourse contexts in which language is used for the purpose of conveying a message. Language is viewed as a complex system, which is greater than the sum of its parts, and thus cannot be broken down into discrete skills that are taught separately. Limited empirical data are available on the effectiveness of these child-centered approaches, with the exception of an investigation of the whole language approach reported by Gillam, McFadden, and van Kleeck (1995) that focused on intervention with older, school-age children. Although the whole language approach has a number of strong advocates, critics have questioned whether this method is effective in addressing syntactic and morphological deficits, namely, language form (Chaney, 1990; Paul, 1995).

Comparison of the Effectiveness of Clinician-Based Approaches

Given this review, it becomes clear that a number of different clinician-based intervention approaches have been shown to be effective in promoting language gains in young children with language impairment. The question arises as to which approach should be selected. Prior comprehensive reviews by Leonard (1981, 1993), as well as a meta-analysis of various intervention approaches by Nye, Foster, and Seaman (1987), have not indicated a single method of choice. A number of investigations have directly compared global intervention programs or components of different approaches in an attempt to address this issue. Several investigations have compared teaching procedures generally associated with distinct theoretical frameworks, namely, imitation versus modeling techniques (Connell, 1987; Connell & Stone, 1992; Courtright & Courtright, 1976, 1979), whereas others have compared variations within a single approach (Ellis Weismer & Murray-Branch, 1989; Ellis Weismer et al., 1993; Olswang, Bain, Dunn, & Cooper, 1983). Studies focused more broadly on comparing entire intervention programs include those by Friedman and Friedman (1980); Cole and Dale (1986); Cole, Dale, et al. (1991); Cole, Mills, Dale, and Jenkins (1991); Camarata et al. (1994); Nelson et al. (1996), and Yoder et al. (1991). These direct comparisons of language-teaching techniques and intervention approaches have often revealed interactions between treatment methods and child characteristics related to cognitive abilities or language aptitude, though conflicting results have been reported (see discussions by Yoder et al., 1991, and Cole, 1995). In summary, while individual studies have sometimes reported findings favoring one approach over another, the intervention efficacy literature as a whole does not support the adoption of any particular method across various language goals and types of children; instead, it suggests that there are a range of viable alternatives. The choice of an intervention approach for a particular child will likely be dependent on a number of factors, including age of the child, severity and type of impairment, presence of concomitant disorders, sociocultural issues, and parental preferences and concerns.

THE IMPACT OF PEER MODELS ON LANGUAGE DEVELOPMENT

There has been increasing interest in the impact of typically developing peer models on children with disabilities. The rationale behind incorporating peer models into programs for young children with language disorders is that the typical language peers can provide models of appropriate language slightly above that of the children with language impairment yet are interested in the same types of play activities and topics as their age level peers. Early experimental evidence was quite encouraging, indicating that typically developing children adjusted their language level when conversing with peers with DD and that children with DD used more complex language when talking with other children who were at a somewhat more advanced developmental level (Guralnick & Paul-Brown, 1980, 1986). However, investigations comparing segregated classrooms with integrated or mainstreamed classes have generally failed to find significant group differences in language development for children with disabilities (Cole, Mills et al., 1991; Jenkins, Odom, & Speltz, 1989; Jenkins, Speltz, & Odom, 1985). Some interesting interactions have been noted, though, between child characteristics and the influence of peer models within these different instructional settings. For example, Cole, Mills et al. (1991) found that among the preschoolers (3-6 years) with mild to moderate DD whom they studied, only those with higher IQ or language scores at pretest made greater gains within an integrated class than a segregated class. They speculated that this finding may relate to the tendency for typically developing children to interact among themselves, which has been reported in investigations of mainstreaming (Rogers-Warren, Ruggles, Peterson, & Cooper, 1981). Presumably, children with milder disabilities would have a greater likelihood of being included in, and therefore benefiting from, interactions with their typically developing peers.

Weiss and Nakamura (1992) examined the influence of typical language peer models within an integrated preschool classroom for children with language impairment. A child-centered approach to intervention was employed in the class to allow observation of naturally occurring interaction patterns. Weiss and Nakamura reported that two of the three typical language peer models spent minimal time engaged in conversation with the children with language disorders. Instead, they tended to seek out adult conversational partners in the room. Based on these findings, it appears incorrect to assume that simply because peer models are available, interactions that lead to productive-language learning opportunities will automatically occur. Instead, it may be necessary to take the initiative in grouping children to ensure that those with language disorders have a chance to benefit from the language models of the typically developing peers.

Using the approach of grouping a typical language peer with a child with language disorders, Robertson and Ellis Weismer (1997) examined the impact of peer modeling on play scripts of children with SLI. Thirty preschoolers participated in their Study 1, including an experimental and control group of children with SLI and a group of age-matched peer models. The treatment involved dyadic play sessions in which children with SLI were paired with a peer model and invited to play house in a specially designed area in their preschool classroom. Verbal scripts for playing house were elicited immediately before and after treatment and at a 3-week follow-up (see Appendix 6-1). Significant differences were found between the play script reports of the experimental and control groups of children with SLI in terms of number of words, appropriate acts, and use of linguistic markers. The second phase of the investigation, employing a multiple baseline design, involved six children with SLI from the control group in Study 1, plus two peer models. Play dyads consisted of either two children with SLI or one child with SLI and a peer model. Findings from Study 2 provided further evidence that interactions with typical language peers (but not an SLI peer) enhanced play scripts in children with SLI.

Although peer models were deliberately paired with children with SLI in the Robertson and Ellis Weismer (1997) study, the peer models received no instructions or training regarding their interactions in the play sessions. Venn et al. (1993), however, explicitly trained peer models in their investigation, in which they taught typical language preschoolers to use, and model, procedures (e.g., "Which one do you want?" "Juice.") within a milieu teaching approach to elicit requests from children with language disorders during snacktime interactions. These results suggest that with clinician modeling and prior practice, typical language preschoolers can provide specific linguistic input to peers with language disorders.

PARENT-BASED LANGUAGE INTERVENTION APPROACHES

The mandate established by federal law PL 105-17: Individuals with Disabilities Education Act Amendments (1997) for family-centered intervention plans for infants and young children, provides additional impetus to carefully examine the efficacy of treatment approaches in which parents assume a central role as intervention agents. Crais (1991) noted that in traditional service delivery models, parents have played a fairly passive role in intervention. She recommended incorporating families in the treatment program to facilitate the generalization of new communication skills to the home setting. Various professionals have suggested that parents be trained to use certain interactive styles and modeling techniques to facilitate their children's language growth (cf. McDade & Varnedoe, 1987; Ratner & Harris, 1994). Weiss (1993) acknowledged the potential value of parents as frequent and interested language interactants and suggested that clinicians work with parents to help them facilitate their child's language use within everyday activities; however, she also warned against unreasonable expectations and pointed out the numerous demands facing many families, which may limit their participation in intervention programs. Paul (1995) has emphasized possible drawbacks to parent-based approaches. These include potential conflicts that may arise when parents assume a teaching role rather than offering the child uncritical support, as well as the need to focus on the form of the message as children acquire more advanced linguistic structures (in contrast to typical communicative exchanges, in which parents focus mostly on meaning). In light of these concerns, Paul (1995) argued that parents are not the intervention agents of choice for establishing new language forms and functions but did suggest that they may prove to be a useful addition to an overall treatment program by facilitating practice within naturalistic contexts. Thus, there seems to be general agreement about incorporating parents in the intervention program, to the extent that they are willing and able, for the purpose of promoting generalization of newly trained language targets. However, debate exists concerning their role as primary intervention agents.

In addition to serving as primary or secondary agents of intervention, another important aspect of the intervention process in which parents can be actively involved is in establishing goals and objectives. Parental input during the intervention-planning phase should result in the identification of language targets that have considerable impact on the child's functional communication across various contexts, as well as promoting joint responsibility for ensuring that the agreed-upon goals are achieved. Research is needed to determine effective strategies for encouraging parental participation in intervention planning and to evaluate the effects of this involvement on treatment outcomes.

Effectiveness of Parent-Based Approaches

Parent-based approaches to intervention are less commonly employed for children with mild language disorders than for those with more severe communication deficits associated with identified developmental disabilities, where the parents may become actively involved in management issues shortly after birth. Nevertheless, it is important to assess the efficacy of this approach for children with mild impairments as well. Several investigations will be reviewed that have examined approaches in which parents served as the primary agents of intervention for toddlers and preschoolers with specific language delay and those with mild DD.

Whitehurst and colleagues (Whitehurst, Fischel, Caulfield, DeBaryshe, & Valdez-Menchaca, 1989; Whitehurst, Fischel, Lonigan, Valdez-Menchaca, Arnold, & Smith, 1991) examined the effectiveness of a parent intervention approach in facilitating language acquisition in toddlers with **specific ex-**

pressive language delay. These children were late talking toddlers with delays restricted to productive language. During biweekly office visits, parents were trained to implement a set of seven assignments in the home using milieu teaching techniques. This program focused on lexical development and early multiword constructions. A notable departure from developmental approaches that was adopted in this program was the initial goal of eliminating children's communicative gesture use. Whitehurst et al. (1991) reported that the parent intervention resulted in significant improvements in the toddlers' expressive language skills compared to a control group who did not receive the treatment. However, they questioned the long-term benefits and importance of early language intervention for this particular population in light of follow-up findings that indicated no significant group differences at 5 years of age on their language assessment measures (but see discussions by Ellis Weismer et al., 1993; Olswang & Bain, 1991; Paul, 1991). The implications of this conclusion will be considered later in the chapter in the section dealing with the role of early language intervention.

Several investigations have explored general stimulation parent-training approaches that have an interaction focus and were designed for preschoolers with mild DD or SLI (Mahoney & Powell, 1988; Tannock, Girolametto, & Siegel, 1992; Weistuch & Brown, 1987; Weistuch & Lewis, 1985). These studies have reported somewhat mixed results. Although they led to changes in maternal interaction styles such that mothers were less directive and more responsive to the children's communication attempts (Tannock et al., 1992; Weistuch & Brown, 1987), the impact on children's language abilities was less clear-cut. Weistuch & Brown (1987) reported significant increases in children's language, as indexed by MLU, for those in the treatment group compared to the delayed treatment control group; however, Tannock et al. (1992) found no significant group differences in children's communication and language skills. Tannock and Girolametto (1992) provided an excellent critical review of parent treatment programs that have followed an interactive model of language intervention involving general stimulation, and they concluded that this approach may be a useful adjunct to other treatment approaches but did not recommend its use as the sole intervention approach for young children with language impairment.

Girolametto, Pearce, and Weitzman (1996) have recently reported positive effects of interactive language intervention that incorporated focused, rather than general stimulation. In this investigation, parents were trained to teach specific target vocabulary to their toddlers, who had specific expressive language delays. Findings indicated that treatment resulted in slower, less complex, and more focused language input for mothers in the experimental group than the control (delayed-treatment) group. More important, beneficial effects were also observed with respect to the experimental children's vocabulary use and early grammatical development compared to the controls. That is, they demonstrated significantly more words in play interactions, had larger overall vocabularies, and used more multiword combinations and early morphemes than children who had not yet received treatment.

Although the majority of parent-based treatment programs target early language acquisition, Fey and colleagues (Fey, Cleave, Long, & Hughes, 1993) have described a focused stimulation intervention program directed at somewhat more advanced grammatical aspects of language. Thirty preschoolers aged 3 years, 8 months (3;8) to 5 years, 10 months (5;10) with SLI or DD who had expressive language delays were randomly assigned to a clinician treatment, parent treatment, or delayed treatment control group. Fey et al. (1993) reported that both the clinician and parent treatments resulted in significant increases in language abilities compared to the delayed treatment control group over a 5-month period, but that gains were more consistently observed for the children in the clinician treatment group than the parent group. Fey, Cleave, and Long (1997) have reported findings from a follow-up investigation based on an additional 5-month intervention phase for 18 of the 30 participants in the original study. Improvements in language abilities were generally not as strong as during the initial phase of intervention; however, larger and more consistent gains were observed for children who received the clinician-based intervention than for those receiving the parent-based intervention.

CONSIDERATION OF LINGUISTIC AND CULTURAL DIVERSITY IN LANGUAGE INTERVENTION

In this section, a brief discussion is provided of issues pertaining to cultural differences in views concerning early intervention, considerations regarding dialectal variation and bilingualism, and culturally compatible teaching approaches for children from diverse backgrounds. For a more in-depth review of multicultural issues related to language intervention, refer to Davis McFarland and Dowell (Chapter 3 of this volume); Miller (1984); Adler (1993); Battle (1993, 1997); Paul (1995); and Kayser (1995).

Taking Into Account the Family's Views

It is important to recognize differing cultural views regarding communication handicaps and the impact that these views may have on a child's participation in early intervention. For example, Harris (1993) pointed out that words to express the concepts of disability or rehabilitation are lacking in many Native American languages, and moreover, that differences in abilities, though noted, are generally more accepted in these cultures. She described an explanation from an Oneida Indian father who said that he viewed the slow development associated with his daughter's neuromuscular disease as a gift from the creator since it allowed him to better appreciate small gains that she made. Within this perspective, it is not necessarily a priority or even desirable to attempt to "remediate" the child's condition. Understanding the cultural background and values of a child's family is essential, given their role in decisions regarding early intervention and potential involvement in the treatment process.

It should also be noted that familial characteristics (i.e., what constitutes the child's family) can vary considerably from one culture to another. In advocating family-centered intervention approaches, Terrell and Terrell (1993) pointed out that African Americans have a variety of family units including extended family systems. In some Native American cultures the practice of shared child rearing is common and other relatives or clan members are instrumental in raising the child; thus, decisions about intervention may be left up to someone other than the parent (cf. Harris, 1993). An effort should be made in intervention planning to consult with, and integrate, all relevant individuals.

Issues Regarding Linguistic Diversity

Language intervention with children from linguistically diverse backgrounds presents a number of special challenges. In working with such children, clinicians should begin from a basis of knowledge and respect. That is, they should attempt to gather as much information as possible about children's dialect or first language and validate its use. This includes developing an appreciation of the sociolinguistic/pragmatic rules concerning the makeup of social interactions (e.g., turn taking), as well as an understanding of nonverbal behaviors such as eye contact, social distance, touch, and gestural use. With regard to validation, it is essential that the clinician acknowledge the importance of the child's language. Along these lines, Terrell and Terrell (1993) warned against targeting dialectal variations in intervention. However, when working with children who have language delays according to the dialect within their own linguistic community, it is useful to also address the language of the majority culture to the extent that code switching is a goal. In discussing the role of monolingual clinicians in the treatment of individuals from minority cultures, Jaurez (1983) suggested that this should include providing in-service training for teachers, aides, and other professionals and consulting with the bilingual instruction team. It is recommended that bilingual clinicians be hired to provide direct intervention; however, this is becoming increasingly difficult given the shortage of bilingual clinicians relative to the growing need (cf. Kayser, 1993).

There is considerable controversy regarding the appropriate language of instruction for bilingual children (cf. Kayser, 1995; Miller, 1984; Ortiz, 1984). Miller (1984) contended that there are no firm guidelines for deciding the language of instruction and suggested that each case should be viewed individually. According to Ortiz (1984), the following factors may help determine the language of choice: preferences of the parent and child, the child's age, intellectual abilities, aptitude for language learning and motivation for learning another language, type and severity of communication problem, how long the child has lived in the United States, and the availability of bilingual personnel. Kayser (1995) reviewed key differences between the bilingual programs in Canada and those in the United States, including differences in the social value afforded to the native language, which impacts on attitudes, self-esteem, identity, and motivation. Bruck (1982) reported that school-age children with language impairment who were enrolled in a Canadian French-immersion program (where bilingualism is viewed as a desirable skill) demonstrated comparable performance to similar children who were educated in their native language. This does not necessarily imply, however, that bilingual children with language deficits whose native language does not have high social value will fare as well. With respect to teaching methods, experimental studies of vocabulary learning by bilingual children have indicated better results under bilingual instruction conditions than under monolingual instruction (Kiernan & Swisher, 1990; Perozzi & Chavez-Sanchez, 1992), and there is some evidence that more rapid learning occurs when words are first taught in the native language and then in the second language (Perozzi, 1985).

Culturally Compatible Teaching Approaches

A child's cultural background will also influence the particular teaching methods that are likely to be most effective. Harris (1993) stressed the need for compatibility between the home and school cultures in terms of various factors that affect learning, including social organization, sociolinguistic variables, and motivation. For example, she noted that in Navajo culture, boys and girls are segregated in play activities, and she suggests that, consequently, intervention groupings that follow cultural mores such as these will be most successful.

A sociolinguistic variable that has been shown to have a substantial impact on learning and for which there is considerable cultural variation is wait time. Wait time refers to the pauses separating speakers' conversational turns, particularly as applied to question-answer sequences between teachers and students in classroom settings (cf. Tobin, 1987). Ellis Weismer and Schraeder (1993) demonstrated the role of wait time in increasing verbal fluency and accuracy of responses to higher-level cognitive questions in interactions between clinicians and children with language-learning disabilities from the majority culture. Consideration of this variable may be even more essential for individuals from certain minority cultures in which silence has special importance. Investigations have revealed that Navajo teachers allow considerably longer wait times than Caucasian teachers and that Pueblo children participate twice as often in classes with longer wait times compared to those with shorter wait times (cf. Harris, 1993). Clinicians should also take into account culturally accepted methods of motivating children and managing behavior during intervention. Harris (1993) reported that findings from the Kamehameha Early Education Program highlighted the high level of respect displayed by Navajo teachers for children's "sovereignty." She pointed out that any explicit attempt to manipulate the behavior of adults or children, including the use of punishment or contingent reinforcement, violates cultural values. Instead of using these procedures, Navajo teachers maintained on-task behavior by circulating quietly throughout the classroom. Similarly, Kayser (1993) noted that Hispanic clinicians working with Mexican American preschoolers made little use of verbal praise and instead used eye gaze and gestures to control behavior. In some cases, clinicians may try certain teaching techniques other than those that are typically associated with a particular cultural group; however, these choices should be made on the basis of reasoned decisions rather than ignorance. Cheng (1993), for example, advocates the use of a meaning-based whole language approach with children from Asian American cultures even though this method may be contrary to the learning and teaching styles of some of these cultural groups, in which direct instruction is more typical.

THE ROLE OF EARLY LANGUAGE INTERVENTION

Ultimately, the question arises as to the role of early intervention for the populations of children who are the focus of this chapter. That is, what do we expect intervention to accomplish? There is debate about the importance of intervention for toddlers with specific expressive language delays given the eventual positive outcomes evidenced by a number of these children (Olswang & Bain, 1991; Paul, 1991, 1994; Whitehurst et al., 1991; Whitehurst & Fischel, 1994). Olswang and Bain (1991) have described differing functions that intervention may serve, including that of facilitation, in which the rate of learning is accelerated without altering the eventual outcome. They have argued for the role of facilitative treatment with late talking toddlers given the potential impact of slow language development on interrelated skills, the effects on the child's social-emotional development and parent-child relations, and the limitations of our measurement abilities in assessing early language problems. For somewhat older preschoolers or children with more comprehensive language difficulties, there is general agreement regarding the need for treatment. Some studies have shown that early intervention can help to close the gap between young children with language impairment and their typically developing peers (cf. Leonard, 1993); however, a number of retrospective and prospective investigations of the link between early language delay and later academic performance have indicated persistent problems (cf. Fey, Catts, & Larrivee, 1995; Leonard, 1993; Paul, 1995). In light of these findings, Windsor (1995) and Fey et al. (1995) recommend that early language intervention should not only address linguistic goals but should also focus more broadly on improving social skills and academic readiness.

CASE STUDY: SIGGI

Siggi's family moved to the United States from Iceland when he was 2½ years old. Shortly after, his parents referred him for an assessment due to their concern about his slow development of Icelandic as well as his difficulty in acquiring English. An assessment by a bilingual speech-language pathologist revealed that Siggi's comprehension in his native language was roughly at age level but that there was a 12-month delay in his expressive skills. Siggi was enrolled in language intervention, which was conducted in his native language for one semester. Following that, language stimulation in English was provided. The family continued to speak Icelandic at home, while Siggi was exposed to English in day-care settings. Although gains were noted in therapy, Siggi's problems with language learning persisted, and he switched day-care programs frequently because of behavior problems that were presumably related to his communication difficulties. When Siggi was 4 years old, an in-depth assessment of both languages indicated comprehension and production delays of 1 to 2 years in Icelandic and English, with somewhat stronger abilities in Icelandic.

At that point, a semester program was implemented to compare the effectiveness of a monolingual approach to that of bilingual instruction in facilitating Siggi's vocabulary development in English (Elin T. Thordardottir, Ellis Weismer, & Smith, 1997). Different sets of home and school words were taught using either monolingual (English only) instruction or bilingual instruction, with the type of treatment being alternated across sessions. A focused stimulation approach was used during monolingual and bilingual instruction, in which repeated models of the target words were provided within meaningful communicative contexts that also contained opportunities for use of the targets by the child. Except for the nature of the linguistic input (English only or both English and Icelandic), the treatments were identical in all other respects, including the kinds of materials and functional tasks that were employed. During monolingual instruction, new vocabulary was presented in English only and comments that Siggi made in Icelandic were either ignored or he was redirected to speak in English. Under the bilingual treatment, vocabulary was presented in English and Icelandic and utterances in both languages were acknowledged and expanded. In order to make a pragmatically valid distinction between the treatments, another adult was incorporated into the intervention sessions. A monolingual, English-speaking adult participated in the monolingual treatment sessions (and served as a cue not to speak Icelandic as she could not understand what was said), whereas another, bilingual adult was included in the sessions in which both languages were used. Production probes of target vocabulary collected at the end of each session indicated that both methods were effective, with similar patterns of learning and levels of accuracy achieved under the two approaches. Given that equivalent outcomes were found for productive vocabulary gains in English with both methods, the bilingual treatment was recommended as the preferred approach for Siggi be-

cause of its potential for also facilitating Icelandic acquisition (which was not measured), as well as improving self-esteem and cultural identity by acknowledging the value of his native language.

CASE STUDY: MIRANDA AND JOEL

Miranda and Joel represent two cases involving different clinical management options for late talking toddlers, where both resulted in positive outcomes in terms of language functioning. As Miranda and Joel approached 2 years of age, they had extremely limited expressive vocabularies, and both sets of parents were becoming concerned about their child's language development. These children (along with two others) were invited to participate in an experimental language stimulation program for late talking toddlers (Ellis Weismer et al., 1993). Just as the program began, when both children were 25 months old, Joel's mother noted that his language skills were "taking off" and decided to adopt a wait-and-see approach rather than have him join the group. She did opt, however, to bring Joel in to the clinic for periodic reassessment of his language skills (which we offered as part of our experimental program). Joel's assessment at 28 months confirmed the family's perceptions about his spurt in language development; in a 3-month period he progressed from a productive vocabulary of 25 words to one of 214 words and advanced from early (MLU 1.00–1.49) to late Stage I (MLU 1.50–1.99) grammatical functioning. Subsequent assessments documented the fact that although Joel had made a slow start in the area of language, he was among those children who catch up to their peers without any special help.

Miranda participated in the 9-month clinician-based language intervention program, which consisted of biweekly sessions involving approximately 45 minutes of group interaction and 15 minutes of individual instruction. Group activities were conducted in a large playroom, following an early childhood classroom format. The goals of this program initially focused on increasing productive vocabulary and later progressed to multiword productions. Variations on a focused stimulation approach were employed under two conditions in which children were provided with multiple models of the language targets within meaningful contexts; in one condition there were no expectations for production of the targets by the children, while the other condition included attempts to evoke spontaneous productions of the targets through manipulations of the environment or conversational exchanges. At first, the children's mothers (and occasionally other caregivers) participated in the activities with the children; they later moved to an observational role as the program continued. This aspect of the program had the added benefit of providing the families with ideas about ways to facilitate language use at home and served as a support network for the mothers to discuss concerns related to their children's communication development. Because we intervened at an early point, we cannot be certain about the extent to which Miranda's language skills may have progressed on their own. It was the case that her vocabulary spurt was not observed until after intervention had begun, and though she responded quite well to intervention with respect to acquiring the targeted forms, at 3 years of age her expressive language, as indexed by MLU, remained slightly below age expectations. However, a follow-up assessment at age 4 years indicated that Miranda as well as Joel exhibited normal-range language abilities, and the children's parents expressed no further concerns.

SUMMARY

Various language intervention approaches are currently used with young children who have specific language delays or language impairment associated with mild DD. There is empirical support for the effectiveness of a number of different clinician-based methods that stem from distinct theoretical frameworks, with no single approach clearly emerging as the intervention method of choice. Factors that may enter into the selection of an intervention approach include the clinician's view of the language-learning process and language disorders, the particular language forms that are being targeted for intervention, and certain characteristics of the child, such as level of cognitive and linguistic functioning, interactive skills, learning style, and cultural and linguistic background. Clinicians are not the only individuals who can provide useful language-learning experiences for children with language deficits; approaches that incorporate peer models or parents have also been successfully employed. The influence of typically developing peer models on children with language disorders has recently received attention. Research indicates that benefits of including peer models in the intervention process are most likely to accrue when the clinician takes an active role in pairing the models with children with language deficits and/or directly teaching the peer models strategies to promote language interactions, rather than assuming that inclusion of peer models will naturally lead to productive exchanges in which appropriate language models are provided. It is generally believed that parents can serve a valuable function in the establishment of treatment goals and objectives and as an adjunct to clinician-based approaches. However, the role of parents as primary intervention agents remains somewhat controversial, and further empirical investigations are needed to examine the efficacy of parent-based approaches. Recently, special attempts have been made to address the intervention needs of children from minority cultures. When working with children from diverse backgrounds, it is important to consider: (a) differing family perspectives concerning early language intervention; (b) issues pertaining to the appropriate language of instruction in the case of bilingual speakers; and (c) the cultural compatibility of teaching methods and materials that are used. Finally, it has been shown that early language intervention is effective in facilitating linguistic development in young children; however, evidence for the persistence of language-related difficulties among children during the school-age years suggests that the focus of this intervention should be broadened to anticipate future areas of concern.

APPENDIX 6: CHILDREN'S VERBAL SCRIPTS FOR PLAYING HOUSE

Peer Model

Time 1 (Pretreatment)
You be a mom. You be a dad. You be a baby. You can do school work and sometimes you can pretend to live at somebody's house. You pretend to be an owl. Sometimes owls live in houses. Or, you could be watchdog or a cat. Sometimes, if you want to, you can bake cookies with a friend. You pretend you are the chef and he wears a big hat that's poofy. Then you go to the store for groceries. There's lots of things like go on summer vacations. But you just pretend, you know. You have to pretend with your friends. You are pretend, you know.

Time 2 (Posttreatment)
You hafta pretend or sometimes you hafta show them how. You know, like Kristin or somebody. Tiffany. Sometimes Tiffany is not a good pretender, but you can show her how to play house. Tiffany can be the baby or something. Then you grow up and play school. The mom can be the teacher or something. You cook food if you play house, if you want to. You make pancakes and French toast sticks for breakfast. I can pretend to eat those bumpy ones, but I don't really like them. Then you wash the dishes. And you dry them too, if, if you want. That's all.

SLI Child—Experimental Group

Time 1 (Pretreatment)
Play with cars and trucks and go outside to the sandbox. (redirect) Trucks. Like a batman car.

Time 2 (Posttreatment)
That good. You play in there. You get the cereal, it Lucky Charms or . . . or . . . or Super Sugar Pops. Use pretend spoons with the mom there. She can be the mom. That Meagan. She the mom there. Then . . . then . . . I be that too. Or I cook it too. That food you cook there. In the pretend stove. But don't eat that food. Just pretend it. Or put on hats. It can be the cop or batman hat.

SLI Child—Control Group

Time 1 (Pretreatment)
Bake. Eat cereal. I got cars, helicopters, trucks. (redirect) Play. I don't know. You play. I don't know. You put dirt in the truck. (redirect) I don't know.

Time 2 (No treatment with peer model)
Us gots to eat. You put it in your mouth. I don't know. You go for a ride. You have a hook. You kill it with a hook. That's all.

REFERENCES

Adler, S. (1993). *Multicultural communication skills in the classroom.* Needham Heights, Mass.: Allyn & Bacon.

Baker, N., & Nelson, K. (1984). Recasting and related conversational techniques for triggering syntactic advances by young children. *First Language*, 5, 3–22.

Battle, D. (Ed.), (1993). *Communication disorders in multicultural populations.* Boston: Andover Medical Publishers.

Battle, D. (1997). Language and communication disorders in culturally and linguistically diverse children. In D. Bernstein & E. Tiegerman-Faber (Eds.), *Language and communication disorders in children* (pp. 382–409). Boston: Allyn & Bacon.

Bricker, D. (1993). Then, now, and the path between: A brief history of language intervention. In A. Kaiser & D. Gray (Eds.), *Communication and language intervention series: Vol. 2. Enhancing children's communication: Research foundations for intervention* (pp. 11–31). Baltimore: Brookes.

Brooks, A., & Benjamin, B. (1989). The use of structured role play therapy in the remediation of grammatical deficits in language delayed children: Three case studies. *Journal of Childhood Communication Disorders*, *12*, 171–186.

Bruck, M. (1982). Language impaired children's performance in an additive bilingual education program. *Applied Psycholinguistics*, *3*, 45–60.

Camarata, S., Nelson, K., & Camarata, M. (1994). Comparison of conversational-recasting and imitative procedures for training grammatical structures in children with specific language impairment. *Journal of Speech and Hearing Research*, *37*, 1414–1423.

Chaney, C. (1990). Evaluating the whole language approach to language arts: The pros and cons. *Language, Speech, and Hearing Services in Schools*, *21*, 244–249.

Cheng, L. (1993). Asian-American cultures. In D. Battle (Ed.), *Communication disorders in multicultural populations* (pp. 38–77). Boston: Andover Medical Publishers.

Cole, K. (1995). Curriculum models and language facilitation in the preschool years. In M. Fey, J. Windsor, & S. Warren (Eds.), *Language intervention: Preschool through the elementary years* (pp. 39–60). Baltimore: Brookes.

Cole, K., & Dale, P. (1986). Direct language instruction and interactive language instruction with language delayed preschool children: A comparison study. *Journal of Speech and Hearing Research*, *29*, 206–217.

Cole, K., Dale, P., & Mills, P. (1991). Individual differences in language delayed children's responses to direct and interactive preschool instruction. *Topics in Early Childhood Special Education*, *11*, 99–124.

Cole, K., Mills, P., Dale, P., & Jenkins, J. (1991). Individual differences in the effects of preschool integration for children with mild and moderate handicaps. *Exceptional Children*, *58*, 36–45.

Connell, P. (1986). Teaching subjecthood to language-disordered children. *Journal of Speech and Hearing Research*, *29*, 481–492.

Connell, P. (1987). An effect of modeling and imitation teaching procedures on children with and without specific language impairment. *Journal of Speech and Hearing Research, 30*, 105–113.

Connell, P., & Stone, C. (1992). Morpheme learning of children with specific language impairment under controlled instruction conditions. *Journal of Speech and Hearing Research, 35*, 844–852.

Constable, C. (1986). The application of scripts in the organization of language intervention contexts. In K. Nelson (Ed.), *Event knowledge: Structure and function in development* (pp. 205–230). Hillsdale, N.J.: Erlbaum.

Courtright, J., & Courtright, I. (1976). Imitative modeling as a theoretical base for instructing language disordered children. *Journal of Speech and Hearing Research, 19*, 655–663.

Courtright, J., & Courtright, I. (1979). Imitative modeling as a language intervention strategy: The effects of two mediating variables. *Journal of Speech and Hearing Research, 22*, 389–402.

Crais, E. (1991). Moving from "parent involvement" to family centered services. *American Journal of Speech-Language Pathology, 1*, 5–8.

Culatta, B., & Horn, D. (1982). A program for achieving generalization of grammatical rules to spontaneous discourse. *Journal of Speech and Hearing Disorders, 47*, 174–180.

Elin T. Thordardottir, Ellis Weismer, S., & Smith, M. E. (1997). Vocabulary learning in bilingual and monolingual clinical intervention. *Child Language Teaching and Therapy, 13*, 215–227.

Ellis Weismer, S. (1997). The role of stress in language processing and intervention. *Topics in Language Disorders, 17*, 41–52.

Ellis Weismer, S., & Murray-Branch, J. (1989). Modeling versus modeling plus evoked production training: A comparison of two language intervention methods. *Journal of Speech and Hearing Disorders, 54*, 269–281.

Ellis Weismer, S., Murray-Branch, J., & Miller, J. (1993). Comparison of two methods for promoting productive vocabulary in late talkers. *Journal of Speech and Hearing Research, 36*, 1037–1050.

Ellis Weismer, S., & Schraeder, T. (1993). Discourse characteristics and verbal reasoning: Wait time effects on the performance of children with language learning disabilities. *Exceptionality Education Canada, 3*, 71–92.

Englemann, S., & Osborn, J. (1976). *Distar Language I and II*. Chicago: Science Research Associates.

Fey, M. (1986). *Language intervention with young children*. Newton, Mass.: Allyn & Bacon.

Fey, M., Catts, H., & Larrivee, L. (1995). Preparing preschoolers for the academic and social challenges of school. In M. Fey, J. Windsor, & S. Warren (Eds.), *Communication and language intervention series: Vol. 5. Language intervention: Preschool through the elementary years* (pp. 3–37). Baltimore: Brookes.

Fey, M., Cleave, P., & Long, S. (1997). Two models of grammar facilitation in children with language impairments: Phase 2. *Journal of Speech, Language and Hearing Research, 40*, 5–19.

Fey, M., Cleave, P., Long, S., & Hughes, D. (1993). Two approaches to the facilitation of grammar in language-impaired children: An experimental evaluation. *Journal of Speech and Hearing Research*, *36*, 141–157.

Friedman, P., & Friedman, K. (1980). Accounting for individual differences when comparing the effectiveness of remedial language teaching methods. *Applied Psycholinguistics*, *1*, 151–170.

Gillam, R., McFadden, T., & van Kleeck, A. (1995). Improving narrative abilities: Whole language and language skills approaches. In M. Fey, J. Windsor, & S. Warren (Eds.), *Communication and language intervention series: Vol. 5. Language intervention: Preschool through the elementary years* (pp. 9–47). Baltimore: Brookes.

Girolametto, L., Pearce, P., & Weitzman, E. (1996). Interactive focused stimulation for toddlers with expressive vocabulary delays. *Journal of Speech and Hearing Research*, *39*, 1274–1283.

Guralnick, M., & Paul–Brown, D. (1980). Functional and discourse analysis of nonhandicapped preschool children's speech to handicapped children. *American Journal of Mental Deficiency*, *84*, 444-454.

Guralnick, M., & Paul-Brown, D. (1986). Communicative interactions of mildly delayed and normally developing preschool children: Effects of listener's developmental level. *Journal of Speech and Hearing Research*, *29*, 2–10.

Halle, J., Marshall, A., & Spradlin, J. (1979). Time delay: A technique to increase language use and facilitate generalization in retarded children. *Journal of Applied Behavior Analysis*, *12*, 431–440.

Harris, G. (1993). American Indian cultures: A lesson in diversity. In D. Battle (Ed.), *Communication disorders in multicultural populations* (pp. 78–113). Boston: Andover Medical Publishers.

Hart, B., & Risley, R. (1980). In vivo language training: Unanticipated and general effects. *Journal of Applied Behavior Analysis*, *12*, 407–432.

Hegde, M. (1980). An experimental-clinical analysis of grammatical and behavioral distinctions between verbal auxiliary and copula. *Journal of Speech and Hearing Research*, *23*, 864–877.

Hubbell, R. (1981). *Children's language disorders: An integrated approach*. Englewood Cliffs, N.J.: Prentice-Hall.

Individuals with Disabilities Education Act Amendments, Public Law 105–17. (1997). Washington, D.C.: Federal Register, June 4.

Jenkins, J., Odom, S., & Speltz, M. (1989). Effects of social integration on preschool children with handicaps. *Exceptional Children*, *55*, 420–428.

Jenkins, J., Speltz, M., & Odom, S. (1985). Integrating normal and handicapped preschoolers: Effects on child development and social interaction. *Exceptional Children*, *52*, 7–17.

Juarez, M. (1983). Assessment and treatment of minority language-handicapped children: The role of the monolingual speech-language pathologist. *Topics in Language Disorders*, *3*, 57–65.

Kaiser, A., Yoder, P., & Keetz, A. (1992). Evaluating milieu teaching. In S. Warren & J. Reichle (Eds.), *Communication and language intervention series:*

Vol. 1. Causes and effects in communication and language intervention (pp. 9–47). Baltimore: Brookes.

Kayser, H. (1993). Hispanic cultures. In D. Battle (Ed.), *Communication disorders in multicultural populations* (pp. 114–157). Boston: Andover Medical Publishers.

Kayser, H. (1995). Intervention with children from linguistically and culturally diverse backgrounds. In M. Fey, J. Windsor, & S. Warren (Eds.), *Communication and language intervention series: Vol. 5. Language intervention: Preschool through the elementary years* (pp. 315–331). Baltimore: Brookes.

Kiernan, B., & Swisher, L. (1990). The initial learning of novel English words: Two single-subject experiments with minority-language children. *Journal of Speech and Hearing Research*, *33*, 707–716.

Kim, Y., & Lombardino, L. (1991). The efficacy of script context in language comprehension intervention with children who have mental retardation. *Journal of Speech and Hearing Research*, *34*, 845–857.

Lee, L., Koenigsknecht, R., & Mulhern, S. (1975). *Interactive language development teaching*. Evanston, Ill.: Northwestern University Press.

Leonard, L. (1981). Facilitating linguistic skills in children with specific language impairment. *Applied Psycholinguistics*, *2*, 89–118.

Leonard, L. (1993). Children with specific language impairment (developmental dysphasia): Treatment. In G. Blanken, J. Dittmann, H. Grimm, J. Marshall, & C. Wallesch (Eds.), *Linguistic disorders and pathologies: An international handbook*.(pp. 262–284). Berlin: de Gruyter.

Leonard, L., Camarata, S., Rowan, L, & Chapman, K. (1982). The communicative functions of lexical usage by language impaired children. *Applied Psycholinguistics*, *3*, 109–125.

Mahoney, G., & Powell, A. (1988). Modifying parent-child interaction: Enhancing the development of handicapped children. *Journal of Special Education*, *22*, 82–96.

McDade, H., & Varnedoe, D. (1987). Training parents to be language facilitators. *Topics in Language Disorders*, *7*, 19–30.

Miller, N. (Ed.). (1984). *Bilingualism and language disability: Assessment and remediation*. San Diego: College Hill Press.

Nelson, K. (1986). Event knowledge and cognitive development. In K. Nelson (Ed.), *Event knowledge: Structure and function in development* (pp. 1–19). Hillsdale, N.J.: Erlbaum.

Nelson, K. E. (1991). On differentiated language learning models and differentiated interventions. In N. Krasnegor, D. Rumbaugh, & R. Schiefelbusch (Eds.), *Language acquisition: Biological and behavioral determinants* (pp. 399–428). Hillsdale, N.J.: Erlbaum.

Nelson, K. E., Camarata, S., Welsh, J., Butkovsky, L., & Camarata, M. (1996). Effects of imitative and conversational recasting treatment on the acquisition of grammar in children with specific language impairment and younger language-normal children. *Journal of Speech and Hearing Research*, *39*, 850–859.

Norris, J., & Damico, J. (1990). Whole language in theory and practice: Implications for language intervention. *Language, Speech, and Hearing Services in Schools, 21,* 212–220.

Norris, J., & Hoffman, P. (1990). Comparison of adult-initiated vs. child-initiated interaction styles with handicapped pre-language children. *Language, Speech, and Hearing Services in Schools, 21,* 28–36.

Norris, J., & Hoffman, P. (1993). *Whole language intervention for school-age children.* San Diego: Singular Publishing.

Nye, C., Foster, S., & Seaman, D. (1987). Effectiveness of language intervention with the language/learning disabled. *Journal of Speech and Hearing Disorders, 52,* 348–357.

Olswang, L., & Bain, B. (1991). Intervention issues for toddlers with specific language impairments. *Topics in Language Disorders, 11,* 69–86.

Olswang, L., Bain, B., Dunn, C., & Cooper, J. (1983). The effects of stimulus variation on lexical learning. *Journal of Speech and Hearing Disorders, 48,* 192–201.

Olswang, L., Bain, B., Rosendahl, P., Oblak, S., & Smith, A. (1986). Language learning: Moving performance from a context-dependent to -independent state. *Child Language Teaching and Therapy, 2,* 180–210.

Ortiz, A. (1984, spring). Choosing the language of instruction for exceptional bilingual children. *Teaching Exceptional Children, 17,* 208–212.

Paul, R. (1991). Profiles of toddlers with slow expressive language development. *Topics in Language Disorders, 11,* 1–13.

Paul, R. (1994). *Clinical implications of the natural history of slow expressive language development.* Miniseminar presented at the American Speech-Language-Hearing Association convention, New Orleans.

Paul, R. (1995). *Language disorders from infancy through adolescence: Assessment and intervention.* St. Louis: Mosby.

Perozzi, J. (1985). A pilot study of language facilitation for bilingual children with language delay: Theoretical and intervention implications. *Journal of Speech and Hearing Disorders, 50,* 403–406.

Perozzi, J., & Chavez-Sanchez, M. (1992). The effect of instruction in L1 on receptive acquisition of L2 for bilingual children with language delay. *Language, Speech, and Hearing Services in Schools, 23,* 348–352.

Ratner, V., & Harris, L. (1994). *Understanding language disorders: The impact on learning.* Eau Claire, Wis.: Thinking Publications.

Robertson, S., & Ellis Weismer, S. (1997). The influence of peer models on the play scripts of children with specific language impairment. *Journal of Speech, Language and Hearing Research, 40,* 49–61.

Rogers-Warren, A., Ruggles, T., Peterson, N., & Cooper, A. (1981). Playing and learning together: Patterns of social interaction in handicapped and non-handicapped children. *Journal of the Division for Early Childhood Special Education, 3,* 56–63.

Rogers-Warren, A., & Warren, S. (1980). Mands for verbalization: Facilitating the display of newly trained language in children. *Behavior Modification, 4,* 361–382.

Schank, R., & Abelson, R. (1977). *Scripts, plans, goals, and understanding.* Hillsdale, N.J.: Erlbaum.

Scherer, N., & Olswang, L. (1989). Using structured discourse as a language intervention technique with autistic children. *Journal of Speech and Hearing Disorders, 54,* 383–394.

Schwartz, I. (1987). A review of techniques for naturalistic language training. *Child Language Teaching and Therapy, 3,* 267–276.

Schwartz, R. (1988). Early action word acquisition in normal and language-impaired children. *Applied Psycholinguistics, 9,* 111–122.

Schwartz, R., Chapman, K., Terrell, B., Prelock, P., & Rowan, L. (1985). Facilitating word combination in language-impaired children in discourse structure. *Journal of Speech and Hearing Disorders, 50,* 31–39.

Shriberg, L., & Kwiatkowski, J. (1982). Phonological disorders II: A conceptual framework for management. *Journal of Speech and Hearing Disorders, 47,* 242–256.

Tannock, R., & Girolametto, L. (1992). Reassessing parent-focused language intervention programs. In S. Warren & J. Reichle (Eds.), *Causes and effects in communication and language intervention* (pp. 49–80). Baltimore: Brookes.

Tannock, R., Girolametto, L., & Siegel, L. (1992). Language intervention with children who have developmental delays: Effects of an interactive approach. *American Journal of Mental Retardation, 97,* 145–160.

Terrell, S., & Terrell, F. (1993). African-American cultures. In D. Battle (Ed.), *Communication disorders in multicultural populations* (pp. 3–37). Boston: Andover Medical Publishers.

Tobin, K. (1987). The role of wait time in higher cognitive level learning. *Review of Educational Research, 57,* 69–95.

Venn, M., Wolery, M., Fleming, L., DeCesare, L., Morris, A., & Cuffs, M. (1993). Effects of teaching preschool peers to use the mand-model procedure during snack activities. *American Journal of Speech-Language Pathology, 2,* 38–46.

Warren, S. (1992). Facilitating basic vocabulary acquisition with milieu teaching procedures. *Journal of Early Intervention, 16,* 235–251.

Warren, S., & Bambara, L. (1989). An experimental analysis of milieu language intervention: Teaching the action-object form. *Journal of Speech and Hearing Disorders, 54,* 448–461.

Warren, S., & Gazdag, G. (1990). Facilitating early language development with milieu intervention procedures. *Journal of Early Intervention, 14,* 62–86.

Warren, S., & Kaiser, A. (1986). Incidental language teaching: A critical review. *Journal of Speech and Hearing Disorders, 51,* 291–299.

Warren, S., McQuarter, R., & Rogers-Warren, A. (1984). The effects of mands and models on the speech of unresponsive language-delayed preschool children. *Journal of Speech and Hearing Disorders, 49,* 43–52.

Waryas, C., & Stremel-Campbell, K. (1983). *Communication Training Program.* New York: Teaching Resources.

Weiss, A. (1993). Planning language intervention for young children. In D. Bernstein & E. Tiegerman (Eds.), *Language and communication disorders in children* (pp. 229–324). Boston: Allyn & Bacon.

Weiss, A., & Nakamura, M. (1992). Children with normal language skills in preschool classrooms for children with language impairments: Differences in modeling styles. *Language, Speech, and Hearing Services in Schools, 23*, 64–70.

Weistuch, L., & Brown, B. (1987). Motherese as therapy: A program and its dissemination. *Child Language Teaching and Therapy, 3*, 57–71.

Weistuch, L., & Lewis, M. (1985). The language interaction intervention project. *Analysis and Intervention in Developmental Disabilities, 5*, 97–106.

Whitehurst, G., & Fischel, J. (1994). Early developmental language delay: What, if anything, should the clinician do about it? *Journal of Child Psychology and Psychiatry, 35*, 613–648.

Whitehurst, G., Fischel, J., Caulfield, M., DeBaryshe, B., & Valdez-Menchaca, M. (1989). Assessment and treatment of early expressive language delay. In P. Aelazo & R. Barr (Eds.), *Challenges to developmental paradigms: Implications for assessment and treatment* (pp. 113–135). Hillsdale, N.J.: Erlbaum.

Whitehurst, G., Fischel, J., Lonigan, C., Valdez-Menchaca, M., Arnold, D., & Smith, M. (1991). Treatment of early expressive language delay. *Topics in Language Disorders, 11*, 55–68.

Windsor, J. (1995). Language impairment and social competence. In M. Fey, J. Windsor, & S. Warren (Eds.), *Communication and language intervention series: Vol. 5. Language intervention: Preschool through the elementary years* (pp. 213–238). Baltimore: Brookes.

Yoder, P., Kaiser, A., & Alpert, C. (1991). An exploratory study of the interaction between language teaching methods and child characteristics. *Journal of Speech and Hearing Research, 34*, 155–167.

CHAPTER 7

Issues in Emergent Literacy for Children With Language Impairments

Joan N. Kaderavek, Ph.D., CCC-SLP
Assistant Professor, Department of Special Education
Eastern Michigan University
Ypsilanti
Elizabeth Sulzby, Ph.D.
Professor, School of Education
University of Michigan
Ann Arbor

Key Terms

conventional literacy
emergent literacy
emergent reading

Overview

Both practical experience and research indicates that there is a relationship between oral language impairment and reading disabilities. Many of the children who experience reading problems in school are also on the caseloads of speech-language pathologists (SLPs). A number of studies have documented that young children with language impairment are at a higher-than-average risk of demonstrating later reading disabilities (Aram, Ekelman, & Nation, 1984; Aram & Nation, 1980; Catts, 1991, 1993). This literature indicates that language impairment may be a basic deficit that affects language function in all its forms—both oral and written.

In this chapter, we explore the concurrent language functioning of preschoolers in specific oral and written language situations. Awareness of the relationship between reading disability and oral language impairment in the school-age population has coincided with newer understandings of the reciprocal nature of oral and written language forms during the preschool years (Cox, 1994; Sulzby, 1985a, 1985b; Teale & Sulzby, 1986). These understandings have been central to research in the field of **emergent literacy**. Emergent literacy theory claims that children show knowledge and ability in written language through oral delivery forms, such as using structures suited to written discourse in an orally delivered version of a storybook while looking at the book's pictures rather than tracking and using cues from print (Sulzby, 1985a, 1994, 1996a). Conversely, children may import features typically suited to oral language situations into their storybook reenactments or their rereadings of scribbled or drawn compositions (Sulzby, 1986).

Integrating the theoretical orientation and concepts central to emergent literacy theory into understandings of oral language development can expand the scope of language remediation services provided to young preschool children. This chapter is designed to aid that process. In this chapter we review the major theoretical concepts and empirical findings central to emergent literacy. Second, we examine oral and written differences in a variety of contexts, including our previous and ongoing work. Finally, we present examples from case study data drawn from our current research and discuss the implications of these data for SLPs who want to incorporate emergent literacy perspectives and practices into their language remediation practices with preschool children.

THEORETICAL ORIENTATION

In our collaborative research program, and in this chapter, we bring together perspectives from speech-language pathology and emergent literacy. Research in the field of speech-language pathology typically has focused on spoken language development of young children, whereas research in the field of emergent literacy has investigated young children's written language development. Researchers in both fields increasingly acknowledge the importance of studying the relationships between oral and written language acquisition. Sulzby (1985a) argues that children develop both oral and written language in an interrelated fashion during the preschool years prior to **conventional literacy**. Such a position suggests that investigation of the reciprocal nature of oral/written language forms during the preschool years is warranted.

Vygotsky's (1978) model of the internalization of speech characteristics from social contexts has typically been used in parent-child interaction theory to mean that the child internalizes the speech characteristics of the more knowledgeable and present adult, usually the parent. Our study acknowledges this part of the Vygotskian model but adds a further acknowledgment of one broader social context of the child-parent dyad—that of the published storybook—or a nonpresent adult writer as mediated through the present adult (the parent). Storybooks, as Teale and Sulzby (1987) have pointed out, have a privileged status within mainstream U.S. and European cultural settings. Bus and her colleagues (Bus & Sulzby, in press; Bus & van IJzendoorn, 1992, 1995; Bus, Sulzby, & van IJzendoorn, 1996) have found, when interviewing Dutch parents, that even those who were found later to read infrequently to children nevertheless strongly asserted that "of course" they read to their preschool-aged children.

Sulzby (1994) claimed that the child's readings also have characteristics of Piagetian-like constructions not totally contained in the parental readings. Sulzby and Teale's (1987) study of parent-child interactions among low- and middle-income Hispanic and Anglo parent-child dyads showed that some, but not all, patterns of emergent storybook readings were seen first in interaction and later in children's independent speech. Our focus in this chapter is upon those language structures from the parental readings that do appear first in interaction and then in the child's independent speech functioning, or the Vygotskian aspect of the Sulzby model. We analyze how this internalization process appears to be similar to, or different from, that which occurs during toy play interactions between parent and child.

In summary, our theoretical orientation is formulated on the basic concept of a reciprocal relationship between oral and written language development during the preschool years. Second, we acknowledge the significance and impact of the parent-child interaction, both in toy play and in storybook interaction. Finally, because of its elevated status within our culture, we suggest that the language surrounding storybooks may be of particular importance for examination and may be particularly relevant to children with communication disorders.

In recent years, much attention has been given to phonemic awareness as a predictor of later reading achievement. This chapter offers complementary research in early literacy development focused on the text and comprehension levels. Phonemic awareness, while a necessary, but not sufficient, condition for reading development, is outside the scope of the current chapter due to space restrictions; however, we urge readers to consult current reviews and studies (Adams, 1990; Catts, 1991, 1993; Scanlon & Vellutino, in press; Scarborough, 1998; Snow, Burns, & Griffin, 1998) in this important area.

EMERGENT LITERACY RESEARCH

In this section, first we review key findings from emergent literacy research along with implications for practice that some researchers have recommended for typically developing young language learners. We also review findings from a small number of studies in which emergent literacy has been studied in children with communication disorders. We then review our own research program in children's **emergent reading** of storybooks, parent-child storybook reading, and elicitation of children's oral and written narratives.

Typically Developing Language Learners

A number of key findings have been identified as important regarding the emergent literacy development of typically developing children. The following is a brief overview.

Finding One. *A literacy-rich environment facilitates literacy development*: Since children learn literacy content in a social context, the literacy environment of young children is critical to their successful literacy/language development (Morrow & Paratore, 1993; Sulzby, 1986). Children become socialized to the functions of literacy in their daily life (Heath, 1983; van Kleeck & Schuele, 1987). Preschool children who show a high interest in literacy activities tend to come from homes and schools where parents and teachers provided a supportive literacy environment (Hiebert, 1994; Morrow, 1983). These environments are not monolithic but vary across individual families and cultural groups (e.g., Anderson & Stokes, 1984; Moll, 1994; Taylor & Dorsey-Gaines, 1988).

Finding Two. *Reading to young children is a significant language-learning tool*: Children learn many aspects of language during storybook reading, ranging from vocabulary to discourse structures. Studies have demonstrated that young children learn vocabulary (Moerk, 1985; Ninio, 1983; Snow & Goldfield, 1983; Whitehurst et al., 1988), syntactical constructions (Snow & Goldfield, 1983), and use of decontextualized language (Snow, 1983; Sulzby, 1985a).

The development of such skills can lead to increased language performance (Chomsky, 1972) and increased achievement in school (Snow, 1983). One meta-analysis indicates that, across studies, parent-preschooler reading is related to outcome measures such as language ability (most specifically, acquisition of the written language register), emergent literacy competency, and reading achievement (Bus, van IJzendoorn, & Pellegrini, 1995).

Finding Three. *Positive language changes occur when children are read storybooks repeatedly:* Repeated reading of a storybook facilitates the child's internalization of written language structures (Sulzby, 1985a; Teale & Sulzby, 1987). Goodsitt, Raitan, and Perlmutter (1988) found that as familiarity with the book increased, the interchanges between parents and children focused more on story content and less on labeling behaviors. Yaden (1988) reported that with repeated reading, children began to ask fewer questions centered around the book's pictures and instead began asking more questions about the meaning of words and the story. Martinez and Roser (1985) suggested that the kinds of questions children asked after repeated readings demonstrated a greater depth of understanding. It has been suggested that reading a book together repeatedly permits a child to assume aspects of the adult language role (Snow & Ninio, 1986). Children of parents who read books repeatedly have been found to begin emergent readings spontaneously (Bus et al., 1996; Sulzby & Teale, 1987).

Finding Four. *Parents use complex language structures during routines such as storybook interactions*: Book-reading routines appear to create a context that is highly routinized (Ninio & Bruner, 1978). There is some evidence that maternal interactive speech during routines is more complex than when experiencing novel objects and activities (Snow et al., 1976; van Kleeck, Gillam, Hamilton, & McGrath, 1997). Thus, book reading appears to create an enriched language environment.

Finding Five. *Different ethnic groups and socioeconomic levels have different* styles *of reading behavior, which impacts child language performance*: Parents can vary greatly in the extent that they use questioning and labeling behaviors during reading interactions (Heath, 1983, 1986; Ninio, 1980). These differences in parents' language performances result in differences in child language behavior. As an example, Anderson-Yockel and Haynes (1994) reported that white mothers asked more questions to their preschooler, which resulted in greater question-answering communications by white preschoolers, whereas African American mothers asked fewer questions, which resulted in a greater incidence of spontaneous verbalizations by the African American preschoolers. SLPs need to be sensitive to these interrelationships and avoid prescriptive approaches that suggest to parents there is only one "right way" to read to their children (Kaderavek & Sulzby, 1995; Sulzby & Edwards, 1993).

Children Who Have Language Impairments

Given the established links between oral and written language among preschoolers developing typically and among school-age children with a history of language impairment, it is important to examine the implications for preschool children with language difficulties. This section will outline a rationale and some principles for intervention in the area of emergent literacy for young children with language impairments.

Principle One. *There is a strong need to support a wide variety of oral language performances to form a foundation for language development, including literacy*: A preschool program that provides for the broadest usage of oral and literacy behaviors will be beneficial for preschool children with language impairment (Schuele & van Kleeck, 1987; Watson, Layton, Pierce, & Abraham, 1994). Early literacy interactions should aim to develop all modes of communication and provide normalizing experiences for children with specific language impairment (Watson et al., 1994). Opportunities for long oral narrative performances allow young African American children, including those with language delays and impairments, to display oral and written language knowledge that might be otherwise overlooked (Hyon & Sulzby, 1994; Sulzby, Branz, & Buhle, 1993).

Principle Two. *Parents' behaviors appear to be different when reading to children with communication impairments*: Parents vary their teaching strategies in response to children's communication status. Pellegrini and colleagues found that parents of children showing typically developing communication skills appeared to be more demanding (high versus low cognitive demands) and use fewer support strategies (e.g., fewer task turns, less nonverbal management) as compared with the strategies used by parents of children with communicative impairments (Pellegrini, Brody, & Sigel, 1985; Pellegrini, McGillicuddy-DeLisi, Sigel, & Brody, 1986).

Principle Three. *Emergent literacy activities may need to be adapted for children who are severely impaired*: Even though children with developmental disabilities or severe speech and physical impairment may have some reduced ability to explore storybooks, all available opportunities including advanced technological solutions, should be explored in order to maintain an enriched literacy environment (Koppenhaver, Coleman, Kalman, & Yoder, 1991; Pierce & McWilliam, 1993). For example, Koppenhaver et al. (1991) have suggested that one way to increase participation by children with severe impairments is to provide communication symbols so that the child can ask an adult to read aloud, request a page to be turned, or ask questions.

Principle Four. *Emergent literacy activities can be used effectively in special education preschool programs*: Katims (1991) examined the effect of using emergent literacy activities in a classroom of preschoolers with handicapping conditions that included cognitive, physical, emotional, behavioral, learning, and developmental disabilities. The emergent literacy activities included daily storybook readings paired with emergent writing activities, as well as the availability of a well-stocked classroom library center. The experimental group was compared with a control group of similar children in a preschool classroom without these emergent literacy activities. It was reported that those children who were exposed to emergent literacy activities demonstrated significant improvement in their ability to interact with books in more sophisticated and varied ways, as compared to the children in the control group.

Many SLPs and teachers who work with young children already engage in many or most of the recommended practices. Others can be encouraged to include positive literacy environments for the children with language impairments on their caseload or in the classrooms they serve. Recommended activities include stimulating communication in all modalities, exposing children to repeated readings of storybooks, and providing many opportunities for emergent writing activities (see, for example, Sulzby & Barnhart, 1992; Sulzby, Teale, & Kamberelis, 1989).

One advantage of incorporating emergent literacy activities such as these into classrooms and clinical practice is that they provide an opportunity for SLPs to observe a child's ability to negotiate the demands of varying oral and written contexts. One aspect that distinguishes oral versus written language production is the varying demands of decontextualization between these contexts. Scollon and Scollon (1981) suggested that written language demands the use of linguistic forms allowing a nonpresent audience to comprehend the text without the context surrounding and/or imagined by the writer at the time of composition. This issue of decontextualization is one that we explore in our research—and it is our research in emergent storybook reading, parent-child storybook elicitation, and children's oral and written narrative productions to which we now turn.

CHILDREN'S EMERGENT STORYBOOK PRODUCTIONS: RESEARCH, ELICITATION PROCEDURES, AND CLASSIFICATION SCHEMES

As we have described, independent emergent book reading elicitations from nonconventional readers allow researchers, teachers, and SLPs to observe the child's shifts between oral-like and more written-like language forms. The protocol we describe here is an outgrowth of Sulzby's research, initiated in 1979, in which she asked young children to "read" from their favorite storybook (Sulzby, 1983).

History of the Sulzby Classification Scheme and Elicitation Techniques

The primary data used to develop the Sulzby Classification Scheme were obtained from 24 kindergartners in a middle to upper-middle socioeconomic status (MSES) suburb of a large midwestern city. The children, whose ages ranged from 4;11 to 5;11, were taking part in a year-long study (Sulzby, 1985b) focusing on emergent reading and writing knowledge. Part of the data for this study (Sulzby, 1985a) included beginning- and end-of-the-year interviews that included a discussion of a well-known book. As the children were taken individually to the interview, each was asked to select a personal favorite book from the classroom library. At the end of the interview, each child was asked to "read me your book." Children's transcribed narrative attempts were content analyzed and classified in a schema from the least mature productions (i.e., picture-governed attempts with story not formed) to independent or conventional readings from print (Figure 7-1).

A second study (also reported in Sulzby, 1985a) tested the scheme with younger children seen more frequently over a year-long investigation. A total of 32 children enrolled in a privately operated day-care center in a suburb outside a large midwestern city took part in the study, at ages 2, 3, and 4, with different numbers of children present for different parts of the study. Half of the children were from lower socioeconomic status (LSES) and half from MSES homes. Along with weekly classroom observations, some of the children were seen quarterly and a subset was seen monthly and videotaped as the familiar researcher asked the child to "read me your book." A variety of books were used, including books read repeatedly in the classroom and "favorite storybooks" sent from home by the children's parents. During the analysis and classification of these younger children's emergent readings, no new categories or sub-categories of reading behaviors emerged. Instead, it was found that (a) the categories appeared to be quite stable, (b) there was reasonable stability across storybooks for individual children, and (c) the behaviors appeared to be developmental in that the patterns differed predictably across ages. Additionally, none of the children, in either the day-care or kindergarten study, were receiving formal literacy instruction, although all were being read to frequently in their care settings. More recently, the Sulzby Classification Scheme has been used reliably with U.S. populations including LSES, white children (Reuning & Sulzby, 1984); LSES white children of Appalachian background (Elijah & Sulzby, 1992); LSES African American children (Elijah & Sulzby, 1992; Sulzby et al., 1993); LSES, Mexican and Mexican American children (Sulzby & Zecker, 1991); and LSES and MSES, Anglo and Mexican American children (Teale & Sulzby, 1987, 1989).

Ideas for Eliciting Emergent Readings

Book selection and the adult's words and affect are very important in eliciting emergent readings from all children, but particularly with children with

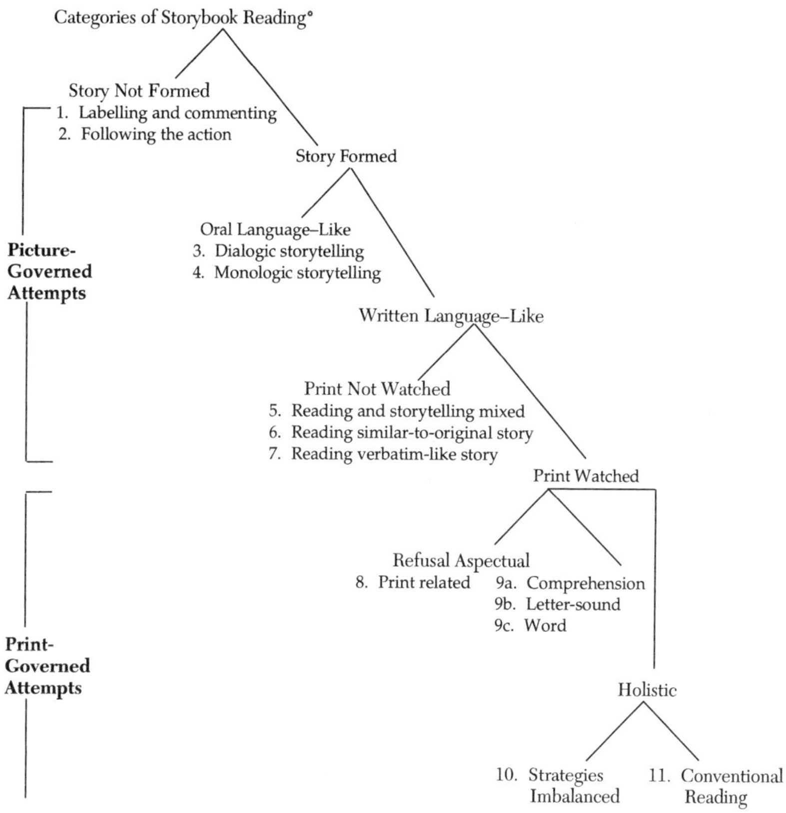

*This figure includes independent reading attempts only:The child is making the reading attempts without dependence.

Figure 7-1. Classification Scheme for Children's Emergent Reading of Favorite Storybooks (From Sulzby, Elizabeth [1985, summer]. Children's emergent reading of favorite storybooks: A developmental study. *Reading Research Quarterly, 20*[4], 458–481. © International Reading Association, Newark, Del. Reprinted with permission.)

language impairments. First, it is important to make certain that the book that is being used for the storybook elicitation is sufficiently familiar to the child. As a rule of thumb we consider a book to be familiar if it has been read to the child on three to four occasions. The book should also be one that the child shows evidence of enjoying through behaviors such as attentive listening, commenting on pictures or story, chiming in, echoing, or completing parts of the reading.

Another book-selection issue concerns the type of book that is used for the elicitation. Sulzby's scheme was developed and used with narrative-type storybooks. (Although it has been used occasionally with other genres, adaptations were necessary, and reliability and validity data are not available.) A narrative story is one that contains characters and a plot. Examples include books such as *Are You My Mother?* (Eastman, 1960), *Clifford, the Big Red Dog* (Bridwell, 1985), and *Where the Wild Things Are* (Sendak, 1963). Research has suggested that by being exposed to complex narratives, children have the opportunity to internalize discourse patterns, whereas with brief pattern books, such as *Brown Bear, Brown Bear* (Martin, 1970), children tend to rely on rote memorization (Sulzby, 1991) and hence show little variation on the Sulzby Classification Scheme.

The instructions that are used to elicit the emergent reading are a second important aspect to be considered. When asking the child to produce an emergent reading, it is important that the SLP use a direct imperative request ("Please read me your book," or "Read me your book."). The SLP must be certain to ask for a reading. If the SLP asks "Can you read me the book?" this comment may be interpreted as calling for a judgment about the child's ability to read. Similarly, if the SLP says, "Tell me the book," or "Tell me about this book," these comments may be interpreted as requests for production of storytelling or an oral narrative.

Many children will eagerly respond to the request to read. Some children will be hesitant. There are some suggestions that may help with this latter situation. First, use plenty of wait time. Wait time is very important with young children when they are asked to perform an unfamiliar task. Attitude is important as well: use a calm tone and convey confidence through tone and glance that the child will begin "reading."

If encouragement is needed, some suggested comments are, "It doesn't have to be like grown-up reading—do it your own way"; or "Try"; or "Give it a try." If the child still refuses, provide support by saying, "Let me read a bit to you," and then read the first page or two to the child. After two or three pages say: "Now it's your turn. You read it to me." If the child continues to refuse, then say, "Let's read it together." At this point, begin an interactive reading at whatever level you feel is best for the child. At an appropriate point at which you feel the child might cooperate, possibly between pages 4 and 6, say, "Now it's your turn. You read it to me." If the child continues to refuse to attempt the task, the behaviors and language observed will nonetheless be helpful in gaining insight about the child's understandings of written language. (This concept will be explored more fully during the discussion of categories of emergent reading.)

Once the SLP or teacher has obtained the emergent reading, it is possible to classify the language produced by the child (Figure 7-1) using an ordinal scale of 1-11. The following is a description of each of the levels of emergent reading, and behaviors and language of children that characterize emergent reading at each level. The Sulzby scheme is applied to the reading as a whole, not to individual utterances or short episodes, although the analysis of smaller elements may help making a decision about the whole. For the SLP, the linguistic analysis of smaller units is important as a separate, but related, type of analysis.

We consider these levels, if gained in a valid manner with good rapport between adult and child, to be relative indicators of the child's development in a specific and important linguistic context; Sulzby (1994) explicitly cautions against interpreting these as stages in the general developmental sense. The levels can be used to indicate literacy progress, but for the SLP, an examination of linguistic usage by the child within the situation is ordinarily of more importance than measuring literacy growth.

Categorization of the Children's Emergent Readings Using the Sulzby Classification Scheme

Transcribe the child's reading, including interactions with the SLP, with notes about the kind of intonation patterns used. Read the transcription carefully and make the categorization based on the structure of the "text" as a whole. The following rubrics concern the structure of the entire reading attempt, not subparts. In contrast with the work of Elster (1994), judgments on subparts should follow rather than precede judgments on the whole. As can be seen in Figure 7-1, the structures are divided by a number of overarching distinctions: whether or not the child is looking at the print or pictures as if they are the source of the reading; whether or not the child's speech sounds like oral or written language; and whether or not the child's speech shows the structure of a story or does not. Further information on this scheme can be found in Sulzby (1985a, 1996a, 1996b).

Attempts Governed by Pictures With Stories Not Formed. Here the child's speech does not sound as if it is a story, but is primarily focused on isolated pictures. Sulzby (1985a, 1994) uses a very rudimentary notion of "story"—of having a beginning, middle, and ending event structure—rather than the full-blown episodic structure of story grammars. The speech is that of face-to-face oral interaction. The child appears to utter speech for each page separately, without integrating the separate pictures into a cohesive story. The most obvious characteristic of this level is that the observer must look at the pictures in the storybook to understand the context of the child's speech utterances; in other words, the speech is very much contextualized to the pictures and face-to-face interaction. The child often looks away from the book to the adult when uttering speech, although he or she may rapidly look back at the book while pointing. It is as if the child were attempting to be sure that the adult was looking at what the child was referring to. When the child makes an aside to comment about the reading event, to change to a different linguistic context such as telling about something happening in the environment or in the child's past, or to ask a question, often the adult cannot be sure that the speech is an aside or part of the storybook reading event. (In later levels, children show appropriate linguistic and paralinguistic markings of asides.) Sulzby divides these "no story formed" reading attempts into two subcategories: labeling and commenting, and following the action.

If a child is producing behaviors that can be classified as labeling and commenting, he or she will point to items on a page of the storybook and give the label or descriptor for that item (e.g., "kitty-cat") or comments about the picture by giving some information ("wash his hand") or even a long sentence ("That's a fighting guy up there.") When the child points, it is usually directly at the picture being labeled or discussed and often with an emphatic punching or tapping motion. It has been observed that the speech of most children during picture-governed attempts is markedly less mature than their general usage. (It should be remembered that these data thus far have come from children without language impairments.)

The second kind of oral production observable at the "story not formed" classification level are those that focus on the action taking place in the pictures, a level called "following the action." Children performing at this level typically point or gesture toward the pictures and talk about the action in the picture in the present tense, as if the action were immediately occurring. Children at this level frequently use their finger to trace the action in the picture, or they may gesture or perform the activity occurring in the picture. Sometimes these reenactments are accompanied by sound effects. In both levels within this category—labeling and commenting, and following the action—the intonation patterns are those of conversational turn taking in oral speech. (Pitch levels from very young children in emergent storybook readings can occasionally be confusing when determining whether the intonation is reading-like or conversational. Young children often use a wide range of pitch, including very high pitch for some key words or phrases; these pitch shifts should not be confused with reading intonation.)

Although the child operating at these levels does not yet sequence the event of the book into a story or decontextualize the language used, the behaviors demonstrated at these early levels demonstrate significant advances in emergent literacy ability. We think this is particularly the case for children with language impairments. When children with language impairments become able to label a storybook picture, they have accepted an important "contract of literacy" (Snow & Ninio, 1986). Snow and Ninio (1986) suggested that when a child comes to understand that "pictures are not things but representatives of things" (p. 126) and that "pictures are for naming" (p. 131), he or she has learned fundamental concepts needed for literacy development.

Some children with language impairments have been observed to use the labeling or following-the-action patterns chronologically later than a child who is developing typically. This suggests that speech-language pathologists and parents need to be particularly sensitive in acquiring books that appeal to a child's interests and level of social-emotional development while continuing to facilitate his or her use of labeling behaviors. Label-type books designed for very young children may not be suitable for a 3- or 4-year-old child with a communicative impairment.

Watkins and Rice (1991) reported that the use of verb particles constitutes a particularly challenging linguistic task for preschool children with language impairments. When a child with a language delay becomes able to use a variety of verbs and verb particles, such as are used in following-the-action reading attempts, a truly important literacy and language milestone has been achieved.

Again, it is particularly important to use books that have a high saliency for a particular child in order to maintain the motivation to perform a task that is difficult. One preschooler with a language impairment whom we observed was especially interested in trains, planes, cars, and trucks, and his mother observed that he would attempt to produce many more verb forms whenever she used storybooks that contained these high-interest items.

Attempts Governed by Pictures, Oral-Like Stories Formed. There are two basic subcategories at this level of emergent reading: dialogic storytelling and monologic storytelling. The basic characteristic of this category is that the speech is intonationally and structurally appropriate to oral, face-to-face recounting of events, either in conversationally structured dialogue or extended discourse.

In dialogic storytelling, it is possible for the listener to infer a weak story line from the child's emergent reading of the book but clarity of the story may be disjointed at times. Usually at the dialogic level, the child looks at the book for more prolonged intervals, this behavior contrasting with that seen at the previous level of "no story formation," in which the child characteristically looked at the listener when giving information. Other behaviors noted to occur at the dialogic storytelling level include the use of "voices" to indicate the various characters and the use of dialogic comments directed toward the listener (e.g., "Look at this").

In addition to these behaviors, the child's sensitivity to the needs of the listener begin to become evident at this level. Although the reenactment is typically contextualized to the picture, the child will begin to use some basic forms that assist in developing the weak story line. This includes the use of present progressive and future tense verbs and a rough story sequence. Two patterns have been detected that will assist the SLP in identifying this structure. Some children create "voices" for characters shown in pictures but rarely use dialogue carriers, such as "he said," or "the bird said to him," to indicate speaker identification. Dialogue may, however, be expressed as indirect quotation, in a typically oral format, "She says she don't wanna." The second pattern is to make conversational overtures and exchanges with the adult in giving the recount.

At the level of monologic storytelling the child begins to tell a complete story, still using characteristics of oral language. Although the story continues to be contextualized to the pictures (which the child assumes both participants can see), the child tells a complete story, without requiring the listener's responses to help "keep it going." The child uses the intonation of face-to-face, oral language, as contrasted with a reading intonation, which will appear at later levels. The child who performs at this level shows ability to sequence the events of a story readily in speech. This level is particularly important for children with language impairments because a relationship has been demonstrated between a child's ability to tell a sequenced story and later reading success (de Hirsch, Janksy, & Langford, 1966).

Sulzby and Zecker (1991) reported that oral monologues are rarely found with middle SES typically developing children in the United States, but are more often detected with LSES and minority children. In a study of LSES Mexican American children, they found a higher frequency of highly developed oral monologues and analyzed internal linguistic structures in these readings, particularly focusing on Spanish reading attempts.

Attempts Governed by Pictures, Written Language–Like Stories Formed. At some point in emergent literacy development, children begin to demonstrate an understanding of written-language conventions. Their reading reenactments at this level fall into three subcategories: reading and storytelling mixed, reading similar-to-original story, and reading verbatim-like story. During reading performances at each of these subcategories, children will demonstrate some written-language linguistic features.

The first subcategory at this level, reading and storytelling mixed, reflects a child's performance that is in transition from an oral production to a production reflecting written-language characteristics. The key feature in these types of reading is fluctuation between speech that sounds appropriate to an oral context and that appropriate for a written context. There should be more than one switch between oral/written forms in the reading attempt. The child's narrative may differ from the actual story, yet the story is recited with a sense of attention to the listener's perspective and some decontextualization. Children from middle SES backgrounds often go from dialogic storytelling to reading and storytelling mixed, skipping monologic storytelling as a level. It can be considered a transition subcategory leading to the next two levels, in which the child sounds like a reader for most of the reading attempt.

If a child performs at the second subcategory, reading similar-to-original story, he or she sounds like a reader while still looking at the pictures as if they were what was read from. Children at this level demonstrate patterns that are very similar to the chosen book. At this level children will decontextualize most of the language that is used and will use reading intonation patterns.

The final subcategory at this level is verbatim-like reading, in which the child shows a marked internalization for stretches of the written text. This level is unique in that the child will appear to self-monitor and self-correct in order to duplicate the remembered text. Children at this level are often described as having "just memorized" the text, but transcripts (Sulzby, 1985a) indicate that the cognitive task is more complex than a verbatim recitation. Instead, the child seems to be attempting to reproduce an internalized representation of the written language contained in the book. Children using the forms of reading similar-to-original story language may sound more reader-like and keep the story closer to the original than do children at the verbatim-like reading level. This is because the overgeneralization and self-correction patterns that help define the verbatim-like reading may lead to some disorganization in local structure and signs of searching for specific wording. The following two examples help to illustrate this phenomenon.

Examples One and Two come from emergent storybook readings of the book *Are You My Mother?* (Eastman, 1960) used in Sulzby (1983, 1996a, 1996b). Children were read this and other storybooks repeatedly in a year-long study conducted in a church-run day-care center. All examples here and in the following sections use pseudonyms for the children. The examples are drawn from pages 22–25 of the book, in which a young bird is in search of his mother, whom he has never seen. He asks each of two animals, a hen and a kitten, "Are you my mother?" In making judgments about emergent literacy, key features of the given book need to be analyzed. In this book, for instance, the key characters, the mother and the baby bird, are introduced specifically in the first few pages; then the baby bird becomes the protagonist throughout the book. The bird is referred to as "he," but young children often overgeneralize the need to give character specification through use of specific nouns or names. In the section these two children are reenacting, the bird is referred to as "he" whereas the new characters are specified by nouns. Additionally, the quoted speech is set off by dialogue carriers after the speech ("he said to the kitten," p. 22).

In Example One, Megan (age 3; 10) gives a similar-to-original reading and, in Example Two, Brian (age 4; 8) gives a verbatim-like reading. Words directly verbatim to the book are shown in capital letters.

Example One:

Megan: Then they CAME TO A KITTEN.
And he said,
"ARE YOU MY MOTHER?"
And THE KITTEN JUST LOOKED AND LOOKED
and looked.
THEN HE CAME TO A HEN—
and said,
"ARE YOU MY MOTHER?"
And the hen said,
"NO-OO."

Example Two:

Brian: CAME TO the kitty.
Said, "ARE YOU MY MOTHER?"
SAID the kitty TO—TO THE, um

(pause, finger in mouth as he appeared to think).

"ARE YOU MY MOTHER?"

said the bird.

THE cat JUST LOOKED at him.

"Are you my mother?"

said—um, said the bird TO THE—HEN.

"NO, I'm a hen."

Megan's similar-to-original emergent reading follows the order of the book and sounds more organized than Brian's verbatim-like example, even though his rendition of the story is classified as the higher of the two. Consistent with a straight-line increase in written language development, he places the dialogue carriers after the speech, in contrast with Megan's preposing of them. Other characteristics illustrate how his usage looks less developed on the surface while actually showing higher development. For example, Brian's emergent literacy knowledge is demostrated in his overgeneralizations about written language structures and his self-corrections, which show evidence of monitoring his speech in relation to an internal model. In the section found in Example Two, Brian overspecifies the dialogue carriers ("said the bird to the—hen"). He attempts to self-correct his attributing the question to the kitty, and he finally gives up and rephrases the question and dialogue carrier.

For a child with a language impairment to reach levels of storybook reenactment containing written-language characteristics such as those shown in the previous three subcategories, he or she not only must understand narrative storytelling structure but must also understand the language differences between oral and written language "codes," within the linguistic community. Tannen (1983) has suggested that children learn to use different language codes or registers depending on the communication goal. Children performing at the written-language level in an emergent storybook elicitation apparently understand the communication goals and perceive the need for increased decontextualization and different linguistic structures when "reading" a book—a milestone in language and literacy development.

Attempts Influenced by Print. The final four subcategories of the classification scheme reflect children's reading reenactments once they demonstrate a fairly stable awareness that it is print that people read rather than the pictures (as was assumed at the previous levels of performance). The levels of reading influenced by print include refusing to read based on print awareness, reading aspectually, reading with strategies imbalanced, and reading conventionally. These categories are very important in the study of the transition into conventional literacy and are discussed at length in Sulzby (1996a, 1996b).

One characteristic indicating a child has become aware of the influence of print is the occurrence of specific "high-level" refusals to read emergently.

High-level refusals are considered a result of the child's awareness of the skills needed for conventional reading. In a high-level refusal, the child might say, "I don't know the words," "I don't know those sounds," or "I can't really read—I was just pretending" (Sulzby, 1985a). In general, the high-level refusals occur in the mature emergent reader as a sudden transition following productions of very complete, written-like storybook reenactments (Sulzby, 1985a).

High-level refusals can be contrasted with low-level refusals, which may result from the child's unfamiliarity with the book, lack of confidence, or difficulty formulating the language to complete the task (a very real possibility for a child with a language impairment). Low-level refusals are shown by the child's repeated silence or head shaking when asked to read and when encouraged. They are also shown by the child's subsequent low level of responsiveness in adult-child interactive reading (Otto, 1984) and continued refusal to take over the reading when told, "Now it's your turn—you read."

Reading aspectually, the next subcategory, is important from a theoretical standpoint (Sulzby, 1996a). Here the child appears to be bringing together knowledge from other interactions with print, including emergent writing, word exploration, and phonologically oriented speech play and instruction. Three types of reading behavior appear to be functionally equivalent, but in all three types, the child focuses on print as the source of the reading. He or she attempts to read from print but focuses on only one or two aspects of the print to the exclusion of other features. Some children give a reading focusing on one aspect, and others switch between aspects. The three aspects are a comprehension focus, a letter-sound focus, or a focus on knowledge of words. Children who focus on comprehension read much like children at a verbatim-like reading level, but they point to the print or look closely at it without tracking it accurately. One child (Sulzby, 1985a) pointed to print left to right, but moved from bottom to top frequently in her reading. When she neglected pointing for stretches, she often added more speech and began to point even after she had covered the semantic content of the story text that had been read to her. Other children sound out text to nonsense words, seeming to ignore the semantic content. Others focus on known words by appearing to search through the text and just list words that sound like a random list ("a, and, the, a, a, the, the, the, too many the's, grandma!") Sulzby (1994) suggested this is an important level of development during which the child is practicing particular aspects of reading in performances that will be integrated in the next levels of reading development.

The final two categories describe print-governed performances during which the child is becoming able to read "holistically" from print (Sulzby, 1985a). In both these levels, the child is tracking the print by pointing or showing evidence of accurate tracking in reproducing a spoken word for most or all printed word units. Most children at this level point, but a close watch of the eyes and record of miscues and self-corrections help verify that it is the text that is being read. The first of these holistic levels is called reading with strategies imbalanced. This type of reading is different from the aspectual level because during reading with strategies imbalanced, the child is able to use a variety of processes to track and decode text. However, at this level the strategies are not completely integrated or flexible. The child may sporadically use "known words" to substitute for unknown words, leave out words, or resort periodically to remembered text versus written text. The final level, reading conventionally, describes reading performances with an increased level of self-regulation and flexibility. When the child at this level makes a mistake, he or she now more adequately self-corrects the errors. Technically, the level is defined by evidence of flexible and coordinated use of the three aspects of reading shown in the two previous levels. Additionally, children at this final level more frequently make comments that indicate awareness of the meaning of the text.

Children who begin to read conventionally may first piece together the aspects of reading with long and complex familiar texts; many of these children soon revert to reading very short and simple books that they had lost interest in previously but now again find interesting because these simple texts are easy to process conventionally. Many children spend much time appearing to "practice" this new skill, particularly orally; others seem to develop fluency quickly and remain with complex texts; and some do both. Children also begin to show interest and pride in reading new or unfamiliar texts and talking about texts they have read.

It is at this final level of conventional level of reading performance that most traditional measures of reading achievement begin. However, the SLP or teacher with an emergent literacy perspective acknowledges the complex patterns of oral and written language understanding that are forerunners of conventional reading. Thus, for the child with a communicative impairment, mastery of yet another language context is an important milestone in language development. This classification scheme for emergent reading can be useful to the SLP as a means of documenting a child's internalization of written language concepts as well as a means of monitoring changes in emergent literacy development over time. A child who struggles in achieving more sophisticated levels of emergent reading may be at particular risk for later reading problems. Some children continue to use emergent reading strategies well into the primary grades, while their peers are becoming proficient conventional readers. Understanding the steps of emergent reading leading to conventional reading can assist in developing a reading intervention program that builds on the child's current written language competencies.

EMERGENT LITERACY ISSUES WITH CHILDREN WITH SPECIFIC LANGUAGE IMPAIRMENT (SLI): CURRENT RESEARCH AND CLINICAL APPLICATIONS

In our most current research (Kaderavek & Sulzby, 1994), we examined the issue of oral-written language contrasts as it occurs with both typically developing 2-, 3-, and 4-year-old children and children of similar ages with language delays. All the children were white children from MSES homes near a middle-sized midwestern city. The data collected from this research permits examination of oral-written language from two different perspectives. First, in order to examine interactive language patterns, we contrast parent-child interactive language as it occurs in a more oral-language situation (toy play) and a more written-language-like situation (storybook reading). Second, in order to examine children's independent language productions, we contrast children's productions of storytelling narratives (a more oral-language task) with children's emergent readings of a favorite storybook (a more written-language task). We will first discuss our observations of parent-child dyadic interactions in storybook reading and toy play contexts.

Parent-Child Storybook and Toy Play Interactions

Research has begun to identify the importance of examining how situational differences affect the behavior and language of the participants. Such variation was demonstrated when comparing children in the two contexts described in the following discussion.

Current Research. As previously mentioned, even young children respond to variations in context and alter their language and behaviors accordingly. For example, Sulzby (1986) demonstrated that 5- and 6-year-old, typically developing children's language performances were different in response to more oral-like tasks (responding to a request to tell a story) versus a more written-like task (responding to a request to dictate a story for an adult to record). Others have demonstrated differences in the interaction and language performance of the participants when comparing father-child versus mother-child conversational dyads of children with SLI (Conti-Ramsden, Hutcheson, & Grove, 1995).

Our research compares toy play and storybook reading interactions for a group of typically developing children and those with SLI. In our preliminary analyses we have been particularly interested in comparing children with SLI who enjoyed storybook reading with other children with SLI who were unwilling participants in book interactions with their parents. Such comparisons may be particularly helpful in understanding the difficulty some children with language delays demonstrate in later reading achievement. To illustrate some of the variation we have noted in this regard, we present data from two preschoolers with language impairments, John and Andrew. Both boys were observed as part of a larger research study over a 3-week period in 12 mother-child in-home interactions. Each was videotaped interacting repeatedly with a storybook and a toy. Although both John and Andrew showed evidence of enjoying their interaction with the toy (a city scene containing small figures of people, cars, pretend mail, and so on), John was observed to enjoy the book *Sam Vole and His Brothers* (Waddell, 1992), whereas Andrew showed some resistance.

All data presented here were obtained during the third mother-child interaction with the city scene or *Sam Vole* storybook. A 4-minute sample was taken from each interaction, with 1 minute being taken from the beginning of the interaction, 2 minutes from the middle of each interaction, and another 1-minute sample from the end of the interaction. In general, storybook interactions lasted 8 to 10 minutes in length whereas toy play interactions lasted for the full 30 minutes allotted. To keep measures such as mean length of utterance from being confounded by the book's text, the language data used for the storybook analysis included only the mother's interactive speech.

John, age 3;1, had been diagnosed as language impaired before being recruited into this study. He had received speech-language therapy prior to his participation in the study, but was not receiving therapy at the time of his in-home observations. In our research assessment protocol, John received a receptive language standard score of 91 (27th percentile rank), which placed his receptive performance within normal limits, and an expressive language standard score of 65 (1st percentile rank), which indicated a severe expressive disorder as measured by the *Clinical Evaluation of Language Fundamentals–Preschool* (Wiig, Secord, & Semel, 1992). Consistent with a diagnosis of SLI, John scored within normal limits, in cognitive performance using a nonverbal intelligence text, and had normal hearing. John's phonological development was within normal limits and he was approximately 90 percent intelligible.

John's spontaneous language was pragmatically and semantically appropriate. His expressive language delay was characterized by immature syntax use and reduced sentence length. These aspects of his language delay are demonstrated in this excerpt (Example Three) from John's third toy play interaction with the city scene:

Example Three:

John: Gas fell down.

Comment: GAS PUMP FALLS OVER.

Mother: Fill 'er up!

John: Oh boy.

John: I buy the gas.

Mother: Does that little boy have any money to pay for the gas?

John: Yep.

Mother: How much?

John: Two.

Mother: Two what?

John: Two gas.

Mother: Oh.
John: All done!
Mother: All done?
Mother: Thank you.
Comment: PRETENDS TO PAY FOR GAS.
John: I welcome.
John: Uh, more gas!
Mother: More gas already?
John: Yep.
Mother: Jeesh!
John: Uh!
Comment: CAR ROLLS DOWN RAMP.
John: Uh!
Mother: Did they get in a car accident?
John: Uh!
John: No.
Mother: Are you sure?
John: No.
Mother: Heres [*sic*] comes the mailman.
John: I want gas.
John: I (unintelligible word), I (unintelligible word) the mail.
John: Stop, gas!
Mother: You want the mailman to get gas?
John: Yeh.
Mother: All right.
Mother: Beep, beep!
Mother: Beep, beep!
Mother: Get out of my way!
John: No.
Mother: It's my turn to get gas.
Comment: PUSHES CAR TO GAS PUMP.
John: My turn get gas!
John: Let me in!
John: Me in too.
John: Me in, mama!
Mother: Huh?

John: That not no nice.
John: That not nice.
Mother: That's not nice.
John: No.

The data for John and his mother during toy play are summarized in Table 7-1. As the data demonstrate, both mother and child participated fairly equally in the toy play context, with John producing about 47 percent of the total utterances and his mother, 53 percent, of which 42 percent consisted of questions. Many of these questions were used to clarify the ongoing play. Some examples included, "Is this a girl baby or a boy baby?", "Is the fireman her Dad?", and "Where does that go?"

The balance of interaction between John and his mother was similar in the storybook interaction as compared to the toy play interaction, with John producing about 44 percent of the total utterances and his mother, producing 56 perent. John's mean length of utterance (MLU) during the storybook reading stayed approximately the same as his utterance length during toy play, as did his mother's. John's type/token ratio (TTR) (a ratio of novel words compared to the total number of words produced) stayed within the same range during both interactions. John's mother's TTR was reduced in book reading, perhaps as a means of scaffolding the book's text to John's level. John's mother produced approximately the same number of questions as she did during toy play, 49 percent. Whereas the majority of her questions during toy play were mostly direct (requiring an answer), now her questions were more evenly di-

Table 7-1. Comparison of Language Data Within Storybook and Toy Contexts for John, a Child With Specific Language Impairment

Storybook Interaction	Toy Interaction
John	
.489 type/token ratio	.454 type/token ratio
46 utterances	62 utterances
44% of utterances	47% of utterances
2.261 mean length of utterance	2.290 mean length of utterance
John's Mother	
.335 type/token ratio	.450 type/token ratio
59 utterances	71 utterances
56% of utterances	53% of utterances
4.627 mean length of utterance	4.127 mean length of utterance
49% questions	42% questions
12 direct	26 direct
17 rhetorical	4 rhetorical

vided between direct and rhetorical (not requiring an answer) types. Some examples of rhetorical questions included, "You think?" and "Is there?" Direct questions included, "Do you think he's scared?", "What are they all doing?", and "Who did he see?" Example Four represents an excerpt from John's storybook interaction.

Example Four:

Mother: Look who has more grass ?

Comment: LOOKS AT THE PICTURE OF SAM HOLDING A SMALL AMOUNT OF GRASS WHEREAS HIS BROTHERS HOLD QUITE A LOT.

Mother: They do?

Comment: JOHN POINTS AT PICTURE OF SAM.

Mother: Look Sam has just a little.

John: Yeh Sam have little.

Mother: 'Cause he's just little.

John: I little.

John: They're big!

Mother: They're big!

Mother: Yeh!

Overall John appeared to enjoy both the toy play and storybook interactions and seemed comfortable initiating comments in both contexts.

We now turn to our observation of a second preschooler with a language impairment, Andrew, age 3;6. Andrew was enrolled in a special preschool for children with language delays through his local school district at the time of his participation in our research. Andrew received a composite receptive language standard score of 84 (14th percentile rank), which indicated that his receptive language abilities were mildly impaired, and a composite expressive language standard score of 50 (below the 1st percentile rank), which indicated a severe expressive disorder as measured by the Clinical Evaluation of Language Fundamentals–Preschool (Wiig et al., 1992). As was required for eligibility in our study, Andrew scored within normal limits in cognitive performance using a nonverbal intelligence test and passed a hearing screening. Andrew had a phonological deficit as well as his language impairment. He was 40 to 50 percent intelligible to a novel listener; however, the investigator was able to understand 80 to 90 percent of his productions after observing him throughout the 3-week period of in-home visits. Andrew was also noted to have a higher-than-typical number of disfluencies characterized by part-word repetitions. No struggle or avoidance behaviors were noted in conjunction with these disfluent behaviors.

As indicated by his MLU in the toy play and storybook interactions, Andrew usually communicated using one- to three-word utterances. He showed deficiency in his use of verb forms, using only the unmarked verbs "do," "get," "go," and "turn," during his 4-minute sample of toy play interaction, and was noted to omit plurals and articles. However, during toy play Andrew took an active part in the conversational interaction, producing 54 percent of the utterances. In fact, he assumed a leadership role within the toy play context by directing his mother's activity and disapproving of certain play sequences that she would suggest. These aspects of his interactive style can be seen in Example Five:

Example 5:

Mother: Am I him?

Andrew: No.

Mother: Or her?

Andrew: No y-you.

Comment: POINTS TO MAIL PERSON.

Mother: I'm the mail lady?

Andrew: M-Mom t-two you.

Comment: GIVES HIS MOTHER TWO FIGURES.

Mother: Two?

Andrew: M-Mom y-you.

Andrew: M-mine.

Comment: SHOWS MOTHER THE FIGURES HE WANTS.

Andrew: 'kay ?

Andrew: 'kay mom?

Mother: 'kay.

Andrew: M-Mom mine lady.

Mother: You're gonna be the lady or you want me to?

Andrew: M-Mom y-you that lady.

Mother: Okay.

Andrew: Vroom.

Comment: PUSHES CAR.

Mother: Here.

Mother: You're going to be these two Andrew?

Andrew: Yes.

Andrew: Mom you go!

Comment: INDICATES MOTHER IS TO DRIVE MAIL TRUCK.

Andrew: Vroom!

The data for Andrew and his mother in the toy play context are summarized in Table 7-2. Andrew's mother produced about 31 percent questions during the toy play interaction, the majority of which were rhetorical in nature. Some examples of her rhetorical questions included, "Should we put it away?" and "Are you sure she can fit?" Some direct questions included, "Where did that baby go now?" and "What do you want me to do with this?"

Whereas Andrew was eager to interact with the toys during his in-home observations, he did not appear to enjoy storybook reading. Andrew's overt behavior at these times consisted of verbalizing loud sighs, slumping down on the couch (sometimes lying down with his head away from his mother or even sliding off the couch), and once, during the book-reading interaction analyzed here, putting his stockinged feet on the book and obscuring the page.

We should note that both John and Andrew were observed interacting with an additional toy and book as part of the larger research project. This second set of items was selected by each subject's mother to make sure that we presented high-interest books and toys. John's and Andrew's reactions were the same in this second set of interactions, demonstrating that these data were not idiosyncratic to a particular book or toy item.

Example Six is illustrative of Andrew and his mother during a book-reading interaction. Rather than selecting an excerpt in which Andrew did not respond at all to his mother's questions (which occurred frequently), the following was chosen because it was one of the segments during which he was most responsive. Even so, Andrew's interaction was quite different than that which occurred during toy play.

Table 7-2. Comparison of Language Data Within Storybook and Toy Contexts for Andrew, a Child With Specific Language Impairment

Storybook Interaction	Toy Interaction
Andrew	
.515 type/token ratio	.396 type/token ratio
21 utterance	57 utterances
18% of utterances	54% of utterances
1.667 mean length of utterance	1.825 mean length of utterance
Andrew's Mother	
.353 type/token ratio	.542 type/token ratio
98 utterances	49 utterances
82% of utterances	46% of utterances
5.347 mean length of utterance	4.0 mean length of utterance
55% questions	31% questions
23 direct	4 direct
31 rhetorical	11 rhetorical

Example Six:

Mother: I forget which one's you.

Comment: MOTHER PERSONALIZES STORY, MAKING ONE CHARACTER (SAM) REPRESENT ANDREW AND OTHER CHARACTERS REPRESENT ANDREW'S BROTHERS.

Mother: Hmmm?

Mother: I don't remember.

Comment: ANDREW POINTS.

Mother: Oh that's you.

Mother: And that's who?

Andrew: Me (whispers).

Mother: Huh?

Andrew: Me (whispers).

Mother: That's you?

Andrew: A (unintelligible word) (whispers).

Mother: Oh that's you this time?

Andrew: Yes (two unintelligible words) (whispers).

Mother: And who's this ?

Andrew: Paul.

Comment: ANDREW'S OLDER BROTHER.

Mother: Paul?

Mother: And who's this?

Andrew: Buddy (whispers).

Comment: ANDREW'S YOUNGER BROTHER.

Mother: Buddy, yeh (laughs) the littlest one!

Andrew: Yeh.

Mother: Yeh.

Mother: Okay.

Mother: You know what else?

Mother: They were eating eggs!

Mother: Does he like to eat eggs?

Andrew: Yeh.

Mother: Yes he does!

Mother: Aah!

Mother: There's the bug people again!

Mother: Look at that.

Mother: Now I wonder if we can find anymore of those guys?
Mother: This guy's sleepin'.
Mother: Does he have (two unintelligible words) (whispers)?
Mother: He's taking a nap (whispers).
Mother: Isn't he?
Mother: He doesn't want any breakfast.

The balance of interaction between Andrew and his mother in the storybook interaction was quite different as compared to the toy play interaction. Andrew's mother's percentage of utterances rose to 82 percent, while Andrew's dropped to 18 percent. Another difference was Andrew's mother's fairly significant increase in question production, to 55 percent as compared with 31 percent during toy play. She used many more direct questions than she had during toy play. Some examples of the direct questions used by Andrew's mother in the book interaction include, "What's another picture you like?", "What kind are those?", and "Why does he do that?"

Andrew's MLU during book reading stayed approximately the same as was produced in toy play, but his mother's MLU rose from 4.0 in the toy play interaction to 5.347 in the book reading interaction. Andrew's use of a greater variety of words increased, as measured by his TTR in the storybook reading, which rose to .515 from a TTR of .396 in toy play. However since he produced only half as many utterances, the smaller sample size during the book-reading may have inflated this ratio. Like John's mother, Andrew's mother's TTR was reduced during the book-reading interaction, indicating the possibility of her attempt to scaffold the book's text to Andrew's language level.

The overarching observation is that the interactive style of John and his mother stayed approximately the same between contexts (as measured by number of utterances produced by John and his mother and number of the mother's questions), whereas these variables changed in Andrew's case (observed loss of balanced interaction and increase in mother's use of questions). Further, the changes occurring for Andrew and his mother during the storybook interaction did not appear to facilitate a positive response. Although these results cannot yet be generalized to the larger population of children with language impairments, our case-by-case examination of these data has made us attentive to the difficulties that emerge for children with language delays when strong contextual shifts occur in parental expectations and language demands. It appears that for some children with SLI, the use of parental practices in relation to the child's development makes the transition from a more contextualized interaction (toy play) to a less contextualized interaction (storybook reading) unrewarding, and sometimes even unpleasant.

In general, when an SLP is faced with a situation like Andrew's, the best suggestion appears to be telling the parent to focus on mutual enjoyment of the storybook rather than using the storybook as a more direct method of "language teaching." Although Andrew's mother's efforts to bring her son into the interaction through direct questioning were well-motivated, this effort did not elicit a positive response from Andrew. This focus on mutual engagement stems from the Vygotskian conceptualization highlighting the importance of mutual engagement and reciprocal interaction in language learning.

These data also suggest that caution is needed in making recommendations about helping parents facilitate mutual engagement in storybook reading. We are concerned about the potential dangers of certain "prescriptive" approaches to educating parents about storybook-reading practices. We are particularly concerned about approaches that would make one set of narrowly defined recommendations for all children.

For example, some researchers in the area of emergent literacy have promoted a method of interactive reading in which parents are trained to use specific questioning strategies with their preschool children (DeBaryshe, 1992; Whitehurst et al., 1994). As part of this training, parents are asked to focus initially on asking what-questions (e.g., "What is this?"), attribute-questions (e.g., "What color is this?), and completion prompts. These are seen as being at a level of "low demand." With older children, parents are asked to increase the level of demand by asking more "distancing questions" (e.g., "how" or "why" questions). Parents are asked to use approximately two to three of these strategies on each page of a storybook.

DeBaryshe (1992) studied 73 low-income children (ages 26 to 60 months) and their parents, of whom 78 percent were African American and the remainder were white. The 25 percent attrition rate found for children and parents who began the study was quite high. The 18 children who dropped out were noted to be significantly different from children who remained in the intervention study. They had significantly lower scores on the Illinois Test of Psycholinguistic Abilities (Kirk, McCarthy, & Kirk, 1968) and were rated by their mothers as not enjoying being read to and not asking for books to be read to them.

This dropout rate could be due to reactions such as we have found with some children with SLI who have disliked being read to and who have responded negatively to their mothers when they used the kinds of questions or the high frequency of questioning that are part of the DeBaryshe (1992) and Whitehurst et al. (1988) procedures. For example, such a recommendation to Andrew's mother might have encouraged her to try even harder to engage Andrew through the use of questions, an avenue unlikely to bring about his increased participation. It is premature to speculate on specific treatment recommendations in cases such as these. However, we can begin the process of understanding how to help children like Andrew by using some basic principles of emergent literacy practice in clinical settings, and it is to these practices that we will now turn.

Clinical Applications. How do these data influence SLPs in regard to the clinical application of emergent literacy perspectives? Most important, these data suggest that there are important reasons to include observation of parent-child book reading interactions into our ongoing work with children with communicative impairments. Speech-language pathologists have always carefully considered the communication dynamics between the child with language impairment and his or her primary caregiver when designing an intervention program. A toy play interaction in which the parent is asked to play with their child while the SLP observes the interaction is a frequently used and valuable observational situation. We would suggest that observation of a shared book reading can provide key and complementary information. But, as noted in Table 7-3, in order to get the most information from a book-reading interaction we must watch repeated book readings over time. It has been reported that children and parents frequently use more sophisticated language and ask different questions with repeated readings (Goodsitt, Raitan, & Perlmutter, 1988; Martinez & Roser, 1985; Snow & Ninio, 1986; Yaden, 1988). Repeated readings are one way in which parents bring the world of written language to children. Our observations of storybook interactions can assist our understanding of a parent's ability to interpret the book's text to his or her child and the child's internalization of these language patterns within a routinized language context.

One of the most significant methods that a parent uses to "negotiate" a book's text to the child's level of understanding is through language scaffolding. Scaffolding has been forwarded as an explanation of how parents interact with their children during storybook reading (Ninio, 1983; Snow, 1983; Sulzby & Edwards, 1993; Teale, 1984). Several aspects of scaffolding appear to be particularly important for a child's emergent literacy development. One

Table 7-3. Guidelines for Setting Up Parent-Child Book-Reading Interactions

1. Pick a narrative-type storybook and avoid brief pattern-type book. A narrative book is one that has characters, a setting, and a plot. Research has demonstrated that with narratives children have the opportunity to internalize complex patterns and written language constructions, whereas with pattern books children tend to rely on rote memorization (Sulzby, 1991).
2. Observe the storybook interaction in the home or provide a home-like setting in your clinic or school. Literacy learning comes about because of the shared pleasure surrounding the literacy event. It's hard for an adult to enjoy the interaction when forced to sit at a table made for young children! Provide a couch or big chair—or even pillows on the floor—to observe the kinds of nonverbal interactions that occur around the storybook reading.
3. Let the parent or child pick the book whenever possible—or if you pick the book, be sensitive to the child's age and interests.
4. Observe more than one reading of the book. Children's concepts of the book will change, and this development will be reflected in their changing comments and questions. Watching repeated readings also allows the SLP to observe the parent's sensitivity to the child's changing levels of understanding.

factor is the parent's ability to encourage the child's verbalizations and to adjust his or her own speech to the child's gradually increasing competence with the written language forms in the storybook. A second factor is the parent's willingness to let the child lead the storybook interaction as soon as he or she is ready to "take charge" of the reading interaction to some extent. In general, many of these scaffolding behaviors appear to change as the child's developmental level and familiarity with the storybook increase (Teale & Sulzby, 1987). Overall, there appears to be a generalized change, from a parental labeling of pictures toward a more frequent occurrence of reading the written text without modification.

A word of caution is needed in regard to tracking parents' changing levels of language scaffolding in their book reading interactions. Although we have observed parents generally moving from picture labeling (e.g., with very young children) to straight reading of the text, these behaviors do not occur in a strict hierarchy. A parent who is effective in engaging his or her child will move freely between levels as the child's interest and attention fluctuate. The implication of this finding is that SLPs will not only want to observe storybook interaction over a period of time but will also observe parents' flexible use of a variety of strategies that are responsive to the type of book, the child's understanding of the ideas contained in the book, and the child's willingness to participate in the book reading on a particular day. A list of the scaffolding interactions frequently seen in parent-child storybook interactions (Kaderavek & Sulzby, 1995) are listed in Table 7-4.

A final note is our finding that all book reading does not have to be "highly interactive" to be successful in accomplishing the goals of engaging children and exposing them to written language. We have observed that in some cases, children actually prefer to have their parent "just read the book," particularly if they are accustomed to being read to and/or as they grow older. In the instance that one is observing a book-reading interaction that is not highly interactive, one can monitor the verbal ("Read another book, Mommy!") and nonverbal indicators (e.g., attending, running to get more books) to assess its success. Additionally, the SLP can (as we do in our research) intermingle parent-child storybook observation with requests for the child to read the book emergently. The emergent readings provide information that helps monitor the child's degree of internalization of the book's language.

Children's Narrative Production: Oral and Written Contexts

In this section we will examine children's production of narratives and their emerging awareness of the differences between oral narratives and written narratives.

Current Research. Our second area of inquiry into oral-written language differences is the examination of the difference between narrative develop-

Table 7-4. Scaffolding Behaviors Frequently Used by Parents During Storybook Reading

1. Labeling and commenting on items in the pictures is one of the behaviors parents demonstrate with very young children during storybook reading. While using this technique, parents often use exaggerated nonverbal communication (gestures, motions, and facial reactions) while naming the pictures.
2. Pausing behaviors are used by parents to provide opportunities for the child to interact during the book-reading exchange. We have observed that pausing seems to function as a means of keeping the child involved in the book without having to question directly or "teach."
3. Parents often use questioning behaviors during book reading. Although questioning can be an effective strategy if not overused, our preliminary data indicate that some language-impaired children do not react favorably to direct questioning during parent-child book reading.
4. Parents often engage in oral dialogue during their storybook reading. Rather than actually reading the book, they will present the story line in an oral form. Clues to this kind of scaffolding are the use of "voices" to indicate the various characters and the use of oral- versus written-language intonation characteristics. At this level the parent may also make connections between the story and situations or vocabulary with which the child is familiar.
5. Sometimes the parents begin to actually read the book but simplify the vocabulary and the syntax of the written text. The intonation patterns of the adult reader may begin to sound like written language—but the parent will alter the text to maintain the child's understanding and interest.
6. Finally, parents begin to read the text verbatim, not in long stretches but in attempts staggered between other scaffolding behaviors. Eventually, the child may ask for the parent to read the entire book verbatim, although we have not yet observed that with our subjects. Parents who read stretches verbatim also often use other internal scaffolding behaviors such as pausing, stopping with rising inflection (to encourage the child to complete the sentence), or stopping to discuss the story when the child appears interested or asks questions.
7. Parents who maintainz a high level of the child's interest and engagement appear to be very sensitive to their child's reactions; they show flexible use of these scaffolding strategies in relation to the child's verbal and nonverbal behaviors.

Source: Kaderavek, J. N., & Sulzby, E. (1994). Literacy contexts and oral language in SLI children. Proposal to National Institutes of Health

ment in a more oral storytelling context versus the emergent reading task developed by Sulzby (1985a). Narratives are particularly important for observation because it has been suggested that narrative discourse development is significantly related to children's emergent literacy (Dickinson & McCabe, 1991) and to successful adaptation to school literacy (Feagans, 1982). This relationship was demonstrated by Roth and Spekman (1986), who found that older children with learning disabilities (who had normal intelligence but had difficulties in reading, written expression, and/or math) had difficulty with the construction of oral narratives.

In our research program we elicit two kinds of narratives, an oral storytelling narrative and an emergent reading, which we consider to be a narrative elicited in a written language context. The protocol to elicit the emergent reading has already been described in this chapter. To elicit the oral storytelling narrative, we use the protocol suggested by Peterson and McCabe (1983). These authors suggest that in order to get a narrative, one needs to tell a narrative. Following this protocol, the adults tell the preschoolers several stories (mostly centering on occasions in which they were hurt or frightened—topics that appear to elicit the best responses from the children) and encourage them to respond with a story of their own (see McCabe & Rollins, 1994, for a recent discussion of this protocol). At least three narratives are elicited from each child and the best narrative obtained is used for analysis.

To illustrate some of the differences in oral versus written-language narrative attempts, we present excerpts from narratives produced by Adam, a typically developing child age 3;5 who participated in our research. Adam's oral narrative appears below (Example Seven). (The ellipsis is used in spoken narratives to indicate a non-final intonation contour; it does not signal an omission.) The investigator told a story about when she was hurt and got stitches and then asked Adam the following question:

Example Seven:

Investigator:	Has anything ever happened to you like that?
Adam:	When I fall down.
Adam:	And when I move the slide this way.
Comment:	MAKES A MOTION WITH HIS HANDS.
Adam:	And I fall down like . . .
Comment:	MOVES BODY IN BIG MOTION.
Adam:	I got stitches right here.
Comment:	POINTS TO THE INSIDE OF HIS CHEEK.

One of the most striking characteristics about this oral narrative was the lack of decontextualization. The narrative was told with motions and incomplete sentences. In fact, this narrative really does not stand alone, but actually appeared to function as a discourse "turn." Overall, it appeared to be a response to the investigator's story about being injured.

According to the narrative assessment protocol (McCabe & Rollins, 1994), Adam's oral narrative above was classified as an end-at-high-point narrative. He did not include the evaluative comments that would reveal the meaning that the event had for him as narrator. Similarly, this narrative did not have any resolution comments that served to wind up the crisis. Although this was not a classic narrative (a classic narrative contains all the features needed for a complete narrative), this kind of end-at-high-point narrative was very good for a child of Adam's age.

Contrast this with the narrative produced by Adam in his emergent reading of the storybook, *Sam Vole and His Brothers.* While Adam read emergently, he stared intently at the pictures, used a quiet voice for "reading" and a louder voice for his comments directed to the investigator, and commented on each picture as he turned the pages. His emergent reading (Example Eight) was as follows:

Example Eight:

Adam: One day we're picking some flowers.

Comment: ADAM USES A QUIET VOICE IN THIS EMERGENT READING EXCEPT WHERE INDICATED.

Adam: And one day, he was break some eggs.

Investigator: Uhhuh

Adam: And the, his brother is breaking some eggs.

Adam: One day, he was stealing some nuts.

Adam: And one day, he was getting some grass.

Adam: And one day, he's give them to his mother.

Adam: And one day, they was too asleep.

Adam: And one day, there's, they was quiet.

Adam: And one day, they goes alone.

Adam: And he singed, and he singed.

Adam: And he goes alone.

Adam: And he jumped.

Adam: And then he go to sad.

Adam: Remember that?

Comment: SAID LOUDER AND DIRECTED AT INVESTIGATOR.

Adam: That is a cricket!

Comment: SAID LOUDLY TO INVESTIGATOR.

Investigator: That's neat.

Adam: That is a cricket!

Comment: SAID LOUDLY WHILE LOOKING AT PICTURE.

Adam: And one day . . .

Adam: And one day he be be he be he be he be very quiet.

Adam: Hey!

Adam: He (unintelligible two words).

Adam: Then he (unintelligible word).

Adam: And then.

Adam: And then he saw his brothers!
Adam: And he saw his brothers.
Adam: And one day . . .
Adam: He and his brother . . .
Adam: And one day . . .
Adam: The bugs are eating!
Comment: SAID TO INVESTIGATOR.
Investigator: Uhhuh.
Adam: And he's (unintelligible word) to eat.
Adam: And he's (unintelligible word) smiling.
Investigator: Everybody's happy!
Adam: The end!

Adam's emergent reading presented here demonstrated characteristics of both written and oral language. Accordingly, using the Sulzby (1985a) Classification Scheme for Emergent Reading of Favorite Storybooks, this emergent reading was classified at the level of "reading and storytelling mixed." Some of the components that demonstrated Adam's switching between the oral (storytelling) and written language (reading) modes in the text in this example included his varying use of verb tense and his vacillation between clear and unclear introduction of characters.

At times Adam used verbs in a manner consistent with written language. Examples of this include his past tense use of "He singed" and "He jumped." Additionally, he used a stative form, as in "He be quiet" (used to describe the characteristics of the protagonist, Sam). In contrast, at other times, Adam used verb forms consistent with oral language use. Examples of this included his use of the present progressive verbs, "He be picking," and "The bugs are eating."

Adam's second vacillation between oral and written forms occurred around his use of varying levels of decontextualization in his character introduction. Adam sometimes used specific, and at other times unspecific, introductions of the characters in the story. For example, toward the end of the story he stated, "And he saw his brother!", a decontextualized form that is characteristic of written language use. (A less decontextualized form would be "And he saw them!") However, an example of a more oral contextualized language form occurred in the initial sentences of the written narrative when Adam stated: "One day we're picking some flowers. And one day he was break some eggs."

It is enlightening to compare Adam's oral (Example Seven) and written (Example Eight) narratives. Several differences are obvious. The first is the difference in length, with the written narrative being quite a bit longer. Second, one can notice the variety of verbs used in the written narrative, in contrast to the verbs "fall," "move," and "got," which occur in the oral narrative. Less obvious, but significant, was Adam's differing decontextualization in the written versus the oral narrative. In fact, had we not elicited both types of narratives, we would have been unaware of his ability to decontextualize. His oral narrative, "And I fall down like . . .", did not reflect his ability to tell a story in a way that permitted a nonpresent listener to understand the gist of what was happening in the narrative.

Finally, it was interesting to note that Adam completed his emergent reading almost completely independently. Other than the few acknowledgments that the investigator made when addressed directly (e.g., "Remember that? That's a cricket."), Adam was able to complete this task alone. This is especially significant when we contrast this emergent reading to that of an older preschooler with language delays who elicited much assistance in his emergent reading (see the case study of "Timmy" in this chapter).

Adam still has some areas that will develop as he moves toward higher levels such as reading-similar-to-original and a verbatim-like story. Most significantly, his ability to decontextualize the story (e.g., introducing the characters first by name and then using pronouns when referring to them) and his ability to re-create longer sentences (that are similar to the written text) will improve. His ability to produce the written narrative that he did at the age of 3½, however, was quite good.

Clinical Applications. The differences in Adam's oral and written narratives have implications for remediation of children with limited ability to produce narratives. It may be that children are able to explore more of the complexities of narrative structure when retelling a story that has been read to them as compared to the demands of creating a novel story in an oral storytelling mode. Future research data and ongoing input from SLPs who use emergent reading activities in their clinical practice will shed further light on the usefulness of emergent reading as a tool to developing increasingly spontaneous narrative productions. However, we feel that even these preliminary data indicated that eliciting children's narratives in response to written, as well as oral, contexts offered a more complete look at their understanding of language and their ability to vary language in response to contextual demands.

This research—along with work being done by other emergent literacy researchers and results of the clinical applications reported by SLPs—will continue to highlight the particular language forms and discourse patterns occurring in relationship to varying oral and written contexts. Overall, our preliminary data suggest that even at the early ages of language development, children and their parents have clearly differentiated the demands of written and oral language contexts. This kind of examination will provide SLPs the opportunity to explore and observe the developing language of young children in even broader arenas.

CASE STUDY: TIMMY

Timmy is a boy aged 4;1 who has been diagnosed with specific expressive language impairment (SLI). He is from an European American, middle-economic level home. Timmy, his parents, his two sisters (ages 13 and 2), and his young brother (age 2 months) live in a two-story, older home in a small town near a midsized midwestern city.

There is no known cause of Timmy's language delay. He was born following an uneventful pregnancy and delivery. Other than his expressive language delay and some articulation delay, Timmy has been typically developing. At 4;1, he performed within normal ranges on a nonverbal intelligence test, and his receptive language abilities tested within the average range. His hearing was also normal. Timmy's utterances ranged from one to six words in length. He obtained a standard score of 3 on the Recalling Sentences in Context Subtest of the Clinical Evaluation of Language Fundamentals–Preschool (CELF-P) and a standard score of 5 on the Word Structure Subtest of the CELF-P. Timmy was within normal limits on all other subtests of the CELF-P.

Timmy's mother first noticed his language delay between 12 and 18 months. She discussed her concerns with her pediatrician, but was told to "wait and see what happens." At age 2½, she had him evaluated at the speech and hearing clinic at a local university, where he went for one semester of therapy. She stated that she was taught to model language for Timmy and decided she would read to him every day, "no matter what."

Timmy's mother described how she began an accelerated program of language stimulation, in consultation with the speech-language pathologist. In the last year and a half she has "talked to him one-on-one all the time," along with daily storybook reading. She said that she feels that if Timmy is interested in a topic, she will try to expose him to whatever they are discussing because he "needs to go out and actively see it."

In describing why she feels storybooks have been particularly important for Timmy, Timmy's mother stated: "Reading brings so many new words into light. Things you normally wouldn't talk about." She indicated that usually she and her son will talk about their most current storybook on and off throughout the day.

Along with his mother's efforts at home, Timmy has benefited from enrollment in a county preschool program for children with developmental delays. His mother indicated that the stimulation of the other children had been particularly important in facilitating Timmy's desire to communicate.

As part of the authors' ongoing research, Timmy was observed over a period of 1 month during storybook reading and toy play interaction and was asked to produce emergent readings (which we consider to be an opportunity to produce a written narrative) and oral storytelling narratives. The following is an example of Timmy's oral narrative. This story was produced in response to the investigator telling him a story of a camping trip she had recently completed. "Wait, first one tell me a me. And my wa. . . . And my. . . . And my my go park. And my Dad. . . . Take me. Da . . . and me. . . . Mayway a park play. . . . With her it come dark up. Go home. And . . . The end!"

(The investigator was assisted in interpreting this story by Timmy's mother. Timmy told about the day that his father took Timmy and his sister, Mayway, to the park. They played. It got dark, and they went home.)

The following example is of Timmy's emergent reading of the book, Sam Vole and His Brothers. *The book had been read to him three times by his mother.*

(Please note that the examiner's repetition of Timmy's utterances is not necessarily a recommended practice. The utterances were repeated because Timmy was fairly unintelligible and the investigator was attempting to assist the transcription process that would occur later.)

Timmy: Uh, two big brothers.

Timmy: One little brother named, my not know.

Inv: Sam?

Timmy: Sam.

Inv: Yeh.

Timmy: Story all himself, only Henry go too.

Inv: Only Henry go too?

Timmy: No.

Timmy: (coughs really hard)

Inv: Wow!

Timmy: Ow!

Inv: Ow, that hurt!

Timmy: Uh, Henry (unintelligible word) pick more more daisies than, my him not know.

Inv: More daisies than . . .

Timmy: My not know.

Timmy: My not know what him name.

Inv: Oh, I don't him name?

Comment: INVESTIGATOR INACCURATELY ATTEMPTS TO IMITATE CHILD.

Inv: Henry?

Inv: Or Arthur?

Timmy: Go.

Inv: Sam, Henry, and Arthur.

Timmy: Sam pick, pick, give, uh daisies, uh, mother.

Inv: Uhhuh.

Timmy: All sleepin', uh, my not, huh, my not know what him name.
Inv: Sam?
Timmy: Sam not sleep.
Inv: Sam not sleep.
Timmy: Uh, go in meadow.
Inv: Uhhuh, go in meadow.
Timmy: Uh, bro . . .
Timmy: Hop.
Timmy: Uh, sad.
Timmy: It bro all himself.
Timmy: All brothers is sad.
Timmy: See, brothers is happy.
Timmy: Vole all home.
Timmy: And vole and vole and vole.
Timmy: Vole, vole, vole, vole, vole.
Timmy: The end.

What is most noticeable about Timmy's emergent reading was that although he struggled to communicate his ideas (and asked for the investigator's help), he also demonstrated a great deal of written language knowledge. First, he was insistent on saying the names of the characters, indicating knowledge of written language's need for decontextualization, even though he had a great deal of difficulty remembering the names. Midway through the story, when he said "All sleeping" he continued to demonstrate that he should be specific and say "Sam not sleep," instead of "But he not," or "Him not." Additionally, he may also have demonstrated some metalinguistic knowledge at the beginning of his emergent reading when he said, "Story all himself," perhaps meaning, "In this story, Sam wanted to go by himself."

When one compares Timmy's oral versus written narratives, one can see differences in length, with the written narrative being quite a bit longer. Although the written narrative is not syntactically more complex, it does appear that his syntax is somewhat more well-formed in the emergent reading as compared to the oral narrative.

We are in the process of studying multiple levels of impact of storybook reading interactions for typically developing children and children with SLI. Initially from these transcripts, one can infer that Timmy's motivation to talk about the stories he enjoys is one avenue for expanding and enriching his language world. The interactions in these two situations provide at least part of what is often called a literacy- and language-rich environment, the kinds of environments that speech-language pathologists increasingly have come to recommend.

SUMMARY

This chapter has provided an overview of emergent literacy issues that relate to the language development of preschool children. Several themes underlie this discussion. First, we illustrated that language performances in young nonconventional readers are not tied to a particular delivery form—in fact, preschool children can demonstrate their understandings of written language concepts orally. We believe that when parents, teachers, or speech-language pathologists use storybooks as stimuli for language production (and much of the time, even when storybooks are not present), children are being asked to illustrate their understandings of written language concepts. This position suggests that those of us who concentrate on oral language development also need to be aware of children's emergent literacy development. Consequently, we highlighted some tasks that enable observers of children's language to more clearly understand and describe their comprehension and use of written language forms.

Second, we described a process that can be used to elicit emergent readings. We provided guidelines for classifying these productions and highlighted some specific language and behaviors important in the process of internalizing written language and becoming conventionally literate. This information can be used to track the development of children through their exposure to repeated storybook readings.

Next, we described parent and child behaviors that occur in both storybook interactions and emergent readings. This information can be useful to teachers and speech-language pathologists in their remediation of children with language impairments and in their efforts to understand how storybook language and behavior might be different than the language and behavior that occur during toy play. In other words, we have attempted to answer the question, "What are we looking for when we observe children and parents interacting with storybooks?" To aid this process, we provided guidelines for setting up parent-child storybook observations and a description of parental scaffolding behaviors that may occur during storybook reading.

Finally, children's narrative language productions during emergent storybook elicitations and oral storytelling were illustrated. Obtaining narratives in a variety of oral and written contexts helps us more carefully monitor children's development of narrative production, their awareness of the need for decontextualization in written language and their ability to use linguistic features suited to oral and written language contexts. Understanding and documenting these changes broadens our perspective of the language capabilities of children we serve.

In conclusion, we feel that one of the most important reasons to include emergent literacy perspectives and methods into clinical practice is that they provide a means for the speech-language pathologist to participate in one of the central features of school instruction, literacy. The SLP's involvement aligns his or her knowledge of the child's oral communication development with understandings of the child's overall language development. If SLPs have a better understanding of a child's oral and written development, we will set up situations that facilitate her or his ability to move between modalities. The resulting interactivity across language forms would be designed to help the child continue to negotiate relationships between oral and written language, which is important for later school success.

ACKNOWLEDGMENTS

The research project (Kaderavek & Sulzby, 1994) has been supported in part by research grant number 1-F32-DC-00185-01 from the National Institute on Deafness and Other Communication Disorders, National Institutes of Health. Portions of this chapter were presented by Elizabeth Sulzby during an invited presentation made at the Annual Convention of the American Speech-Language-Hearing Association, Anaheim, California, November 1993, entitled "Implications of Emergent Literacy for Language Assessment."

REFERENCES

Adams, M. (1990). *Beginning to read: Thinking and learning about print.* Cambridge, Mass.: MIT Press.

Anderson, A. B., & Stokes, S. (1984). Social and institutional influences on the development and practice of literacy. In H. Goelman, A. Oberg, & F. Smith (Eds.), *Awakening to literacy* (pp. 158–184). Portsmouth, N.H.: Heinemann.

Anderson-Yockel, J., & Haynes, W. O. (1994). Joint book-reading strategies in working-class African American and white mother-toddler dyads. *Journal of Speech and Hearing Research, 37,* 583–593.

Aram, D., Ekelman, B., & Nation, J. (1984). Preschoolers with language disorders: 10 years later. *Journal of Speech and Hearing Research, 27,* 232–244.

Aram, D., & Nation, J. (1980). Preschool language disorders and subsequent language and academic difficulties. *Journal of Communication Disorders, 13,* 159–179.

Bridwell, N. (1985). *Clifford, the big red dog.* New York: Scholastic.

Bus, A. G., & Sulzby, E. (1996). Becoming literate in a multicultural society. To appear in J. Shimron (Ed.), *Literacy and education: Essays in memory of Dina Feitelson.* Norwood, N.J.: Hampton Press.

Bus, A. G., Sulzby, E., & van IJzendoorn, M. H. (1996). *Children's internalizations from repeated storybook readings: A study of emergent literacy and attachment.* Manuscript.

Bus, A. G., & van IJzendoorn, M. H. (1992). Patterns of attachment in frequently and infrequently reading dyads. *Journal of Genetic Psychology, 153,* 395–403.

Bus, A. G., & van IJzendoorn, M. H. (1995) Mothers reading to their 3-year-olds: The role of mother-child attachment security in becoming literate. *Reading Research Quarterly, 30,* 998–1015.

Bus, A. G., van IJzendoorn, M. H., & Pellegrini, A. D. (1995). Storybook reading makes for success in learning to read: A meta-analysis on the intergenerational transmission of literacy. *Review of Educational Research, 65,* 1–21.

Catts, H. W. (1991). Early identification of reading disorders. *Topics in Language Disorders, 12,* 1–16.

Catts, H. W. (1993). The relationship between speech-language impairments and reading disabilities. *Journal of Speech and Hearing Research, 36,* 948–958.

Chomsky, C. (1972). Stages in language development and reading exposure. *Harvard Educational Review, 42,* 1–33.

Conti-Ramsden, G., Hutcheson, G. D., & Grove, J. (1995). Contingency and breakdown: Children with SLI and their conversations with mothers and fathers. *Journal of Speech and Hearing Research, 28,* 1290–1302.

Cox, B. E. (1994). Young children's regulatory talk: Evidence of emerging metacognitive control over literary products and processes . In R. B. Ruddell, M. R. Ruddell, & H. Singer (Eds.), *Theoretical models and processes of reading* (4th ed., pp. 733–756). Newark, Del.: International Reading Association.

DeBaryshe, B. D. (1992). *Early language and literacy activities in the home* (U.S. Department of Education Field Initiated Studies Program. Final report for the project). University of North Carolina, Greensboro. (ERIC Document Reproduction Service No. ED 351 406)

de Hirsch, K., Jansky, J. J., & Langford, W. S. (1966). *Predicting reading failure.* New York: Harper & Row.

Dickinson, D. K., & McCabe, A. (1991). A social interactionist account of language and literacy development. In J. Kavanaugh (Ed.), *The language continuum* (pp. 1–40). Parkton, Md.: York Press.

Eastman, P. D. (1960). *Are you my mother?* New York: Random House.

Elijah, R., & Sulzby, E. (1992, April). *From emergent reading to conventional literacy: LSES black children's storybook reading.* Paper presented at the annual meeting of the American Educational Research Association, San Francisco.

Elster, C. A. (1994). Patterns within preschooler's emergent readings. *Reading Research Quarterly, 29,* 402–418.

Feagans, L. (1982). The development and importance of narratives for school adaptation. In L. Feagans & D. Farran (Eds.), *The language of children reared in poverty* (pp. 95–116). New York: Academic.

Goodsitt, J., Raitan, J. G., & Perlmutter, M. (1988). Interaction between mothers and preschool children when reading a novel and familiar book. *International Journal of Behavioral Development, 11,* 489–505.

Heath, S. (1983). *Ways with words.* Cambridge: Cambridge University Press.

Heath, S. (1986). What no bedtime story means: Narrative skills at home and school. In B. Schieffelin & E. Ochs (Eds.), *Language socialization across cultures* (pp. 97–124). New York: Cambridge University Press.

Hiebert, E. H. (1994). Becoming literate through authentic tasks: Evidence and adaptations. In R. B. Ruddell, M. R. Ruddell, & H. Singer (Eds.), *Theoretical models and processes of reading* (pp. 391–413). Newark, Del.: International Reading Association.

Hyon, S., & Sulzby, E. (1994). African-American kindergartners' spoken narratives: Topic associating and topic centered styles. *Linguistics and Education, 6,* 121–152.

Kaderavek, J. N., & Sulzby, E. (1994). *Literacy contexts and oral language in SLI children.* Proposal to National Institutes of Health.

Kaderavek, J. N., & Sulzby, E. (1995). *Parent-child joint bookreading: Analytic procedures.* Manuscript submitted for publication.

Katims, D. S. (1991). Emergent literacy in early childhood special education: Curriculum and instruction. *Topics in Early Childhood Special Education, 11,* 69–84.

Kirk, S. A., McCarthy, J. J., & Kirk, W. D. (1968). *Illinois Test of Psycholinguistic Abilities.* Urbana: University of Illinois Press.

Koppenhaver, D. A., Coleman, P. P., Kalman, S. L., & Yoder, D. E. (1991). The implications of emergent literacy research for children with developmental disabilities. *American Journal of Speech-Language Pathology, 1,* 38–44.

Martin, B. (1970). *Brown bear, brown bear, what do you see?* New York: Holt.

Martinez, M., & Roser, N. (1985). Read it again: The value of repeated readings during storytime. *The Reading Teacher, 38,* 782–786.

McCabe, A., & Rollins, P. R. (1994). Assessment of preschool narrative skills. *American Journal of Speech-Language Pathology, 3,* 45–56.

Moerk, E. L. (1985). Picture-book readings by mothers and young children and its impact upon language development. *Journal of Pragmatics, 9,* 547–566.

Moll, L. C. (1994). Literacy research in community and classrooms: A sociocultural approach. In R. B. Ruddell, M. R. Ruddell, & H. Singer (Eds.), *Theoretical models and processes of reading* (pp. 179–207). Newark, Del.: International Reading Association.

Morrow, L. M. (1983). Home and school correlates of early interest in literature. *Journal of Educational Research, 76,* 221–230.

Morrow, L. M., & Paratore, J. (1993). Family literacy: Perspectives and practices. *The Reading Teacher, 47,* 194–200.

Ninio, A. (1980). Picture-book reading in mother-infant dyads belonging to two subgroups in Israel. *Child Development, 51,* 587–590.

Ninio, A. (1983). Joint book reading as a multiple vocabulary acquisition device. *Developmental Psychology, 19,* 445–451.

Ninio, A., & Bruner, J. (1978). The achievement and antecedents of labeling. *Journal of Child Language, 4,* 1–22.

Otto, B. (1984). *Evidence of emergent reading behaviors in young children's interactions with favorite storybooks.* Unpublished doctoral dissertation, Northwestern University, Evanston, Ill.

Pellegrini, A. D., Brody, G. H., & Sigel, I. E. (1985). Parents' book-reading habits with their children. *Journal of Educational Psychology, 77,* 332–340.

Pellegrini, A. D., McGillicuddy-DeLisi, A. V., Sigel, I. E., & Brody, G. H. (1986). The effects of children's communicative status and task on parent's teaching strategies. *Contemporary Educational Psychology, 11,* 240–252.

Peterson, C., & McCabe, A. (1983). *Developmental psycholinguistics. Three ways of looking at a child's narrative.* New York: Plenum.

Pierce, P. L., & McWilliam, P. J. (1993). Emerging literacy and children with severe speech and physical impairments (SSPI): Issues and possible intervention strategies. *Topics in Language Disorders, 13,* 47–57.

Reuning, C., & Sulzby, E. (1984). Emergent storybook reading in high and low literacy background children. *National Reading Conference Yearbook, 34,* 310–319.

Roth, F. P., & Spekman, N. J. (1986). Narrative discourse: Spontaneously generated stories of learning-disabled and normally achieving students. *Journal of Speech and Hearing Disorders, 51,* 8–23.

Scanlon, D. M., & Vellutino, F. R. (in press). A comparison of the instructional backgrounds and cognitive profiles of poor, average and good readers who were initially identified as at risk for reading failure. *Scientific Studies of Reading.*

Scarborough, H. S. (1998). Early identification of children at risk for reading disabilities: Phonological awareness and some other promising predictors. In B. K. Shapiro, P. J. Accardo, & A. J. Capute (Eds.), *Specific reading disability: A view of the spectrum* (pp. 77–121). Timonium, Md.: York Press.

Schuele, C. M., & van Kleeck, A. (1987). Precursors to literacy: Assessment and intervention. *Topics in Language Disorders, 7,* 32–44.

Scollon, R., & Scollon, S. B. K. (1981). *Narrative, literacy, and face in interethnic communication.* Norwood, N.J.: Ablex.

Sendak, M. (1963). *Where the Wild Things Are.* New York: Harper Trophy.

Snow, C. E. (1983). Literacy and language: Relationships during the preschool years. *Harvard Educational Review, 53,* 165–189.

Snow, C. E., Arlman-Rupp, A., Hassing, Y., Jobse, J., Joosten, J., & Vorster, J. (1976). Mothers' speech in three social classes. *Journal of Psycholinguistic Research, 5,* 1–20.

Snow, C. E., Burns, M. S., & Griffin, P. (1998). (Eds.). *Preventing reading difficulties in young children.* Washington, D.C.: National Academy Press.

Snow, C. E., & Goldfield, B. A. (1983). Turn the page please: Situation-specific language acquisition. *Journal of Child Language, 10,* 551–569.

Snow, C. E., & Ninio, A. (1986). The contracts of literacy: What children learn from learning to read books. In W. H. Teale & E. Sulzby (Eds.), *Emergent literacy: Writing and Reading* (pp. 116–138). Norwood, N.J.: Ablex.

Sulzby, E. (1983, August). *Children's emergent abilities to read favorite storybooks.* Final report to the Spencer Foundation. Unpublished manuscript, Northwestern University, Evanston, Ill.

Sulzby, E. (1985a). Children's emergent reading of favorite storybooks: A developmental study. *Reading Research Quarterly, 20*(4), 458–481.

Sulzby, E. (1985b). Kindergartners as writers and readers. In M. Farr (Ed.), *Advances in writing research: Vol. 1. Children's early writing development* (pp. 127–199). Norwood, N.J.: Ablex.

Sulzby, E. (1986). Writing and reading: Signs of oral and written language organization in the young child. In W. H. Teale & E. Sulzby (Eds.), *Emergent literacy: Writing and reading* (pp. 50–89). Norwood, N.J.: Ablex.

Sulzby, E. (1991). Assessment of emergent literacy: Storybook reading. *The Reading Teacher, 44,* 498–500.

Sulzby, E. (1994). Childrens emergent reading of favorite storybooks: A developmental study. In R. B. Ruddell, M. R. Ruddell, & H. Singer (Eds.), *Theoretical models and processes of reading* (4th ed., pp. 244–280). Newark, Del.: International Reading Association.

Sulzby, E. (1996a). Roles of oral and written language as children approach conventional literacy. In C. Pontecorvo, M. Orsolini, B. Burge, & L. Resnick (Eds.), *Early text construction in children* (pp. 25–46). Hillsdale, N.J.: Erlbaum.

Sulzby, E. (1996b). [Transcripts and field notes to accompany Sulzby Classification Scheme for Emergent Storybook Reading]. Unpublished raw data.

Sulzby, E., & Barnhart, J. (1992). The development of academic competence: All our children emerge as writers and readers. In J. W. Irwin & M. A. Doyle (Eds.), *Reading/writing connections: Learning from research* (pp. 120–144). Newark, Del.: International Reading Association.

Sulzby, E., Branz, C. M., & Buhle, R. (1993). Repeated readings of literature and LSES black kindergartners and first graders. *Reading and Writing Quarterly, 9,* 183–196.

Sulzby, E., & Edwards, P. A. (1993). The role of parents in supporting literacy development. In B. Spodek & O. N. Saracho (Eds.), *Language and literacy in early childhood education* (pp. 156–177). New York: Teacher's College Press.

Sulzby, E., & Teale, W. H. (1987, November). *Young children's storybook reading: Longitudinal study of parent-child interaction and children's independent functioning.* Final report to The Spencer Foundation, University of Michigan, Ann Arbor.

Sulzby, E., Teale, W. H., & Kamberelis, G. (1989). Emergent writing in the classroom: Home and school connections. In D. Strickland & L. Morrow (Eds.), *Emerging literacy: Young children learn to read and write* (pp. 63–79). Newark, Del.: International Reading Association.

Sulzby, E., & Zecker, L. B. (1991). The oral monologue as a form of emergent reading. In A. McCabe & C. Peterson (Eds.), *Developing narrative structure* (pp. 175–214). Hillsdale, N.J.: Erlbaum.

Tannen, D. (1983). Oral and literate strategies in spoken and written discourse. In R. W. Bailey & R. M. Fosheim (Eds.), *Literacy for life: The demand for reading and writing* (pp. 79–96). New York: Modern Language Association.

Taylor, D., & Dorsey-Gaines, C. (1988). *Growing up literate: Learning from inner-city families.* Portsmouth, N.H.: Heinemann.

Teale, W. H. (1984). Reading to young children: Its significance for literacy development. In H. Goelman, A. Oberg, & F. Smith (Eds.), *Awakening to literacy* (pp. 110–121). Portsmouth, N.H.: Heinemann.

Teale, W. H., & Sulzby, E. (1986). Emergent literacy as a perspective for examining how young children become readers and writers. In W. H. Teale & E. Sulzby (Eds.), *Emergent literacy: Writing and reading* (pp.vii–xxv). Norwood, N.J.: Ablex.

Teale, W. H., & Sulzby, E. (1987). Literacy acquisition in early childhood: The roles of access and mediation in storybook reading. In D. Wagner (Ed.), *The future of literacy in a changing world* (pp. 111–130). New York: Pergamon.

Teale, W. H., & Sulzby, E. (1989). Emergent literacy: New perspectives on young children's reading and writing development. In D. Strickland & L. Morrow (Eds.), *Emerging literacy: Young children learn to read and write* (pp. 1–15). Newark, Del.: International Reading Association.

van Kleeck, A., Gillam, R., Hamilton, L. & McGrath, C. (1997). The relationship between middle-class parent's book-sharing discussion and their preschoolers abstract language development. *Journal of Speech and Hearing Research, 40,* 1261–1271.

van Kleeck, A., & Schuele, C. M. (1987). Precursors to literacy: Normal development. *Topics in Language Disorders, 7,* 13–31.

Vygotsky, L. S. (1978). *Mind in society: The development of higher psychological processes.* Cambridge, Mass.: Harvard University Press

Waddell, M. (1992). *Sam Vole and his brothers.* Cambridge, Mass.: Candlewick Press.

Watkins, R. V., & Rice, M. L. (1991). Verb particle and preposition acquisition in language-impaired preschoolers. *Journal of Speech and Hearing Research, 34,* 1130–1141.

Watson, L. R., Layton, T. L., Pierce, P. L., & Abraham, L. M. (1994). Enhancing emerging literacy in a language preschool. *Language, Speech, and Hearing Services in Schools, 25,* 136–145.

Whitehurst, G. J., Arnold, D. S., Epstein, J. N., Angell, A. L., Smith, M., & Fischel, J. E. (1994). A picture book reading intervention in day care and home for children from low-income families. *Developmental Psychology, 30*(5), 679–689.

Whitehurst, G. J., Falco, F. L., Lonigan, C. J., Fischel, J. E., DeBaryshe, B. D., Valdez-Menchaca, M. C., & Caulfield, M. (1988). Accelerating language development through picture book reading. *Developmental Psychology, 24,* 552–559.

Wiig, E. H., Secord, W., & Semel, E. (1992). *Clinical Evaluation of Language Fundamentals–Preschool.* New York: The Psychological Corporation.

Yaden, D. B. (1988). Understanding stories through repeated read-alouds: How many does it take? *The Reading Teacher, 41,* 556–566.

CHAPTER 8

Language Intervention for Prelinguistic and Nonverbal Children

Mary Blake Huer, Ph.D., CCC-SLP
Professor
California State University
Fullerton

Key terms

aid
augmentative and alternative communication (AAC)
strategy
symbols
system
technique

Overview

It is a familiar scenario. Parents postpone seeking language intervention for their nonverbal preschool child because she or he is "just a late talker." If the preschool child is severely physically challenged in addition to being language impaired, most clinical resources will be focused on the physical challenge first rather than on the language delay. Unfortunately, the years will pass and the child will continue to be nonverbal. Valuable time is lost that could have been devoted to language intervention by providing a rich communication environment to foster the development of alternatives, other than speech, for communication (e.g., sign language or the use of a communication board) or facilitating the development of language through "augmentation" of residual speech and language skills (e.g., electronic communication displays with voice output).

Birth to 5 years is a critical period for the language development of all children, whether physically or cognitively challenged or not. Given appropriate language intervention, a child with disabilities may demonstrate the beginning of mastery of communication during this period and prepare for exciting conversations with all their future communication partners. Thus, it is important that language stimulation be provided for all children during the early years, even when it appears that physical and/or cognitive challenges are too great to overcome.

The purpose of this chapter is to focus on early language intervention for prelinguistic and/or nonverbal children who are severely physically and/or cognitively challenged. Critical needs for early language intervention are identified. Several issues related to language intervention for the young child who uses **augmentative and alternative communication (AAC)** will be discussed. Throughout this chapter the term *augmentative and alternative communication (AAC)* will refer to "an area of clinical practice that attempts to compensate (either temporarily or permanently) for the impairment and disability patterns of individuals with severe expressive communication disorders" (American Speech-Language-Hearing Association [ASHA], 1989, p. 107). The variety of augmentative and alternative communication systems that are appropriate for the preschool population will be described (see Appendix 8-1). **System** selection criteria for choosing AAC technology for preschoolers is included. Finally, several clinical case examples are presented throughout the chapter for additional self-study.

NEEDS FOR LANGUAGE INTERVENTION WITH PRELINGUISTIC AND NONVERBAL CHILDREN

Language provides a means for communication between two or more persons. At birth, a child's parents or caregivers begin the process of developing communication with the child.

Establishing communication takes time for all children and their caregivers. If a child experiences a physical challenge and/or some cognitive delay, communication development often takes a little longer because physical challenges and/or cognitive delays present additional impairments, which must be dealt with by the child as well as by the caregivers at the same time that communication is developing. Many parents and professional practitioners do not yet have a knowledge base to identify and promote the development of forms of communication other than speech. If speech is not emerging, however, alternatives for communication must be developed. Indeed, AAC methods have been used with infants as young as 4 to 6 months (Hanrahan, Ferrier, & Jolie, 1987; Reinhartsen, Edmondson, & Crais, 1997).

Underlying the communication process is an elaborate language system, which begins to be evident during the prelinguistic stages and continues to develop even for nonverbal children. That is, the language system provides the means through which communication may occur. While the language system provides the means, the culture of the individuals communicating determines the code that will be recognized. "The code may be in the form of words, gestures, facial expressions, formal signing systems or pictorial symbols that act to signal the communicative intent of the interaction. Where a spoken code cannot be used, alternative symbolic systems can be taught as a means to augment existing vocal abilities" (Butterfield, 1994, p. 13).

Augmentative and alternative communication (AAC) users may be identified as a cultural group. In other words, there is a cultural framework for communication in the nonverbal population. An understanding of this framework allows one to identify the communication patterns that are shared by young nonverbal children and their partners. The underlying rules that govern the communication patterns form the "code" for expression. Parameters of the communication code include a means of communicating, something to communicate, reasons for communication; and someone with whom to communicate. Zangari (1994) describes an integrative approach to AAC assessment and intervention that incorporates each of these four parameters. Language intervention for AAC, then, incorporates strategies for identifying these four parameters in order to provide appropriate communication for the prelinguistic and/or nonverbal child. That is, language intervention examines the following issues:

1. Why does a young child communicate? There are several reasons for communication.

2. What do young prelinguistic and/or nonverbal children say? They do have vocabularies.

3. How do nonverbal children communicate if they cannot speak? There are alternatives.

4. With whom do prelinguistic and/or nonverbal children communicate? They can communicate with facilitators.

NEEDS FOR COMMUNICATION

Young children begin to communicate immediately after birth. Early communication serves several purposes: to express basic wants and needs, to respond to the expectations of caregivers, and to react to stimuli in one's environment. Later communication development allows us to practice expressing one's linguistic competence, to play with others, and to exercise power over daily life events. In the case of the prelinguistic child, there is an expression of physical states like hunger, pain, and sleepiness. Older children continue to develop expressive language skills in order to communicate choices, preferences, and other communicative functions. Communication partners, whether it be a parent or friend, expect children to participate in the communication dyad from infancy onward.

The Roles for Functional Communication

Young children with disabilities appear to "use" language differently than do typically developing children. The source of the apparent differences is not clear (e.g., the language system or the communicative acts), and there continues to be little available research (Linfoot, 1994). Of course, the very nature of augmentative and alternative communication appears different (e.g., using communication boards versus speech). Nevertheless, the needs, or roles, for communication are the same: to request objects, actions, and attention. It is the means of representation that differ for the nonverbal child. Our knowledge is slowly expanding as researchers explore such topics as the development of intervention strategies to facilitate prelinguistic communication skills and the role of context on the early communicative functions noted in augmented communicators. There continues to be a need for the study of early language intervention with nonverbal children in order to determine the relationships between pragmatic functions and discourse role and to establish what is necessary for functional communication with children with severe communication challenges.

The Function of Language for Play and Social Participation

Children with cognitive and/or physical challenges need to play with toys, with peers, with family, and with friends. Often primary caregivers do not know how to play with children who are not following typical developmental profiles for physical, cognitive, and language development. Young children using AAC often have different patterns of play and alternative experiences with toys and games and with the manipulation of objects than do other children. Thus, the patterns of early language development observed in children using AAC may be different, even during activities intended to promote socialization with peers, than those patterns noted in able-bodied children. Sometimes physical limitations prohibit playing with toys their peers enjoy. Children with cognitive and/or physical challenges are sometimes not enrolled in preschool programs because of the extra care and specialized facilities that may be required. Early language intervention programs offer children the opportunity to play and socialize. Teachers and therapists work with parents to provide training. Practitioners are knowledgeable about issues of access to special equipment and/or services. Early language intervention programs often provide group experiences for young children in therapy. Nonverbal children attending early language intervention programs are encouraged to play and socialize with their peers as they develop language.

Language Empowers Nonverbal Children

Language is a tool that empowers even a very young child. Because the literature has noted that persons who are disabled are perceived and treated differently (Damico, 1994), it is not unreasonable to assume that young children with severe disabilities may face greater challenges that will impact their future lives from social factors than from their physical or cognitive inadequacies. Providing early language intervention may preclude the assignment of stereotypical identities (i.e., stereotypes such as passive, helpless, and incompetent) to nonverbal children during their early years.

The development of early expressive language provides for participation in the simplest daily living activities. Maximizing every child's participation through daily communicative exchanges provides for the development of early language skills and for becoming "an active" rather than a passive partner in communication. Linguistic competence promotes self-confidence and builds self-esteem as young preschoolers develop their social skills, prepare for first educational experiences, and meet early cognitive challenges. Parents, siblings, caregivers, friends, and teachers expect children to acquire language. When language is delayed, participation in life's activities is delayed as well. Progressively, severely physically challenged children who are nonverbal find themselves left out during play activities, lose their motivation to participate, lack interest, and become increasingly dependent on caregivers. The elimination of opportunities for social participation and play is painful for all communication partners—and it is unnecessary. The acquisition of language provides one tool that can empower physically challenged, formerly nonverbal children during the early, formative years.

Expectations for Communication Across Cultures

Early language intervention is mandatory for young toddlers who are severely physically and/or cognitively challenged. Through early language intervention, the child using AAC acquires the "code" through which she or he will begin to participate in communicative interactions. The expressive codes of the nonverbal child may be different from those of the child's able-bodied peers. The methods for expressive communication with nonverbal children will probably differ from those of the child's parents or siblings. However, clinical experience has proven that families and practitioners can expand their own communication repertoires, given the proper training. The cultural framework for communication with nonverbal children is learnable.

It also becomes important to recognize that many young children with severe disabilities reside in homes with families of ethnic backgrounds different than those of mainstream European Americans. There is already an expectation, especially in educational settings, that practitioners learn the language codes of other cultures because young children with cognitive and/or physical challenges need to acquire the language code that is reflective of their culture. In essence, young nonverbal children warrant early language intervention so that they may be prepared for intentional communication with others within their own cultures, as well as across cultures. An understanding of multicultural communication within the educational setting is necessary to foster communication within, as well as between, cultural groups.

NONSYMBOLIC VERSUS SYMBOLIC COMMUNICATION

Most children can be attributed with having "something to say." Although the content of a child's message and extent of her or his linguistic knowledge may range from a simple form to a complex structure, most users of AAC are capable of some communication. It is the means of representation of the message and the vocabulary utilized that establish the continuum of nonsymbolic to symbolic communication.

Let us examine the transition of a child from prelinguistic to linguistic levels. In a prelinguistic child who is learning to communicate, one might observe preintentional primitive forms of communication, for example, idiosyncratic behaviors that are initially interpreted and understood only by the caregivers (Butterfield, Linfoot, & Arthur, 1994). Gradually the prelinguistic child will exhibit behavior that appears to be more goal-directed and conventional, such as directing eye gaze to one of two toys to request a particular toy. As the child moves along the continuum, she or he will develop intentional conventional forms of communication (e.g., pointing, waving "bye-bye," shaking head "no"). In addition, the prelinguistic child will typically acquire vocabulary that signals "something." Here is where nonverbal and speaking children differ. As speaking children acquire words, nonverbal children acquire other **symbols**.

In the field of AAC, there is a common division between nonsymbolic communication (prelinguistic) and symbolic communication (nonverbal). That is, prelinguistic communication is nonsymbolic; nonverbal communication is symbolic. As children using AAC advance in their perceived language development, they move from nonsymbolic forms of communication toward symbolic forms. Prelinguistic forms of communication include attention to preparatory training conditions (von Tetzchner & Martinsen, 1992), and nonsymbolic expressions (Siegel-Causey & Guess, 1989). Examples of preparatory skills include: "eye contact, direction of gaze, attentiveness, sitting still, behavior chains, imitation and motor skills" (von Tetzchner & Martinsen, 1992, p. 137). Attention to the full range of nonsymbolic expressions warrants careful examination of a child's affect, body movements, vocalizations, responses to touch, visual responses, and gestures. One example of an excellent program for enhancing nonsymbolic communication was presented by Siegel-Causey and Guess (1989), who suggested five instructional guidelines for increasing a child's communication effectiveness: "Developing nurturance; enhancing sensitivity; increasing opportunities; sequencing experiences; and utilizing movement" (p. 23). Through developing explicit guidelines and strategies, these authors direct practitioners through supportive programs to develop communication.

Excellent descriptions are available in the literature for determining extent of development of prelinguistic (nonsymbolic) communication functions (Butterfield et al., 1994; Letto, Bedrosian, & Skarakis-Doyle, 1994; Mar & Sall, 1994; Warren, Yoder, Gazdag, Kim, & Jones, 1993). Practitioners evaluating young children's expressive language systems should observe the extent of development of prelinguistic communication before rushing to develop an expensive and elaborate AAC system.

DEVELOPMENT OF INITIAL VOCABULARY: SYMBOLIC COMMUNICATION

Just as able-bodied children begin to acquire their first words, so do AAC users enrolled in early language intervention programs. AAC users, however, need extra assistance in acquiring "first words." Typically, a parent, teacher, or clinician makes a decision regarding the best symbolic system for representation of the child's first words. AAC users do not typically communicate through speech; therefore, alternative expressive signals, including symbols, need to be supplied early. Symbolic communication incorporates verbalizations (when present), sign language, photographs, objects that represent vocabulary, pictures, and graphic systems to represent concepts or activities. Symbolic forms represent the nonverbal, but expressive, language skills of children who are unable to speak. Nonverbal children acquire symbolic forms as verbal children acquire words.

It is mandatory that young nonverbal children be supplied with an alternative to spoken first words as soon as possible in order that they may play with, and convey messages to, their communicative partners. Based on results from a child's initial assessment, clinicians, in collaboration with parents and caregivers, begin to map out a plan for depicting the AAC users' "first words." An initial plan may include idiosyncratic gestures, simple signs, photographs to which the child might point, or an array of symbols. Separate from, but simultaneous with, the determination of the most appropriate symbol set for representation of basic vocabulary, the choice of vocabulary must also be determined early.

Selecting vocabulary for young toddlers is no easy task. Fried-Oken and More noted that "the vocabulary selection process is so influenced by sociolinguistic, biologic, and psycholinguistic variables that it is often difficult to find the starting point" (1992, p. 52). A review of the literature and current practices indicates that vocabulary decisions are often based on developmental data using typical language acquisition as a model. Some teachers and clinicians rely on spoken language samples from preschool children who are able-bodied or samples from nonspeaking device users. Parent inventories and case study data have become important data banks for vocabulary selection. Professionals selecting an early vocabulary set should probably make reference to several composite vocabulary lists representing words utilized by young children, nonspeaking children, and adult users (Beukelman, Jones, & Rowan, 1989; Beukelman, McGinnis, & Morrow, 1991; Fried-Oken & More, 1992; Yorkston, Dowden, Honsinger, Marriner, & Smith, 1988). Such references form an important data pool from which beginning vocabularies may be selected for young children who are users of augmentative and alternative communication. Each of these four articles includes extensive appendices with word lists for vocabulary selection.

Yorkston et al. (1998) summarized the usefulness of composite vocabulary lists: "Composite vocabulary lists afford the opportunity to sample from a range of vocabulary sizes, . . . prevents the clinician from 'guessing'. . . [and may be] obtained from users who are matched along a number of dimensions reflecting language capability and environmentally dictated communication needs" (1998, p. 202). Beukelman, Jones, & Rowan (1989) examined word usage by nondisabled preschool peers, recording more than 2,800 words for each of the preschool children in the study. In their findings, "45.1% of the total language sample is represented by the 25 most frequently occurring words, 60% by the 50 most frequently occurring words, and 85% of the total language sample . . . by the 250 most frequently occurring words" (p. 245). Thus, "a substantial portion of the total communication sample [was] represented by a limited number of words" (Beukelman et al., 1989, p. 245).

Marvin, Beukelman, and Bilyeu (1994) investigated vocabulary-use patterns of nondisabled, preschool-aged children at home and at preschool. Their findings were similar to the Beukelman et al. (1989) study in that children tended to use a core of only 25 words in school or home settings and a core of 250 words, which accounted for the majority of the frequently occurring words, in both settings. What was interesting in the Marvin et al. study was the finding that "a significant portion (one third) of the vocabulary selected for one context, such as home, may not meet the child's communication needs in another context, such as school" (1994, p. 233). Vocabulary selection thus must take into account both concepts that may be shared across settings and vocabulary that will be specific to different settings. Clinical planning during vocabulary selection should ensure an efficient and functional AAC system.

Based on the research described here and my own clinical experience, teachers or speech-language pathologists might select early words (symbols) for an AAC user with reference to those concepts that are:

1. frequently used by young children, able-bodied or physically challenged, as reported in the literature;
2. developmentally appropriate according to the known order of acquisition by young children;
3. frequently found across published composite word/phrase lists collected from different demographic samples and organized by structure and content;
4. identified through environmental inventories and interviews with parents and teachers;
5. representative of unique settings and contexts, including words that reflect, and are sensitive to, issues of cultural diversity.

Clinical experience has proven that often the initial vocabulary set that is selected serves as a "starter set" of concepts, words and messages, from which an AAC user's personalized vocabulary set will grow. Young children who use AAC with their parents, teachers, and therapists will gradually customize the vocabulary in order to appropriately meet the needs of all communication partners.

CONVEYING MESSAGES THROUGH AUGMENTATIVE COMMUNICATION SYSTEMS

Augmentative and alternative communication as a practice is often associated with technology. It is false to assume, however, that all AAC is dependent on technological devices. According to Arthur (1994), technology support has been a major contributor to bridging the gap between a person's "drive to convey a message and the delivery of that message to a listener. However, as our definition of communication has broadened beyond the boundaries imposed by language, so the role of technology has changed" (p. 178). Arthur noted two reasons for this shift: (1) communication is a multimodal process (i.e., one communicates through speech, facial expressions, gestures, smiles, etc.), and (2) we are becoming more adept at recognizing "existing communication abilities" in the children with whom we interact. We can no longer afford to arbitrarily select AAC systems for consumers; rather we must build on existing communication skills within each user and move outward toward the expansion of those skills. Thus, AAC systems, developed for individual children, may or may not include technology or devices.

By definition, AAC systems include several different components. An AAC system is a collection of separate components, each of which has been carefully selected to enhance communication for a specific individual. Because the design or selection of an AAC system results from a collection of clinical decisions, it is important that all practitioners understand the choices typically available within systems.

The American Speech-Language-Hearing Association (ASHA, 1991) defined an AAC system as "an integrated group of components, including the symbols, aids, strategies, and techniques used by individuals to enhance communication" (p. 10). Beukelman and Mirenda (1992) listed four components, "symbol, aid, strategy, and technique," as the critical elements that form the basis for all AAC interventions. With regard to the preschool child, symbols might include pictures, gestures, objects, or signs that the child utilizes as a method to represent basic concepts. The physical unit through which the child transmits messages is the child's **aid**, namely, "a physical object or device used to transmit or receive messages (e.g., a communication book, board, chart, mechanical or electronic device, or computer)" (ASHA, 1991, p. 10). A **strategy** is the way in which the child uses symbols and aids to enhance communication. Strategies may be self-discovered by the child or taught by a clinician or parent. Finally, the **technique** will be the means through which the child transmits messages, for example, through direct selection of a photo on a communication board, through signing, or through a device that scans each row and column of items on the board.

Because there may be some overlap between the four components within an AAC system used by a young child, several examples of the four components are provided in Table 8-1 for clarity. As the child becomes a more sophisticated AAC user, the four components overlap to a diminishing extent and the entire AAC system becomes more complex. Such systems are beyond the scope of this chapter. Interested readers may contact the manufacturers listed in Appendix 8-1 to order copies of catalogues in which more complex systems are described.

AAC SYSTEM SELECTION CONSIDERATIONS

The selection of an AAC system is a process, as no two children with severe communication impairments and physical disabilities are alike. Each child presents an array of communication needs, offers a diversity of communication functions, and is in an environment with multiple communication partners, each having his or her own communication patterns and styles. If the child comes from a culturally diverse background, the parameters for selection of an AAC system are even broader. With these complex factors in mind, how should one approach selection of a system?

Initial Assessment

Practitioners should be cautious in approaching an AAC assessment. They must not equate the concept of an augmentative and alternative communication system with technology. AAC best practices do not always include the

Table 8-1. Components of AAC Systems for Preschool Users—Selected Examples

Symbols	Examples	Type
Gestures	fine or gross body movements	unaided symbol
Vocalizations	involuntary or voluntary sounds	unaided symbol
Manual sign system	first designed for deaf population	unaided symbol
Real or miniature objects	associated with actual referent	aided symbol
Photographs	color, black and white	aided symbol
Picture Communication Symbols	line drawings	aided symbol
Picsyms	visual-graphic symbols	aided symbol
Selection Techniques	**Examples**	**Access**
Direct selection	direct indication of choice	eye gaze, finger, hand
Scanning	user waits till choice available	circular, linear, group
Aids	**Examples**	**Type**
Chart-based	retrieval is encoded or fixed	static or dynamic
Communication board	displays objects, symbols, pictures, words, other	fixed or dynamic
Strategies	**Examples**	**Source**
Adaptive play	spontaneous games, voluntary fun	Musselwhite, 1986
Using microswitches	adapting battery-operated toys	Goossens' & Crain, 1986
Remnant books	scraps from activities saved in photo album	Musselwhite, 1990
Miniboards	limited context communication displays	Goossens' & Crain, 1986

selection of assistive devices. It is often the case that young children requiring AAC intervention utilize a "light tech" or "no tech" approach during the early stages of intervention, and they may never need an AAC system that utilizes technological components. While not all children utilizing AAC techniques require technology, many young children immediately benefit from the use of technology as a part of their AAC system. Therefore, take the time to perform a complete initial assessment to determine the need for the AAC system (see Huer, 1987). It is mandatory that the professional have sufficient information before selecting an AAC system. Thus, the clinician approaches the initial assessment with the intent of answering several important questions and prepared to compile basic information about the child's skills, including observations across the following 15 areas:

- Auditory perception and memory
- Visual memory and perception
- Cognitive skills, including the ability to handle codes
- Environmental constraints and attitudes/experiences within the home, school, and community, including support services/persons
- Suitability of graphic systems, including traditional orthography, pictures, symbols, and so on
- Gross and fine motor skills
- Hand use skill, including finger dexterity
- Interactive language skills across partners and situations
- Methods of access to system/technique
- Mobility
- Paralinguistic aspects of language, such as facial expression and natural gesture
- Positioning/seating needs for the potential AAC users as well as for the technique or system
- Receptive and expressive language
- Speech (phonetic inventory)
- Efficiency of present communication, across partners

Careful observation of skills across the 15 areas allows the practitioner an opportunity to compile basic information regarding the child's competencies. Such information is constantly referenced when moving to the second phase of assessment, namely, "fitting" an AAC system to the child.

"Fitting" Technology to the Young Child

Consider that the initial assessment reveals that one is working with a child who is functioning at a prelinguistic, nonsymbolic level. If these are the findings, then technology will probably not be warranted until the child demonstrates intentional learning or begins to use conventional forms for expression. On the other hand, it might be the decision by the clinician that "light tech" devices should be introduced, such as switches, for play or for early choice-making and establishing goal-directed behaviors (see Warren & Reichle, 1992). There are excellent resources for introducing technical interfaces to young, prelinguistic children. The purpose of this section, however, is to examine the process for selecting technology for nonverbal, symbolic communication.

Assuming, after the initial assessment, that technology will be utilized with the young child, what is the next step? The process through which decisions are made is based on literature that addresses the selection of nonelectronic or electronic devices for AAC users (Cook & Coleman, 1987; Fishman, 1987; Rosen & Goodenough-Trepagnier, 1989; Vanderheiden & Lloyd, 1986). Although these authors did not target the young preschool child specifically, they proposed a process through which any AAC system might be selected. In brief, there are approximately 25 mutually exclusive parameters to consider in the decision-making process. Because there is a wealth of information within these four sources, a summary of each follows, with appropriate modifications and adaptations regarding the selection of technology for young preschool children.

Hierarchy of Decision Making. Cook and Coleman (1987, p. 154) outlined a systematic methodology for matching a child's skills and or needs to augmentative communication systems. Reflecting expertise in engineering, they place great emphasis on the characteristics of the device. Through comprehensive tables of communication goals and questions regarding a child's needs, they lead the practitioner through a seven-point hierarchy of decision making. Applications of their hierarchy with a young child include:

1. an assessment of the symbol systems utilized by the child,
2. the methods by which the child selects symbols,
3. the method of cognitive selection,
4. the required format for output from the child's system,
5. the child's projected vocabulary size,
6. the methods through which the child manipulates vocabulary,
7. the actual specifications for design and construction of the child's system, e.g., color, size, weight, need for mounting, and so forth.

Especially useful are Cook and Coleman's (1987) lists of "critical questions" (p. 160). The authors guide the practitioner through questions pertaining to a nonverbal child's conversational objectives with peers and strangers. System needs for drawing and beginning graphic skills are also addressed through questions. For the practitioner who may be interested in reviewing some of the information presented within the full text of the article, a few examples from their critical questions follow:

- Should an explanation of system use be provided for listeners?
- Are there any size and/or weight restrictions based on child's abilities?
- What types of items, events, activities are most important to the child?
- How large or loud does the output need to be?
- Will the system be moved to different environments?

- Is there a need to aid positioning of the body, arm, hand, or writing materials?
- Is there a need for enlarged characters?
- Would a prestored vocabulary be desirable?
- What subjects are covered in the preschool?
- Will the system be used both at home and at school or will it remain at home? (pp. 160–161)

Cook and Coleman's (1987) article concludes with two case studies, which are examples of their decision-making process. Each case summarizes the choices made for the individuals, with a rationale for each choice made within each step of the hierarchy. Interested practitioners should refer to the article for additional details.

Crucial Dimensions for AAC Components. Fishman (1987), a practicing augmentative communication specialist, outlined 10 crucial dimensions for the assessment of augmentative components. Fishman's list is a reflection of expertise developed after years of questioning while practicing and is complementary to Cook and Coleman's (1987) hierarchy. Each list contributes important components to the decision-making process for the selection and "fit" of technology. Practitioners selecting communication aids will find this work invaluable.

Often, practitioners request a list of questions that should be asked when selecting a system. Fishman's list of 10 components follows, with examples of the types of questions that should be asked before prescribing a particular AAC system for a young preschool child:

1. Intelligibility of messages—Will communication partners understand the child's messages when the device is used?
2. Rate of message production—What are the future requirements for speed of speaking and writing by the device?
3. Assertability—Will the child need to interrupt during conversations?
4. Independence in producing messages—Will the child be able to use the device when a familiar partner is absent?
5. Ability to project—Will the child be able to be understood from across the room?
6. Display permanence—Can the child create a message to show to a communication partner at a later time?
7. Correctability of messages—Can the child correct mistakes?
8. Accessibility—Where will the device be positioned during the child's day?
9. Openness/expandability—Will it be possible to add to the vocabulary within the system?

10. Flexibility—How difficult will it be to transport the system?

These 10 questions were not taken directly from Fishman (1987) but rather are presented as an example of an application of Fishman's work. Practitioners should refer to the case examples within Fishman (1987) for more complete information.

Computerized System for Prescribing AAC Devices. Utilizing a software program, Rosen and Goodenough-Trepagnier (1989) developed a system for prescribing augmentative communication devices. According to the authors, "special-purpose assessment instrumentation has been developed to perform the motor-assessment tasks required by the (Prescription) Guide to estimate expert rate" (p. 51). In an attempt to eliminate "trial-and-error assessment of client performance with devices," the authors report their work on a system that scores "devices for their suitability for a client" (p. 51). Due to the quantitative nature of the reported work, the present form of their equation is not provided within this chapter. However, the "fourteen functional categories of needs used in (the) Benefit calculation" (p. 59) are reported: "flexibility and operation, portability, ease of learning for user, communication rate, menu flexibility, reliability, electronic output, appearance, privacy, ease of setup, ease of learning for receiver, ease of maintenance, environmental control functions, and unlimited vocabulary" (p. 59). According to the authors, these 14 categories were derived during the development of the system with reference to answers to a 155-item questionnaire.

Practitioners should begin to see a pattern in the types of categories that have appeared across the three references for selection of AAC systems. It is critical that the components that are common to each list be examined for the significance that each contributes to the decision-making process for young children. Although the process of selecting technology may begin during the preschool years, it continues through adulthood. Thus, some of the decisions that practitioners will make during the early years must take into account what will be expected from the child in her or his later years. Technology is too expensive to fail to carefully plan for the future. Preschool children soon grow up and attend school. Thus, clinicians must determine how an AAC system might grow with the child.

Requirements and Functional Dimensions for AAC Components. In a comprehensive chapter describing communication systems and the components of systems, Vanderheiden and Lloyd (1986) offered two outstanding compilations of the literature. In a checklist of "requirements of an overall multi-component communication system" (p. 54), multiple requirements within nine broad categories were listed for use by practitioners during an assessment. The nine categories might be utilized to develop a series of questions that would prove useful to practitioners working with nonverbal children. The checklist may be utilized during an assessment of a young child, or may prove useful during a team meeting that focuses on projected programmatic needs for AAC intervention. The types of questions that might be developed include:

1. Does the proposed system provide a range of functions for communication?
2. How would the system (technique) fit into the child's life?
3. Is the technique usable across all communication partners?
4. Where may the child use the system?
5. How does the system restrict the child when communicating?
6. How much more effective does the system make the child as a communicator?
7. Does the system grow with the child?
8. How does the child feel about the system?
9. Can the child's family afford to purchase and/or maintain the system?

These questions and many others must be asked by AAC specialists when evaluating and selecting assistive technology. Practitioners may want to review the original source and develop decision-making protocols of their own for use with their clients.

Twenty-one "functional dimensions of individual system components" (p. 60) were outlined by Vanderheiden and Lloyd (1986). Each of 21 dimensions was defined, followed by a summary of the importance or impact of each dimension. The 21 dimensions may be used by practitioners who need to evaluate the usefulness of a specific component within the context of a child's total AAC system. The criteria from which practitioners may select, for incorporation into a child's system, include: "openness, speed, assertability, display permanence, projection, correctability, expandability, portability, position independence, independence, intelligibility/obviousness, appropriateness, durability, total cost, cosmesis, materials/practice compatibility, similarity, training, adaptability, interdevice compatibility, and computer compatibility" (p. 60). Although beyond the scope of this introductory chapter, these 21 criteria form the foundation from which the process of device selection should occur. That is, we cannot afford to select devices because they seem attractive and useful—we must select assistive technology because it matches specific needs.

The task of selecting technology for the nonverbal child who uses AAC can seem overwhelming because it is difficult to project into the future and even more difficult to find funding sources if you make a mistake during the selection process. The four resources described in this section should be utilized to help sort through the numerous decisions to be made when selecting AAC systems for the young preschool child. Each author has had years of experience, and therefore offers invaluable guidelines for those who are inexperienced.

In summary, there are two steps when selecting an AAC system: (1) collect initial data through complete observations of all skills, and (2) fit the child with an appropriate AAC system that matches the needs identified during the initial assessment.

INTERVENTION FOR THE YOUNG CHILD WHO USES AUGMENTATIVE AND ALTERNATIVE COMMUNICATION

Assuming that an initial assessment has been completed (see Huer, 1987) and it has been determined that augmentative and alternative communication is appropriate, there are several immediate decisions that face the speech-language pathologist or special education teacher with regard to language intervention. First, in the case of a young child who is nonverbal, there must be a plan to develop expressive language through strategies in addition to speech. Thus, considerable attention is paid to all alternative forms for expression, such as gestures, sign languages, pointing to pictures on a communication board, and so forth. The intervention plan should also address ways to augment residual vocalizations and nonverbal communication developing in the young child. Several case studies are included within this chapter as examples of selection between gestures versus communication board use. In general, no two clients are alike. AAC intervention is a process in which each child's needs are evaluated and a plan of action begins. With most young nonverbal children, the first plan of action involves working with the child's caregivers.

Stimulating Communication Development Through Involvement of Caregivers

Young children are expected to develop communication skills according to predictable developmental sequences. When nonverbal children demonstrate atypical communication patterns that place them at risk for expressive language development, professionals can help their primary caregivers take advantage of their time and thus optimize communication development. Billeaud (1995) offered tips for helping families promote development of prelinguistic skills from 6 to 12 months. By the age of 6 months, babies usually have a variety of communication partners and have experiences with "nonverbal (e.g., postural, gestural, touch, glance), vocal (e.g., crying, intonational variations), or verbal (words) interactions" (p. 47), to which they are beginning to attach meaning. Teachers as well as speech-language pathologists may need to collaborate with family members about expectations for the emergence of communication and the need to provide experiences to motivate the child to become a better communicator.

Billeaud (1995) noted the importance of explaining the distinctions between the terms "communication," "language," and "speech" to primary caregivers and suggested the following specific techniques to be taught to foster communication development: "attribution of meaning to the child's actions; self-talk; parallel talk; vocal play; simple games with incidental phonations, e.g., 'gotcha'; assisting with direction of the child's eye contact; sensory stimulation; therapeutic positioning; coaching the immediate family and their designees in working at the child's level of ability; and facilitating effective communication between parent and service providers" (pp. 50–51). One area that warrants particular attention is positioning. Optimal positioning facilitates communication development. Positioning is critical to accessing assistive technology, communication boards, and all other forms of AAC. Without the proper positioning, children may have no or limited access to optional AAC. Attention to positioning is critical to language intervention for the nonverbal and physically challenged.

Literacy Development for Preschoolers Who Use AAC

An additional means for ensuring the development of appropriate vocabulary is through careful attention to the early literacy experiences of preschool children. Although it is beyond the scope of this chapter to comment in detail on literacy issues (see Chapter 7 for a complete discussion of the issues related to literacy and language learning in a preschool language environment), literacy is an important issue in language intervention for the young child who uses AAC. Light, Binger, and Kelford Smith (1994) have provided an excellent summary of the literature on early literacy development for preschoolers who use AAC. Their report focuses on story-reading interactions between preschoolers who use AAC and their mothers. The results of their study indicate that children may participate less frequently during story-reading interactions than do mothers. Children may have less means to participate as they rely on unaided modes of communication when they do interact. There apparently is a lack of access to effective means to communicate when children sit in their mothers' laps or sit beside their mothers in chairs. Such positional constraints impact the mother's abilities to read eye gaze and facial expressions. Story reading does foster the goal for establishing social closeness and the development of closer interpersonal relationships between participants. Suggestions for clinical and educational activities proposed by Light et al. (1994), as well as the review of the literature and references listed therein, make this a valuable resource for professionals concerned with AAC use among preschoolers.

Expressive Language Development

It is always the case that AAC practices build on those traditional expressive language skills (speech) that are present. However, often the speech segments and single words produced by children with severe physical disabilities are not sufficient for communication. Thus, AAC "augments" the residual communication that is functional for the young child. That is, one issue that must be addressed is how a young AAC user might express a message through sign, gesture, pointing, hitting a switch on an electronic device, or making another "expressive signal" (which might also include speech or meaningfully inflected vocalizations). One of the early issues in language intervention for the very young child becomes how to develop expressive language through symbolic forms.

In essence, the issues in language intervention for the young child using AAC focus on what should be selected for training and how to support language development through what was selected. To provide a specific example: Suppose a clinician determines that a child might utilize an electronic device with voice output for expression. In this example, the "what" focuses on the various issues surrounding the introduction of an electronic device. If a clinician selects an electronic device with voice output for expressive language, then she or he must develop a plan to aid expressive language development. Exactly how the clinical plan is implemented includes a consideration of issues such as vocabulary storage, selection of symbol sets, determination of best methods for access and retrieval, portability of the device, and type of voice that will best match the preschool child's personality. Multiple issues immediately face the clinician or teacher providing AAC services to young children. Refer to the case studies in this chapter for explicit examples of the interplay between decisions regarding technology and those regarding vocabulary.

Interactive Language Skills

More broadly, beyond those issues previously mentioned, there are additional factors that are critical to the development of language. Young children need to develop competence in interaction (discourse). Simply providing alternative forms for expression, specific vocabulary, and voice output does not directly lead to interaction. Issues pertaining to the development of interactive skills in young children who are AAC users include strategies for initiation and turn taking. Young children with physical disabilities do not always initiate as much as other children. Children who are AAC users are often known to be very passive communicators. Physical movement may be limited; involvement in the upper and/or lower extremities may prevent typical initiation patterns like pointing, gesturing, grabbing, and pulling. Involvement of the laryngeal muscles may prevent spontaneous vocalizations, which are normally under voluntary control of the child. With AAC users, most of the communicative exchanges focus on attention to a child's hands, a communication board, or voice output from an electronic device. The typical signals for turn taking, such as eye gaze, eye contact, and physical movements, are different for able-bodied children during individual turns than for children with disabilities.

Explicit activities to facilitate early interaction skills can be found in works by Kraat (1985) and Dunst (1981), who offer numerous suggestions for activities that facilitate a young child's "wanting" to initiate communication. Examples of the strategies that these investigators described include:

1. not giving the child her or his turn during a game—instead pause to see what the child will do.

2. have the adult play with the child's favorite toy in front of the child.

3. request that the child play with a toy that the child dislikes.

4. remove the batteries from a favorite toy so that it stops working after the child has started playing.

5. place the child's favorite toy just out of reach but in her or his line of vision.

6. sit silently next to the child but do not interact or establish eye contact with her or him.

These activities have been proven useful for the professional who wishes to begin to teach the young preschool and school-age child to initiate communication.

Language and Communication Activities: Examples

Skilled speech-language pathologists have developed numerous activities to facilitate language development in the nonverbal child (Burkhart, 1993). Several examples of activities for young children are listed in the following sections (Stewart, personal communication, February 1, 1991).

Early Morning Routines. Routines for morning might include activities such as discussing past events (e.g., What did you do last night?). Daily schedules might be discussed. Activities that pertain to the bus, the ride to school, home, taking off of coats, weekend trips, the schedule for the day, and so forth may be utilized to elicit requests for help, to ask *wh-* questions, and to describe meaningful events. The language objectives of initiation, maintaining and shifting topics, and use of multiple modes for communication can be reinforced and monitored during this time. Natural consequences should be used as reinforcements as much as possible.

The Group Speech Therapy Session. Group sessions may be used for drill and practice when introducing new signs, symbols, or technology, or they may be set up to enhance spontaneous communication. The session can be designed to be flexible, or it can be structured to meet the objectives that are determined during the conference with the parents. During a very structured program, the speech-language pathologist leads the group while the educational assistant helps those students with special physical needs to participate.

The speech room may be designed for structured receptive training on one day, and on alternate days may be "set up" to enhance spontaneous communication. There are several ways to sabotage a room to encourage spontaneous communication from children. Toys may be placed on shelves out of reach. A "where" board might be constructed near the door with all the places in the building represented, as well as all of the teachers and children with whom the children in therapy come into contact. A daily schedule and several miniboards can be made available near activity areas that have been loaded with "hidden" symbols, toys, clues for games, and other problem-solving activities.

Snack Activities. Snack activities may incorporate the speech-language pathologist, teacher, educational assistants, and other students who have been trained in AAC. There are numerous activities that may focus on natural communication and interaction during mealtimes. Snacktimes provide excellent opportunities to teach initiation and requesting strategies. Mealtimes offer additional "opportunities for sabotage," which provide motivation and fun for the children (e.g., give the child an unopened carton of milk, forget to give eating utensils, or serve food not requested).

Training Partner Facilitators. Training peer partners has become a critical area, which must be addressed within a program of intervention. Partners can serve an invaluable role in the development of communication. Throughout each day, partners can provide opportunities for communication. Able-bodied children who have observed or received training in multimodal communication may recognize the communicative symbols or signs and respond to the AAC user in the hallways or lunchroom. They may be trained to use cues for elaboration and expansion. They may assist in identifying communication breakdowns during the day. They may offer the speech-language pathologist increased time for drill and training with communication boards or technology with individual AAC users. Young computer "hackers" love to assist AAC users in acquiring skill on their new computerized devices. Some older "buddies" may provide a link with the AAC user and the community, outside school hours. Most important, AAC buddies serve as models for other students.

Parents. Parents have been included within early intervention programs through weekly meetings to discuss current issues in AAC, to provide updates on available techniques for communication, and to share problems, successes, and follow-up. A home/school notebook is often utilized to describe particular activities the child enjoyed at home or in school. New vocabulary trained or needed is recorded in the weekly notebook. The notebook serves as a diary for some parents to record the progress, or lack thereof, in communicating. Frustrations of the speech-language pathologist, parents, teacher, and child may be communicated immediately in order to facilitate a check on the system as needed.

Some speech-language pathologists have set up an AAC resource room for parents and professionals as a part of their program. A variety of materials, books, videotapes, tests, and commercial brochures from manufacturers have proven useful for management within preschools. As videotapes, books, and journals are acquired by professionals within individual programs, a monthly "reading" club might be formed in order to benefit everyone in contact with the young preschool child.

CASE STUDY: JOEY

Joey was a child aged 2;7, who had been diagnosed with severe Goldenhar syndrome, Type III, which resulted in multiple facial anomalies, including left facial cleft, no hard palate, no left facial bones, and no left eye or ear. His mother reported that 2 of his series of 11 planned surgeries had been completed. Receptive language testing during the initial assessment resulted in a language age equivalent of 36 months; expressive language testing placed Joey's productive skills at approximately 18 to 21 months. Other testing indicated apparently normal hearing in the right ear, age-appropriate motor skills, and normal cognitive development.

Joey's mother requested immediate augmentative and alternative communication therapy to minimize the receptive/expressive gap that was emerging due to the need for many surgical procedures. In addition, it was apparent that Joey's facial structure anomalies adversely affected his speech production mechanism. Therefore, AAC programming for this typically developing, active child with severe facial anomalies was planned for the interim period before surgical repair would be completed.

Because of Joey's medical needs, it was particularly important to establish a close working relationship with the parents. During the initial parent conference, it was readily apparent that Joey needed a representational system for depicting expressive vocabulary because his speech production mechanism was severely involved. Together, the speech-language pathologist and family compiled lists of words that had to be accessible within the vocabulary sets to be selected. It was especially critical that Joey be able to communicate with persons in the medical community as his visits there were so frequent and answers directly from Joey to the doctors and nurses were so critical. It was also highly relevant to note that Joey's speech production skills (phonetic inventory) were developing at an accelerated rate with each new surgery. It was important to observe and plan for Joey's speech development within the overall intervention program, so that eventually, the AAC techniques would be eliminated as speech production skills increased through surgical techniques.

Several of the commercially available picture (symbol) sets were presented to the family. Joey favored the Mayer-Johnson Picture Communication Symbols and the Touch 'N Talk communication stickers (available from Don Johnston Developmental Equipment). The two symbol sets were recorded as preferred. Mini-communication boards were planned. In addition, Joey's mother was taking a class in sign language and had begun to teach him some signs. A dictionary of the signs that Joey knew was compiled. Finally, spoken words that were in Joey's repertoire and were intelligible to strangers were listed. Within the first 2 months, a listing of all of Joey's words, signs, pictures, and symbols currently used (or to be used) for expressive communication was compiled as a baseline from which to work. A communication board was designed with reference to each of the techniques through which Joey would communicate. Redundant symbols were removed from the planned layout of the board (and miniboards); because Joey signed or verbalized a few words, it was unnecessary to place these on the communication board.

During the same time frame, the speech-language pathologist provided education regarding the technology that was available for augmenting a young child's communication. The speech-language pathologist discussed the 10 crucial dimensions (Fishman, 1987); the 14 categories (Rosen & Goodenough-Trepagnier, 1989); the seven-point hierarchy (Cook & Coleman, 1987); and the 21 functional dimensions (Vanderheiden & Lloyd, 1986) often reviewed when considering technology. In short, multiple examples of a variety of techniques that might be relevant to Joey's needs were presented. Following a series of questions and answers during conferencing, it was determined that the relevant criteria for Joey's initial system should include a system that incorporated direct selection techniques, had a speech output, was light weight for portability by Joey, provided for prestorage of selected vocabulary, was accessible in multiple environments, provided for assertability and correctability, provided for independence when Joey wanted to communicate, was easy to learn, would require a minimum of training before use, and could be expanded as Joey grew. Other, secondary features, such as cost, were also noted.

The speech-language pathologist and parents reviewed videotapes depicting several commercially available devices (see Appendix 8-1) and selected two devices as potential systems that met the criteria selected to meet the child's needs. A consultant from the company was invited to demonstrate the equipment and to provide Joey and his parents with a hands-on trial. Joey and his parents, along with the speech-language pathologist, picked an assistive device and software that met the criteria and that Joey himself liked. A decision was made to order the communication device in approximately 6 months. Toward that objective, the symbol systems that had been selected were reviewed. In order to help Joey make the transition toward assistive technology, the symbols on his communication board and the overlay of the assistive device were laid in a similar way. The symbol system to be used on the device and the symbol systems preferred during early conferences were ordered so as to offer Joey the following advantages: a "planned layout" for a communication board and/or the device; opportunities for interaction with multiple symbol sets that offered unique vocabularies; practice in direct selection of the same symbols that would appear on the device; immediate receptive training of the "new" symbol system, which would be utilized for representation of expressive language; a plan for the future transition from communication board to electronic device; and "simulated experiences" in learning one component of the new system, vocabulary selection. The miniboards and the communication boards were planned with similar layouts in order to minimize the future effects of switching between the boards and the device.

Within 3 months, an expressive vocabulary was accessible to Joey; a device had been selected for introduction 6 months later; and a trial period of management was established through a rented device. Intervention strategies that focused on Joey's use of the new system for requests, confirmations and denials, and other selected speech acts were introduced. After each surgery, the intervention plan was reexamined and adjusted as necessary.

CASE STUDY: MARTHA

Martha was a preschool child diagnosed with spastic cerebral palsy with quadriplegia.

Results of an initial assessment indicated the following: single word intelligibility (5%); a few paralinguistic skills (facial expressions, intonations, vocalizations); questionable receptive language score (vocabulary, approximately 2 years); expressive language (estimated 12 months); cognitive skill (understands cause-and-effect); fine and gross motor skills very limited (learning to pick up spoon during feeding; uses adapted splints and grips); a few consonants (bilabials) and vowels in phonetic inventory; three picture communication board; very supportive parents.

On meeting this child and the family it was immediately apparent that measures of receptive and expressive language functioning as well as presumed cognitive skills were not conclusive due to the child's physical disability. Martha appeared to be the typical "difficult-to-test" child. It was important, therefore, to immediately have the preschool staff work together with the parents and with other professionals to establish a solid team. Martha's multiple needs warranted consulting with the speech-language pathologist, teacher, physical therapist, occupational therapist, biomedical engineer, seating specialist, doctor, nurse, computer specialist (for adapting input and/or interface options), and other communication partners in Martha's life. Not all these professionals were within the preschool system and accessible for a group conference. It was important, therefore, for the speech-language pathologist to establish lines of communication with them in order to better determine the exact nature of Martha's multiple needs. Through interviews with Martha's parents, it was possible to access medical records and to contact several of the relevant professionals who were familiar with Martha.

The initial plan for establishing therapy for Martha started with the collection of baseline data regarding Martha's multiple modes of communication. Her parents and preschool staff, including the speech-language pathologist, were asked to create a dictionary of Martha's expressive communication signals. Specifically, the parents, and preschool staff were asked to record the "words" often spoken by Martha, her idiosyncratic gestures, and the paralinguistic functions of language noted around the home or school. Examples of each type of expressive communication signal were provided to the parents and preschool staff by the speech-language pathologist. Next to each expressive signal (i.e., word or gesture), all participants were instructed to record the "assumed meaning." Multiple meanings were recorded, as appropriate. If Martha used the signal more than once, a tally mark was made in the dictionary beside the signal in order to show frequency of use and to eliminate redundancy of entering the same signal over and over in the dictionary. Because the siblings as well as the mother and father were very supportive of the preschool programming, each family member was asked to make her or his own dictionary of all Martha's expressive signals. In addition, the parents and preschool staff were asked to videotape a few of their interactions with Martha.

Over a several-week period, Martha's expressive repertoire was compiled, and the consistency of use of expressive signaling was observed across communication partners. As the weeks passed, the communication partners were instructed to change some of Martha's routines to encourage her to communicate through a specific signal, and to encourage a range of signal use. At the end of several weeks, the compiled information indicated that Martha had very few expressive signals. In addition, it was revealed that Martha's partners interpreted her expressions differently, and that Martha was inconsistent when expressing her intent. Based on these data, it was apparent that a "base" of communication signals did not exist on which an expressive communication program might be built. The few consistent, intelligible expressive signals were compiled into a list to be added to additional expressive programming, when available.

Simultaneous with the team's review of the dictionary data and videotape segments, the speech-language pathologist presented six representational systems for depicting vocabulary. After a careful review of each vocabulary set with the parents and child, the Core Picture Vocabulary (available from Don Johnston Developmental Equipment) was selected.

During those sessions where vocabulary was reviewed, it was noted that physical access for direct selection warranted further review. The physical therapist volunteered to make a T-shaped pointer for use in direct selection. The need for an overhead sling and/or arm support was discussed. A comprehensive assessment of fine and gross motor skills was initiated within the context of diversity of techniques for access.

At the initial conference, Martha's parents expressed an interest in an electronic device. Therefore, some conference times were allocated to the viewing of videotapes depicting available technology. The speech-language pathologist discussed the 10 crucial dimensions (Fishman, 1987); the 14 categories (Rosen & Goodenough-Trepagnier, 1989); the seven-point hierarchy (Cook & Coleman, 1987); and the 21 functional dimensions (Vanderheiden & Lloyd, 1986) often reviewed when considering technology. In addition, Martha was provided with opportunities for "hands on" practice with assistive technology.

Based on the discussions regarding technology and the observations of Martha interacting with various devices and switches, it was determined that her immediate needs for communication programming included the consistent development of a receptive vocabulary set, further examination of alternatives for physical access to a communication board or device, and a structured program of remediation to establish consistency of response.

Martha's communication program focused on receptive and expressive vocabulary selection, communication board design and layout, establishment of a consistent response for direct selection utilizing the right hand with adapted pointer, and the modeling of selected speech acts of requesting and responding. Selected strategies from Kangas and Lloyd (1988) were introduced to facilitate the development of language and cognition. In addition, the classroom, lunchroom, and home were frequently "sabotaged" to facilitate increased initiation. Decisions regarding purchase of technology were postponed for six months.

CASE STUDY: EDDIE

Eddie was a 5-year-old preschooler diagnosed with Williams syndrome. Initial assessments reported that Eddie had a receptive language age equivalency of 4 years. He had limited verbalizations, however, and poor imitation skills. He was reported to be a very social child and to use some gesturing and pointing. He was ambulatory, with some gross and fine motor coordination problems. Finally, the assessment reports noted that Eddie was highly distractible and had a short attention span.

The clinician's initial objective was to develop an expressive vocabulary for Eddie through the selection of an appropriate symbol system. The second objective was the development of an interactive communication board that was also portable. At the initial meeting with the child, there existed limited means for the expression of content. Although Eddie verbalized and gestured, his communicative attempts were not readily intelligible to strangers. He was very active, easily distracted, and often moved about the room to examine objects.

During the first week with Eddie, the speech-language pathologist constructed a wall chart with a 2-inch symbol for "outside." When Eddie entered the room, the speech-language pathologist physically assisted him in pointing to the symbol and then they went outside to play. Each day Eddie entered the preschool classroom the speech-language pathologist added a new symbol to the wall chart, prompted Eddie, and provided an appropriate reinforcement.

After the first week, Eddie differentiated between the symbols and began requesting.

The speech-language pathologist constructed a notebook with the newly learned symbols for Eddie's use and arranged a meeting with the parents and an educational assistant in the preschool. At the conference, the symbol system was described and a plan of action was devised by the group. The educational assistant agreed to encourage communication during snacktime, on the playground, and in the hallways using the new communication book. The educational assistant trained Eddie's "typical" peers to communicate using the book and to respond to Eddie when he used it. The parents agreed to take Eddie to places on request, such as to Grandma's, a fast food restaurant, and the grocery store.

Three months after the initial plan was devised, portability was seen to be a problem because Eddie was misplacing the communication book often. The speech-language pathologist devised a "trucker's style" wallet and attached it to Eddie's belt. A home/school notebook was implemented for communication between the preschool and home. The parents used the notebook to report activities of the week and listed symbols that were needed for Eddie's communication book. The communication book provided opportunities for Eddie to communicate with his peers. (He was even invited to a birthday party.) Eddie's expressive vocabulary and interaction skills became intelligible both around the home and at preschool.

CASE STUDY: CAROLYN

Carolyn was a preschooler diagnosed as "trainable mentally retarded." She appeared as a noncompliant, hyperactive, highly distractible child whose behavior interfered even with informal testing strategies. Some idiosyncratic gesturing and limited signing were observed. Her receptive language skills were approximately 3 years (presumed). At the initial meeting with Carolyn, it was evident that a behavior modification program was needed. In addition, it was determined that the first objective for therapy would be the introduction of a symbol or sign technique for meeting expressive vocabulary needs. A second objective of therapy was the further development of paralinguistic behaviors and appropriate pragmatic language skills.

During the initial meeting, it was noted that Carolyn's predominant means for expression was through gesturing and sign. Although Carolyn demonstrated good imitation of sign, her fine motor difficulties led to adaptations of several signs. She was quite active, frequently threw toys presented by the speech-language pathologist, often moved away from the task, and became easily frustrated.

As it appeared that Carolyn's behavior problems might be related to her frustration with communication, the speech-language pathologist developed a management plan that incorporated training of symbols in place of sign, and a variety of group language activities. The symbols were targeted for Carolyn's expressive communication needs. The objectives of the group activities included behavior modification, attention to selected speech acts, and the introduction of basic strategies during discourse.

The speech-language pathologist built on Carolyn's activity level by designing "places to go" within the preschool building. A cue was presented: "Where do you want to go?" When Carolyn touched a "place" symbol, the speech-language pathologist and Carolyn went to that place. If Carolyn had another place in mind, conversational repair strategies could be modeled by the speech-language pathologist. "Food" symbols were introduced during snack and lunch times, following the prompt "What?"

During the group language activity, current preschool events were discussed. Carolyn liked to play "teacher" and lead the group by touching symbols and the days and months on calendars. The modeling by the other students in the language group assisted Carolyn in acquiring more appropriate turn-taking skills. As playing the "teacher" was highly reinforcing, Carolyn's behavior improved considerably in her attempts to receive a turn.

Carolyn's behavior modification program emphasized control. Control of Carolyn's behavior was facilitated by an observation that Carolyn liked to control others. Carolyn rejected a communication board and symbols placed within a folder. However, when the board was reconstructed on a clipboard similar to the ones used by the preschool staff, Carolyn accepted the communication clipboard and carried it around the preschool grounds proudly.

As Carolyn liked the feeling of control, favorite activities were frequently sabotaged in order to prompt selected speech acts and to practice discourse. One such routine centered around a candy machine. Carolyn had to request "money," point to the machine's location, and then point to the candy she wanted. Frequently the candy machine was "broken." Often sent in the wrong direction, Carolyn also had to clarify direction. The candy was packaged so that it was difficult to open. Thus, Carolyn had to repeatedly request assistance.

SUMMARY

A brief overview of several issues pertaining to augmentative and alternative communication programming appropriate for young children with severe physical challenges and/or cognitive impairments was presented. Issues pertaining to the identification of prelinguistic (nonsymbolic) communication were outlined, and selection criteria for choosing the most appropriate vocabulary for nonverbal children were compiled. An overview of augmentative and alternative communication systems commercially available for preschool populations was provided (Appendix 8-1), and crucial dimensions for selecting between assistive technology were discussed. The case studies offer additional self-study.

Augmentative and alternative communication therapy incorporates an integrative approach to assessment and intervention (Zangari, 1994). Critical factors necessary to all intervention practices include attention to reasons for communication, a means to represent vocabulary and express intent, strategies through which messages may be communicated, and the communication styles and patterns of each child's communication partners. Language intervention for prelinguistic and/or nonverbal children is multidimensional. Much of the current practice is based on decision making along a continuum. The approaches to practice follow an "if-then" model. The outcomes of clinical practices in AAC are improving as our knowledge bases and clinical case studies expand.

APPENDIX 8: PUBLISHERS AND MANUFACTURERS OF AUGMENTATIVE AND ALTERNATIVE COMMUNICATION EQUIPMENT AND MATERIALS FOR THE PRESCHOOL CHILD USING AAC

Ablenet Inc., 1081 Tenth Avenue S.E., Minneapolis, MN 55414-1312, (800) 322-0956. A variety of switches for access to electrical games and appliances, toys, mounting systems, adapters, ranging from $12.00 to $54.00 up.

Crestwood Company, 6625 N. Sidney Place, Milwaukee, WI 53209-3259, (414) 352-5678. Interactive talk-back and voice/sound activated aids, $22.00 up; Opticommunicator, $59.95.

Don Johnston Developmental Equipment, Inc., P.O. Box 639, 1000 N. Rand Road 115, Wauconda, IL 60084-0639, (708) 526-2682 or (800) 999-4660. The Nonspeech Test, $195.00 (for language assessment); Core Picture Vocabulary, $28.00 (160 words); Switches, mounts, adapters, light technology, call for pricing; Circletime Tales Deluxe, $95.00 (CD-ROM program); Ke:nx 3.5, $780.00 MAC based (computer interface).

Imaginart Communication Products, 307 Arizona Street, Bisbee, AZ 85603, (800) 828-1376. Pick 'n Stick Primary Pack, $28.00 (96 stickers); Touch 'n Talk Communication Board, $15.00; Eye-Com Board, $39.95.

IntelliTools, Inc., 55 Leveroni Court, Suite 9, Novato, CA 94949, (800) 899-6687. IntelliKeys Keyboard, $395.00 up (variety of software available).

Mayer-Johnson Company, P.O. Box 1579, Solana Beach, CA 92075-1579, (619) 550-0084. Picture Communication Symbol Books I–III, $45.00–$49.00; *Engineering the Preschool Environment for Interactive, Symbolic Communication,* by Goossens´, C., Crain, S., & Elder, P., $40.00 (202 pages); *Communication Displays for Engineered Preschool Environments, Books I and II* by Goossens´, C., Crain, S., & Elder, P., $129.00 (multiple displays); *Total Augmentative Communication in the Early Childhood Classroom,* by Burkhart, L., $29.95 (284 pages); *Preschool AAC Checklist* by Henderson, J., $19.00 (116 pages); Boardmaker™ 3.0, $399.00 (produces communication displays on Macintosh).

Prentke Romich Company, 1022 Heyl Road, Wooster, Ohio 44691, (216) 262-1984 or (800) 262-1984. Delta Talker, $4,995 (call for other products).

Sentient Systems Inc., 2100 Wharton, Suite 630, Pittsburgh, PA 15203, (412) 381-4883 or (800) 344-1778. Dynavox, $4,995–$7,995 (color or BW, different memory capacities); Dynavox 2 DOS Software $995, MAC Software $995.

Southeast Augmentative Communication Publications, 2430 11th Avenue North, Birmingham, AL 35234, (205) 251-0165. *Communication Displays for Engineered Preschool Environments, Preschool Display Book 1,* $69.00 (Matrix-16, Horsehoe/Rotary-13); *Preschool Display Book II,* $69.00 (Matrix-36, Matrix-32); *Engineering the Preschool Environment for Interactive Symbolic Communication,* $40.00 (18 months to 5 years developmentally); *Utilizing Switch Interfaces With Children Who Are Severely Physically Challenged,* call for pricing (316 pages).

TASH, Inc. (Technical Aids and Systems for the Handicapped), Unit 1-91 Station Street, Ajax, Ontario, Canada L1S 3H2, (905) 686-4129 or (800) 463-5685. Switches, mounting hardware, keyguards, and alternative keyboards, ranging from $30 to $400 and up.

Words+, Inc., 40015 Sierra Highway, Building B-145, Palmdale, CA 93550, (800) 869-8521. MessageMate 20, call for pricing.

Zygo Industries, Inc., P.O. Box 1008, Portland, OR 97207-1008, (800) 234-6006. AD-2 "Tiny Tot" Pointer, $160.00 (headpointer); The MACAW "Family" of Products, call for pricing.

REFERENCES

American Speech-Language-Hearing Association. (1989). Competencies for speech-language pathologists providing services in augmentative communication. *Asha, 31,* 107–110.

American Speech-Language-Hearing Association (1991). Report: Augmentative and alternative communication. *Asha,* 33(Suppl. 5), 9–12.

Arthur, M. (1994). Communication instruction in the 1990s: An overview of future directions. In K. Linfoot (Ed.), *Communication strategies for people with developmental disabilities: Issues from theory and practice* (pp. 177–197). Baltimore: Brookes.

Beukelman, D. R., Jones, R. S., & Rowan, M. (1989). Frequency of word usage by nondisabled peers in integrated preschool classrooms. *Augmentative and Alternative Communication,* 5(4), 243–248.

Beukelman, D. R., McGinnis, J., & Morrow, D. (1991). Vocabulary selection in augmentative and alternative communication. *Augmentative and Alternative Communication, 7*(3), 171–185.

Beukelman, D., & Mirenda, P. (1992). *Augmentative and alternative communication: Management of severe communication disorders in children and adults.* Baltimore: Brookes.

Billeaud, F. (1995). Communication development from 6 to 12 months: Helping families promote skills in late infancy for babies at risk for atypical development. *National Student Speech-Language-Hearing Association Journal, 22,* 47–52.

Burkhart, L. (1993). *Total augmentative communication in the early childhood classroom.* Eldersburg, Md.: Author.

Butterfield, N. (1994). Play as an assessment and intervention strategy for children with language and intellectual disabilities. In K. Linfoot (Ed.), *Communication strategies for people with developmental disabilities: Issues from theory and practice* (pp. 12–44). Baltimore: Brookes.

Butterfield, N., Linfoot, K., & Arthur, M. (1994). Enhancing communication in functional settings: Putting research into practice. In K. Linfoot (Ed.), *Communication strategies for people with developmental disabilities: Issues from theory and practice* (pp. 198–212). Baltimore: Brookes.

Cook, A. M., & Coleman, C. L. (1987). Selecting augmentative communication systems by matching client skills and needs to system characteristics. *Seminars in Speech and Language, 8*(2), 153–167.

Damico, S. (1994). Empowering nonvocal populations: An emerging concept. *National Student Speech-Language-Hearing Association Journal, 21,* 31–44.

Dunst, C. J. (1981). *Infant learning: A cognitive-linguistic intervention strategy.* New York: Teaching Resources Corporation.

Fishman, I. (l987). *Electronic communication aids selection and use.* Boston: College Hill Press.

Fried-Oken, M., & More, L. (1992). An initial vocabulary for nonspeaking preschool children based on developmental and environmental language sources. *Augmentative and Alternative Communication, 8*(1), 41–56.

Goossens´, C., & Crain, S. (1986). *Augmentative communication intervention resource.* Wauconda, Ill.: Don Johnston Developmental Equipment.

Hanrahan, L., Ferrier, L., & Jolie, K. (1987, November). *Infants, caregivers and augmentative communication: We must intervene earlier.* Paper presented at the American Speech-Language-Hearing Association Annual Convention, New Orleans.

Huer, M. B. (1987). 1986 ISAAC Round Table Discussion—Formal assessment tools: What we have, what we need. *The ISAAC* [International Society for Augmentative and Alternative Communication] *Bulletin, 10,* 14–17.

Kangas, K. A., & Lloyd, L. L. (1988). Early cognitive skills as prerequisites to augmentative and alternative communication use: What are we waiting for? *Augmentative and Alternative Communication, 4,* 211–221.

Kraat, A. W. (1985). *Communication interaction between aided and natural speakers: A state of the art report.* Toronto: Canadian Rehabilitation Council for the Disabled.

Letto, M., Bedrosian, J., & Skarakis-Doyle, E. (1994). Application of Vygotskian developmental theory to language acquisition in a young child with cerebral palsy. *Augmentative and Alternative Communication, 10,* 151–168.

Light, J., Binger, C., & Kelford Smith, A. (1994). Story reading interactions between preschoolers who use AAC and their mothers. *Augmentative and Alternative Communication, 10,* 255–268.

Linfoot, K. (Ed.). (1994). *Communication strategies for people with developmental disabilities: Issues from theory and practice.* Baltimore: Brookes.

Mar, H., & Sall, N. (1994). Programmatic approach to use of technology in communication instruction for children with dual sensory impairments. *Augmentative and Alternative Communication, 10,* 138–151.

Marvin, C., Beukelman, D., & Bilyeu, D. (1994). Vocabulary-use patterns in preschool children: Effects of context and time sampling. *Augmentative and Alternative Communication, 10,* 224–236.

Musselwhite, C. (1986). *Adaptive play for special needs children: Strategies to enhance communication and learning.* San Diego: Singular Publishing.

Musselwhite, C. (1990, August). *Topic setting: Generic and specific strategies.* Paper presented at the Sixth Biennial Conference of the International Society for Augmentative and Alternative Communication, Stockholm, Sweden.

Reinhartsen, D., Edmondson, R., & Crais, E. (1997). Developing assistive technology strategies for infants and toddlers with communication difficulties. *Seminars in Speech and Language, 18*(3), 283–301.

Rosen, M. J., & Goodenough-Trepagnier, C. (1989). The Tufts-MIT prescription guide: Assessment of users to predict the suitability of augmentative communication devices. *Assistive Technology, 1,* 51–61.

Siegel-Causey, E., & Guess, D. (1989). *Enhancing nonsymbolic communication interactions among learners with severe disabilities.* Baltimore: Brookes.

Vanderheiden, G., & Lloyd, L. (1986). Communication systems and their components. In S. W. Blackstone (Ed.), *Augmentative communication: An introduction* (pp. 49–161). Rockville, Md.: American Speech-Language-Hearing Association.

von Tetzchner, S., & Martinsen, H. (1992). *Introduction to symbolic and augmentative communication.* San Diego: Singular Publishing.

Warren, S., & Reichle, J. (1992). *Causes and effects in communication and language intervention.* Baltimore: Brookes.

Warren, S., Yoder, P., Gazdag, G., Kim, K., & Jones, H. (1993). Facilitating prelinguistic communication skills in young children with developmental delay. *Journal of Speech and Hearing Research, 36,* 83–97.

Yorkston, K. M., Dowden, P. A., Honsinger, M. J., Marriner, N., & Smith, K. (1988). A comparison of standard and user vocabulary lists. *Augmentative and Alternative Communication, 4*(4), 189–210.

Zangari, C. (1994, November). *An integrative approach to AAC services: A framework for assessment and intervention.* A paper presented at the Meeting of the American Speech-Language-Hearing Association, New Orleans.

CHAPTER 9

Sensory Integration Treatment for Children With Language Impairments

Tracy Murnan Stackhouse, M.A., OTR
Children's Hospital
Denver
Sarah K. Scharfenaker, M.A., CCC-SLP
Children's Hospital
Denver

Key Terms

adaptive response
arousal
dyspraxia
praxis
proprioception
sensory integration (SI)
sensory modulation
suck/swallow/breathe (SSB)
tactile
vestibular

Overview

Many children with language impairments have sensory integrative problems that complicate their communication difficulties. This chapter will explore the bidirectionally dependent relationship between language and **sensory integration (SI).** The effect of SI disorders on language is an important construct to observe in children with language impairment, and having this knowledge will enable the entry-level therapist to provide state-of-the-art intervention. A mini-course in SI theory within the context of occupational therapy is given, along with a brief neurologic review. This information is then applied to communication disorders with case studies to illustrate the clinical features of these ideas. The intent in this chapter is not to provide detailed assessment and intervention guidelines for professionals to use with children with SI deficits, but to facilitate an understanding of SI principles and to encourage professionals to seek further information and consultation with occupational therapists for the "how" and "what" of assessment and treatment.

SENSORY INTEGRATION

Sensory integration (SI) is a theory of brain-behavior relationships that is also a primary frame of reference used for assessment and intervention within the field of occupational therapy. While the treatment theory was originally formulated by Dr. A. Jean Ayres for use with school-age children with learning disabilities, the theory has grown and developed for use across ages and diagnoses. Clinical practice indicates strong support and efficacy of this treatment process; however, empirical studies continue to be needed to support this expanding practice area. This chapter will focus on early intervention using SI as a framework for understanding and intervening with children with a wide variety of communication disorders. However, to understand the breadth of application of SI theory, it is necessary to explore the context in which SI is applied, that being within the practice of occupational therapy (OT).

Occupational therapists (OTs) bring a broad spectrum of scientific and theoretical information to their practice. Because the framework of occupational therapy is focused on human occupation, the spectrum of OT practice necessarily crosses all age, cultural, and setting boundaries. Fundamental to occupational therapy intervention, then, is engagement of the client in active participation with activities or occupations that are selected to specifically address each individual's unique needs—the needs that brought them to intervention (Keilhofner, 1995). SI is an example of an OT model of practice that views the individual holistically and is based on neuroscientific principles, making it a sound frame of reference for OT practitioners. The neuroscientific underpinnings of SI are complemented by the theory's strong regard for typical development and the influences of play and social cognition. SI places strong emphasis on the process of influencing the nervous system, and it utilizes children as guides of their own actions to exert the most meaningful functional changes in the therapeutic process (Keilhofner, 1995). Ayres (1979, p.135) was careful to emphasize that her theory was based on how sensations *and the responses to them* are what cause the brain to develop. This critical feature of response—or, more accurately, **adaptive response**—is vital to understanding how SI forms a frame within the broader scope of OT.

"O.T. has defined itself as a profession that encompasses human performance components that serve as the basis for occupational performance areas. Performance components and occupational performance areas are influenced strongly by a person's age, state of development, sociocultural background, and environment" (Kramer & Hinojosa, 1993, p. 24). Consequently, you may encounter an occupational therapist practicing in a geriatric setting, a corporate wellness facility, an AIDS treatment program, a community recreation center, a local hospital or specialty treatment center, a community mental health facility, a jail, a school, or a client's home. The spectrum covers physical, cognitive, and mental health disabilities, along with concerns for life management, play, skills, and overall developmental needs. The entire age span is covered, working from pregnancy, through infancy and childhood, into adolescence, adulthood and geriatrics. This is exciting for OT practitioners, but often confusing to medical, school, and lay staff, as well as to the general public. It is beyond the scope of this chapter to further define OT practice; however, mindfulness that SI is a part of OT practice is critical to the scope of the chapter.

Communication is fundamental in our assumptions about human occupation. We depend totally on communication, in its many forms, in order to benefit, enjoy, and contribute to our human culture. Communication is at the crux of what makes us fully human (Vygotsky, 1978). Disordered sensory processing can affect communication (Ayres & Mailloux, 1981) in such a way as to alter a person's ability to carry out daily life roles (Paul, Cohen & Caparulo, 1983). For a child, these roles include that of infant family member growing into child, sibling, playmate, friend, explorer, learner, student, citizen, and future independent person.

The focus of this chapter is on pediatric intervention, specifically in the birth to 5-year age range. Early intervention in pediatric occupational therapy has been transformed in many aspects by the work of Dr. A. Jean Ayres and her theory of sensory integration (Parham & Mailloux, 1996). Children receiving OT will typically have their needs assessed and addressed using a wide variety of frameworks. A child who struggles to use his or her hands efficiently, creating stress with academic performance, needs to learn strategies to adapt for the short term. Intervention also needs to be geared at changing the foundations of the difficulty so that in the long term the problem no longer needs the adaptation. In a quality pediatric program, all aspects of the reason for referral are covered. Given this, it is unusual for a child to receive intervention from only one aspect or theory base while involved in pediatric OT. Pediatric OTs utilize this range of information to affect human development through occupation. Interventions based in sensory-processing theory are very powerful (Ottenbacher & Short, 1985), and often the focus of a child's intervention. Sensory integration provides a broad developmental perspective about how the brain develops the capacity to perceive, learn, and organize behavior (Parham & Mailloux, 1996). Ayres (1972) defined sensory integration as the organization of sensory input in the brain for emitting adaptive responses. Adaptive responses range from scratching when you feel an itch to learning to refine a golf swing—and on to assertively dealing with a difficult or intimidating situation. Adaptive responses can occur automatically with rehearsed patterns, such as driving a car on a familiar route, or can require split-second precision, such as veering around a child who runs out in front of the vehicle. Adaptive responses develop using internal and external feedforward and feedback loops of sensation and thought, as might be illustrated in the process of learning to drive with a standard transmission for the first time. Challenging adaptive responses at the "just right" level are fundamental to SI intervention and were part of the brilliant constructs of the art of therapy that Ayres originated. Ayres was concerned with detailing as many aspects of sensory integration as she could. She developed the primary tests and methods for evaluating and treating the disorders, carried out formal and informal research on these aspects, and continually wrote about and taught her emerging theories. She mentored many colleagues in the full gamut of her work, and she encouraged people to continue the work and never stop asking questions in an effort to lead it forward. See Fisher, Murray, and Bundy (1991) for a detailed accounting of Ayres's contributions to our understanding of the foundations of sensory integration.

Ayres Model of Sensory Integration

Sensory integration is multifaceted. It is a neurological process, a theory of sensory processing related to behavior as well as an intervention (i.e., assessment and treatment) frame of reference. Sensory integration theory is an expansion of sensorimotor developmental theory, originated by Piaget, with its roots in the study of neurobehavioral development (Parham & Mailloux, 1996). Sensory integrative theory is unique in its application of how basic sensory systems affect and influence skill and function. Ayres's widely distributed flowchart is an excellent reference for beginning to visualize the process of sensory integration (Figure 9-1). (The flowchart is presented in a linear manner for simplicity's sake. The actual process of sensory integration would be better represented in a hologram, as it truly is a three-dimensional, spiraling, dynamic process.) Note the presence of more than the five basic senses in the first column (Figure 9-1). Ayres's theories brought to light the influences of less well-known sensory systems and broadened our understanding of how sensation is fundamental to higher-level skill development. While auditory and visual systems are the focus of many behavioral, cognitive, and learning theories, SI theory focuses on how the "hidden senses"—the **vestibular sense**, **proprioception**, and the **tactile sense**—are the precursors to visual and auditory development and to most end-product behaviors, including communication (Ayres, 1979; Ayres & Mailloux, 1981).

According to Kandel, Schwartz, and Jessell (1991), "sensory systems are not only our means for perceiving the external world, but are also essential for maintaining **arousal**, forming our body image, and regulating movement (p. 339)." These are some of the principles on which sensory integration is based.

The SI flowchart should be studied at each level to foster understanding of the concept of SI. It is clearly described in Ayres's 1979 book, *Sensory Integration and the Child* (on pages 59–65). The following is a brief overview of the diagram for beginning to understand Ayres's concepts. Emphasis is placed on the relationship of each level of the chart to the end product of communication. The interested reader is encouraged to study Ayres's writings for detailed information.

Level I. In Figure 9-1, the basic sensory systems are presented to the far left of the diagram. They form the first level of the sensory integrative process. The major sensory systems are defined as follows:

1. Tactile (touch) are the sensations we receive from our skin receptors. They tell us about the type of touch we are feeling (light or crude), about temperature, pain, and specific nuances in texture and location of the stimulus. Touch gives us the physical contact we need to learn, love, and thrive in our complex world (Ayres, 1964; Montague, 1981). From infancy, touch is one of our most important sensations; it has a direct impact on our early relationships, which ultimately form the foundation for interaction and emotional readiness for communication on every level. Ayres's factor-analytic studies also defined a functional linkage between central nervous system tactile processing and the development of motor planning (**praxis**) (Ayres, 1985).

2. Proprioception is the sense we receive from our muscles and joints about where and how our bodies are positioned and moving through space. This is

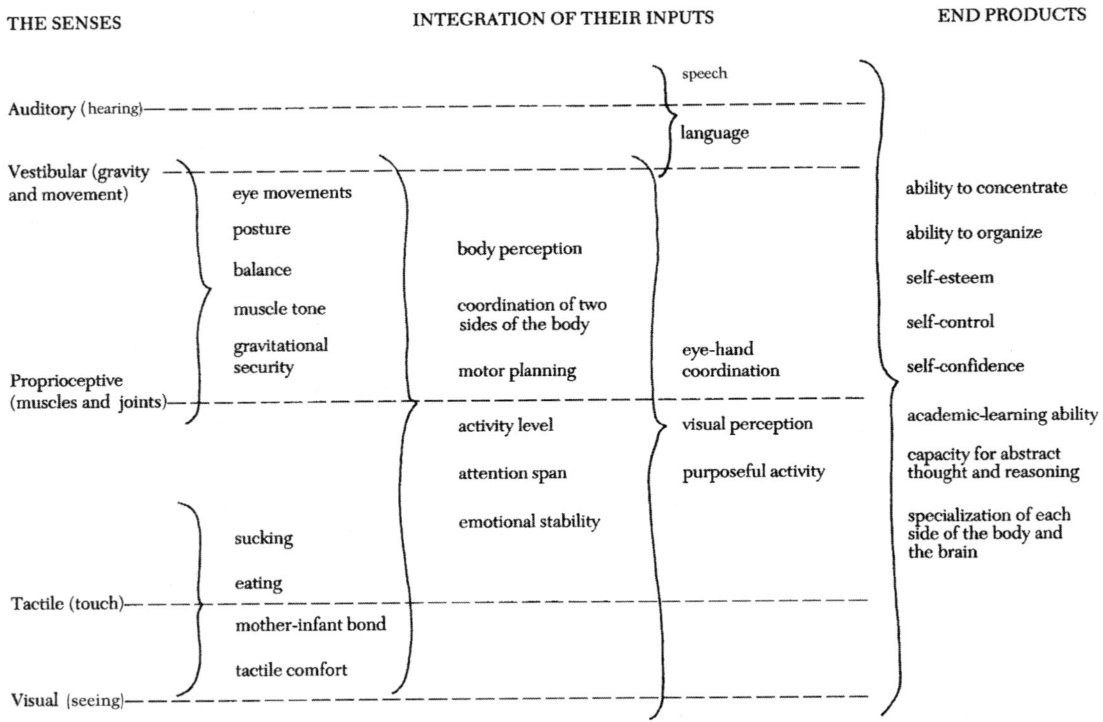

Figure 9-1. The Senses, Integration of Their Inputs, and Their End Products. (From Ayres, A. [1972b]. *Sensory integration and learning disorders*. Los Angeles: Western Psychological Services. Used with permission.

perceived, either cortically or subcortically, as a merged sensation with our movement sense (vestibular) and our vision. It is through this parallel, redundant sensory processing that we develop our body scheme and balance capabilities. In our oral structures, information from proprioceptors and tactile sensations helps us to coordinate complex suck, swallow, and breathing patterns, feeding patterns, and speech production.

3. The vestibular system has peripheral receptors located in the inner ear, which respond to gravity and movement of the head/neck complex. The peripheral information travels along the eighth cranial nerve with the auditory nerve until they bifurcate; then the vestibular system functionally "marries" the proprioceptive system in the brain stem. Together, they provide organization and structure for the other sensory systems and for incoming and outgoing central nervous system information. The vestibular system is popularly thought of as the balance center, a purpose it serves, both literally and figuratively. The vestibular system has wide influence on our arousal state, general organization, posture and muscle tone, and the development of coordination of the body in space and during movement. It is highly interconnected with the visual system as well. As a result, it influences visual motor and perceptual skills.

Level II. The next level of the sensory integrative process starts to represent the functional implications of sensation in the nervous system. Ayres (1979) referred to this as the primary level of integration. Postural control is a product of parallel redundant sensory processing in the vestibular, proprioceptive, and visual systems. With well-developed postural control, the child is able to move about and explore the environment, thus receiving the beginnings of the rich input necessary to develop language concepts. Postural support is also the foundation for adequate breath support.

According to Oetter, Laurel, and Cool (1991), in **suck/swallow/breathe (SSB)**, sensorimotor integration is critical to these early developmental building blocks, which form the basis on which meaning, use, and preference for future experience and interaction will be laid. Any disruption in the ability to register, process, and integrate sensorimotor information will distort these early patterns of interaction. The suck/swallow/breathe (SSB) synergy represents one of the earliest forms of sensorimotor integration and self-regulation (see also Wolf & Glass, 1992).

The coordination of SSB encompasses complex internal and external environmental demands. The development of this synergy results in a framework that contributes to many aspects of interaction and communication. The ability to grade and vary the SSB pattern allows the infant to:

- Eat in a manner that supports growth and bonding, and develop oral, neck, and trunk musculature.
- Achieve and maintain appropriate alertness levels through nonnutritive sucking, grading of respiration, biting, crunching, chewing, and licking—

all of which support development of healthy, comfortable, and predictable sleep-wake cycles and allow appropriate orienting and attending behavior (postural, visual, and auditory).

- Clear the eustachian tubes in the ears, nasal, and throat passages, as well as the bronchial tubes and lungs, in order to prevent chronic ear and/or upper respiratory conditions. This is achieved when sucking creates both a seal and a vacuum in the oral cavity.
- Facilitate coordination for binocular vision, which supports visual regard of facial expressions, near and far objects and activities, and visual orientation to sound.
- Achieve automatic swallowing of excess saliva to prevent drooling and enhance intelligibility of sound production.
- Provide a defined oral space in which the palate, cheeks, lips, tongue, and teeth develop in a way to support adequate speech sound production. This is developed by muscle tone and stability/mobility patterns in the jaw, tongue, lips, and cheeks.
- Develop a sense of midline, or center, which influences state regulation and postural control for attention and nonverbal communication.
- Develop adequate breath support for producing sound, volume control, intonation, articulation, and length of utterance.
- Develop visual regard, monitoring, and direction of hand activity for manipulating objects, play, and tool use.

Integration of physical contact, which occurs in this second level of the SI process, is most saliently understood in studies related to parent-infant bonding. Bonding gives an infant the first experiences of him- or herself as a physical being, and tactile-emotional attachment is critical to development (Montague, 1981; Stern 1985). Early bonding and feeding experiences are also a primary means of early communication.

Level III. The third level of the sensory integrative process reflects the ever-merging functional components that ultimately culminate in human adaptation/response to produce the last level of occupational performance components, or the end products of sensory integration.

According to Ayres (1979), "tactile, vestibular and proprioception are the building blocks for emotional stability" (p. 62). With disordered sensory processing, "the child is much more likely to react poorly to the environment" (p. 62). Consequently, some children are hard to engage whereas others are overly eager to please. Some withdraw whereas others appear to be hyperactive.

Some children may act disorganized because they feel that way inside, more physically than emotionally. These children often are described as not knowing where their bodies are in space. They have deficient "maps" of their body and how to use them. They have trouble planning, organizing, and sequencing their actions. This problem is called **dyspraxia** (Ayres, 1985).

The final two levels of the SI flowchart reflect the continually developing complexity of sensorimotor interaction that results in human performance. As Ayres (1979) carefully pointed out:

> SI is a continuously flowing process, each level of integration makes the next level possible. Before a child can understand words, he must be able to pay attention to the speaker. Before he can form words, he must have good sensory information from his mouth. The auditory-language center of brain also needs sensations from the vestibular system. Thus, speech and language depend on integration of auditory . . . and vestibular systems. (p. 63)

The last level of the flowchart is only applicable at school age. If there are irregularities in previous levels, then resultant disorders at this final adaptive response level become apparent. Disorders in these end-product behaviors are the most observable, yet without an understanding of the underlying layers, these disorders are often labeled as disabling. Occupational therapists have refined the art of observing behavior at the far right of the flow chart and then through careful assessment are able to look back through the levels to determine what might be helpful to address the disability. Ayres (1972, 1989) spent much of her research time developing assessment tools to assist in this process.

Ayres does not include communication or cognition as an end product of SI. However, for the purposes of this chapter, we will consider them as fitting in at this last level of the process of SI. Communication and cognition are complex, high-order, emergent abilities that result from multiple simple processing interactions (Elman et al., 1996). In a hierarchically derived system, communication and cognition result naturally as a culmination of the levels of processing described in Ayres's original model. Communication and cognition are implicitly included in the Ayres model (1972, 1975), and her later work reflected this (Parham & Mailloux, 1996), although Ayres did not update her linearly organized chart to reflect this change in thinking. Table 9-1 describes the relationship and flow of the neurological sensory processing systems to communication and cognition. As with all complex schemas, this is an attempt to map the system in two dimensions but it must be thought of in three dimensions to fully understand the complex, multidirectional interrelationships represented in the linear presentation. The diagram is also useful to remind us that sensory systems are organized in parallel and hierarchical fashion (Kandel et al., 1995).

Sensory sensitivity is an abbreviated way of referring to the process of sensory stimuli becoming sensory information for use in the nervous system. Sensory systems extract four basic attributes from the stimulus: modality (quality), intensity, duration, and location. These attributes combine to produce adequate sensory stimulus for detection. This is known as the sensory threshold phenomenon. When detectable criteria are reached, the signal is fired and

Table 9-1. Hierarchy of Attributes Related to Human Communication

	Communication and cognition	
	Interaction	
	Exploration	
	Memory functions	
	Attention functions	
	Sensory motor drive	
	Arousal	
Discrimination		Value/relevance
	Sensory processing	
	Sensory sensitivity	

Source: Windeck, S. L., & Laurel, M. (1989, March). A theoretical framework combining speech-language therapy with sensory integration treatment. *Sensory Integration Special Interest Newsletter, 12*(1). American Occupational Therapy Association, Inc., Bethesda, Md. Adapted with permission.

processed according to its modality and type of information it is bringing to the nervous system (Kandel et al., 1995).

Discriminative sensory input is that input that usually leads to conscious perception or to impact motor control (Kandel, Schwartz & Jessell, 1995). Each sensory system has the role of providing information to our brains to give us the qualities that inform or help us learn and know what it is we are encountering. This is discriminative information. In our touch (tactile) systems, discriminative information tells us the details about which finger is which and conveys information about the feeling and intention associated with, for example, a gentle caress.

Sensation gives information about the importance and relevance of the information as well. Classically, this was thought of as the protective or survival information system. This is best described when thinking of sensation encountered that is harmful and from which we withdraw in order to "survive." Conversely, we seek out pleasant sensation—a hug, a pleasant smell, or texture—to enhance our mood and level of comfort. These seeking/avoiding responses are parallel processes that give us distinctly different information. The information can be traced through different brain centers. Sensory integrative theory has evolved to cluster around two major branches referred to as sensory discrimination and **sensory modulation**.

Sensory discrimination includes patterns of functioning that are emergent processes based in discrete sensory processing. This includes, but is not limited to, the large cluster of praxis, bilateral motor coordination/integration and sequencing, visual and tactile space and form perception, eye/hand coordination and auditory language processing. Many of these are outlined in the third level of the SI flowchart (Figure 9-1).

Sensory modulation is less well defined, but includes sensory seeking and avoidance, sensory defensiveness, and problems with self-regulation, which is the capacity to maintain an alert and aroused state appropriate for the conditions and demands of the environment. Figure 9-2 shows the classic arousal curve originated by Hebb, which is usually associated with autonomic nervous system arousal (Hebb, 1949; Pribram & McGinnis, 1975). There is an inverse "U" relationship between arousal level and optimum function. The best functioning occurs in the middle range, known as the "optimal state" or "just right" level of arousal. On either the up or down side of this range, function is limited by, respectively, a state of over- or underarousal.

The best early childhood education and intervention programs typically include multisensory learning experiences. This is because enhanced sensory experiences help children to learn and have usually been thought of as influencing the discriminative or learning sensory systems. However, having the right amount of stimuli without overload creates the environment conducive to learning. Such a "just right" environment enhances learning much as op-

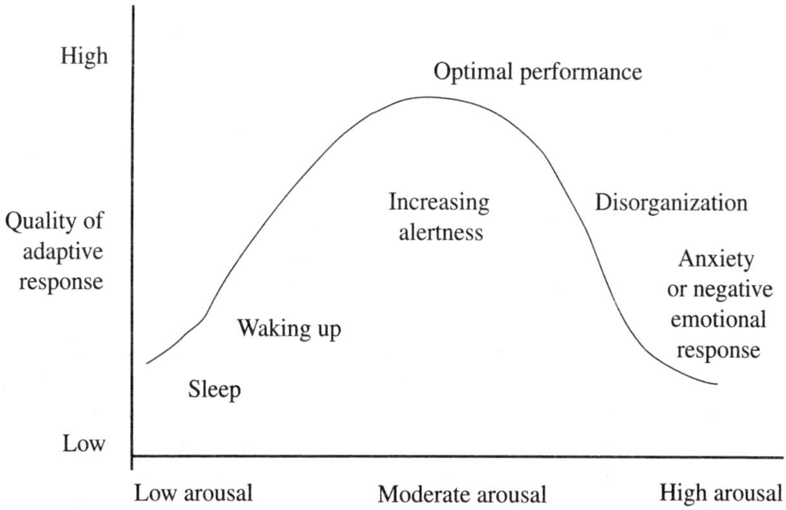

Figure 9-2. Classic Arousal Curve. (From Kimball, J. [1993]. Sensory integrative frame of reference. In P. Kramer & J. Hinojosa [Eds.], *Frames of reference for pediatric occupational therapy* [pp. 87–131]. Baltimore: Williams & Wilkins. Used with permission.)

portunities for rich exploration do. The SI approach suggests a balance between having many choices in a "stimulating" environment and a calm, organized space that fosters learning.

Sensory experience sets our nervous system's capacity to attend and influences memory functions as well. With an appropriate amount of sensory input, the nervous system is organized and moves along, through intrinsic wiring, to motivate or drive us to explore, interact, and learn. This drive toward exploration is directed at the environment, the task at hand, and the interaction occurring given the task and environment. This is all reciprocally dependent on communicative and cognitive abilities.

SI DYSFUNCTION RELATED TO COMMUNICATION

Communication is a product of our life experiences, and more specifically, our sensory experiences. According to Adler: "There is a reciprocal relationship among perception, concept, and language. One's perceptual and conceptual abilities influence and enhance language development and conversely new terminology enhances one's conceptual development" (1983, p. 18).

The development of communication involves a sequence of events that are hierarchical in nature but also reciprocal. Simplified, the process goes something like this: (1) one perceives sensory experiences within the environment and makes appropriate adjustments to these experiences; (2) recognition and discrimination of these sensory experiences occur; (3) conceptual development takes place as information is categorized and classified; and (4) symbolic behavior emerges, allowing for communication (Owens 1988, p. 343).

Bloom and Lahey (1978) summarized the relationship between incoming sensory information and language learning:

> Another aspect of perception that is logically related to language learning is attention to and integration of separate sensory stimuli from different modalities. It would seem that visual and tactile features of input from the context must be attended to and integrated with auditory impressions, if the interactions between content/form/use are to develop. That is, children need to experience the objects and events referred to by the speech that they hear in order to hear the coding relationship between meaning and sound. (p. 535)

In discussing early perceptual development, Moerk (1977) reported that "communication has as a prerequisite a relatively fine discrimination ability on the part of the communicating subject" (p. 67). Discrimination of all incoming sensory information and of essential versus nonessential information is important in making sense of our world. Once this has been accomplished, we can make judgments about our perceptions and store that information in memory for later reference. Some children are unable to screen out unwanted incoming sensory information. Unfiltered sounds, tactile perceptions, and visual stimuli can then become overwhelming, causing the child to shift into a fear ("fight or flight") mode. This may be manifested behaviorally by the child shutting down emotionally or acting out in a manner apparently inappropriate to the perceived situation (Wilbarger, 1991). These children perceive sensory information as threatening and unsafe, and therefore interactions with their environment and their subsequent sensory experiences are disrupted.

Communication development, with its early prerequisites based in development through sensory experiences may then be disorganized. "Language . . . mapped on disordered sensorimotor experiences will reflect that disorder" (Oetter, Richter, & Frick, 1993, p. 10). Sensory-processing problems are one of the many contributing factors to language disorders (Culatta, 1978). Affected individuals may have severe or mild sensory-processing problems, and not all children with difficulties will have concomitant language problems. However, based on what we know about the importance of typically developing sensory experiences and their relationship to language, the assessment of sensory-processing skills in relationship to language impairment cannot be overlooked.

Understanding the importance of sensory processing is integral for a complete understanding of language development and disorders. Speech-language pathologists who grasp the relevant concepts are better able to provide a more comprehensive, global, and inclusive treatment program for their patients. However, the benefits of SI therapy to language have not been well documented in research literature (Densom, Nuthall, Bushnell, & Horn, 1989). Many studies try to show a cause-and-effect relationship between SI therapy and language skills; however, SI theory does not intend this effect. SI therapy addresses sensory processing, which is the foundation of the hierarchy of communication development (see Table 9-1).

SI therapy does not profess to change academic or language functioning or any other end product. It may, however, have an *effect* on these skills as SI therapy works upon their foundations via the neurosensory processes. These processes are, necessarily, interdependent and therefore influence other, emergent processes including language and academics.

In the following pages, we hope to make the reader aware of how sensory integration deficits may manifest themselves in language impairment. We will discuss the specific areas and subcategories of sensory modulation and self-regulation and how disruption in these areas may contribute to specific language and speech problems. The information presented is based on clinical observations and experiences. Case studies (from our clinical experience) are used to illustrate these relationships.

Sensory Modulation Related to Communication

Sensory modulation disorders were defined earlier in the chapter as involving difficulty in screening essential from nonessential information. For example, a child may have difficulty screening out background noises in the classroom, with subsequent difficulties in attending to relevant and important information. Maintaining appropriate alertness is a function of sensory modulation (Kimball, 1993). Some children appear "unavailable" or passive in their play and interactions because they fail to appropriately utilize sensory information to orient and direct their attention toward their active environments. These two examples illustrate the main categories of modulation disorders: sensory defensiveness and poor self-regulation. Clinical experience shows us that sensory modulation may have several communication correlates, which are discussed next.

Sensory Defensiveness. "A tendency to react negatively or with alarm to sensory input that is generally considered harmless or non-irritating is typical of sensory defensiveness. Common symptoms may include oversensitivity to light or unexpected touch, sudden movement or overreaction to unstable surfaces, high frequency noises, excesses of noise or visual stimuli and certain smells" (Wilbarger & Wilbarger 1991, p.3). Oversensitivity or overgathering of sensation in any or all of the sensory systems may create such overstimulation that persons with sensory defensiveness are typified by avoidant, aversive, or negative responses to sensory input and can easily cycle into fear, fight-or-flight, and freeze responses because of the autonomic nervous system connections to this part of sensory processing. Defensiveness in the tactile system makes physical and social contact difficult to tolerate. The learning of social rules, boundaries, and interaction is easily impacted by this disorder, resulting in difficulties in pragmatic skill and early play development (Oetter et al., 1993). Hypersensitivity in the tactile system orally makes oral experiences related to talking, feeding, and physical contact difficult to manage. Marshalla (1994) reported that some children have tactile difficulties with production of specific sounds, such as fricatives, due to the unpleasant feel of the sound in the mouth (Alexander, Boehme & Cupps, 1994; Morris, 1981). Three influential clinicians have published separate, but convergent, views on how oral motor skills specific to feeding develop through infancy and toddlerhood to produce the patterns necessary for speech production (Alexander, 1987; Morris, 1981; Pinder, 1987). When these patterns are avoided secondary to hypersensitivity, they have a detrimental effect on this skill development. Affolter (1991, p. 162) reports that children with difficulties in tactile-kinesthetic input have a disordered sequence of their language development, with some children producing longer sentences before the typical sequence of one- and two-word phrases. These children may also skip the babbling stage. Affolter used her observations to support different developmental sequences of language performance among sensory disordered children.

Oversensitivity in movement systems results in difficulties tolerating normal movement experiences. Children who are afraid to swing, climb, and typically explore early childhood environments exemplify this. Within the occupational therapy field, this phenomenon is referred to as gravitational insecurity and temperamental development of shyness and anxiety. The inhibited exploration of the environment that results from movement hypersensitivity affects the quality of early perceptual experiences, impacting the early acquisition of perceptual-conceptual knowledge necessary for language development.

Hypersensitivity in the auditory system is another feature of sensory defensiveness. Background noise is particularly difficult to filter out. Inability to do so leads to distractibility, and listening, especially in an academic or social setting, becomes quite a difficult task. In severe cases, avoidance of what most people consider normal levels of environmental noise is demonstrated. Affected children have been observed to cover their ears, hunch their shoulders, or make their own "white noise" in an attempt to dampen noxious auditory stimuli. Many children physically hide to avoid the bombardment.

Auditory attention and discrimination are well defined as prerequisites to phonological and language development (Dodd, 1995). The child who is diagnosed with auditory hypersensitivity will often avoid the aversive stimuli of typical social environments, where competing and distracting background noise is hard to control. When unable to avoid such an environment, the child will find it difficult to maintain attention to relevant stimuli. In these situations, it becomes difficult to screen out essential from nonessential auditory information. The concentration needed to attend to language and to develop communication as a life skill is affected by the defensive process. Auditory defensiveness may mask developing language and phonological skills and make them unavailable for use until the hypersensitivity has been treated. Wilbarger (personal communication, 1995) reports the unfolding of previously hidden language development in the weeks following intensive intervention for sensory defensiveness.

The auditory and visual systems serve as our primary anticipatory systems (Gordon, 1992), meaning that we see or hear what is going on around us and then adjust our physical and social responses prior to engaging in interactions. Children who demonstrate visual hypersensitivity will decrease the amount of scanning and tracking they have to do in their environment. This, in turn, affects how efficiently they are able to anticipate and plan their repertoire of social and motor activities.

Defensiveness in auditory or visual systems decreases our effectiveness as social participants. The most overt expression of visual defensiveness is gaze aversion. Most simply, decreased eye contact often signals that a person is visually overwhelmed. Belser and Sudhalter (1995) have studied the relation between gaze avoidance and social anxiety. In a study of children with Fragile X Syndrome (FXS) who had significant sensory-processing disorders, they were able to demonstrate that less deviant language occurs when the stress of social interaction through eye contact is diminished. They compared children with FXS to children with Down syndrome and Attention Deficit Hyperactivity Disorder (ADHD) and found that FXS children who demonstrated physiological hyperarousal issues showed deviant language, including perseveration and tangential speech. The other groups in the study lacked the hyperarousal variable and did not demonstrate these deviant language patterns. This study supports the hypothesis that maintenance of eye gaze during conversation may cause significant hyperarousal in males with FXS, resulting in social avoidance and deviant language. Following up on the notion of hyperarousal difficulties, Miller and colleagues (in press) have documented multisensory hyperarousal in subjects with FXS using measures of electrodermal response (EDR) to a sensory challenge paradigm. The findings offer further support for sensory defensiveness and sensory modulation disruptions in this population.

CASE STUDY: BOBBY

Bobby is a 4-year-old boy with a diagnosis of FXS. Typical of this diagnosis, he struggles with many aspects of sensory-processing disorders, including sensory defensiveness and dyspraxia. His language has been slow and tedious in its development. These problems have been addressed in a therapeutic manner since he was 18 months old.

The first 2 years of Bobby's life were extremely stressful. Bobby had significant trouble learning to manage sucking. He was irritable nearly all of the time, and would only sleep for 1 to 2 hours at a time. His parents were exhausted and frustrated, and they started to have trouble managing the stress in their lives to such a degree that they began to consider separating from each other. Bobby's inability to be soothed and his trouble with feeding and sleeping persisted for several years. He was very rigid in the types of interaction he could tolerate. His mother was able to sort out little of this on her own, even though she and Bobby had managed to form a bond. However, she felt depressed and anxious regarding her role as mother/nurturer. Once Bobby was diagnosed with FXS and the family was able to access appropriate intervention, the situation quickly started to improve. The relief experienced because of having specific information regarding the serious difficulties that had been present served as the first step in the intervention process. Bobby's mother could finally understand her son on a new level, and she stopped feeling such painful emotional responsibility for his troubles. Treatment began with focusing on Bobby's sensory modulation difficulties. Within 6 weeks his sensory defensiveness was resolved to the point that he increased oral exploration by accepting and enjoying his first solid foods. He started to sleep for up to 5 hours at a time during the night. His motor skills started to blossom as Bobby found enjoyment in movement experiences for the first time, thus uncovering his drive to explore. With this increased freedom, he started to respond to verbal prompts and showed beginning receptive language abilities. Given these foundations, treatment shifted toward his sensory discrimination disorders. Addressing praxis in oral and gross motor areas was a priority.

With Bobby's defensiveness significantly decreased, his attention to language and playful interaction markedly improved. Although he continued to have difficulties with oral and verbal dyspraxia, his verbal imitations and approximations started to emerge. Given these foundations, treatment shifted toward his sensory discrimination disorders, including oral and somatosensory discrimination, and ideation during playful exploration, which emphasized expressive language development.

Self-Regulation

Disorders in self-regulation relate to trouble with managing sensory input and how the resultant overresponsive, underresponsive, or varying responses to sensory input affect arousal levels. Overarousal is typified by either overactivity or protective shutting down and withdrawal behavior when sensory overload occurs. Underarousal is typified by delayed, slow, or passive response to the environment. These responses are the most common and simple to understand. There are several other clusters of self-regulatory problems associated with sensory modulation disorders; interested readers are referred to Greenspan and Wieder (1993).

Language in children with difficulties managing arousal states can look deviant. Children who easily move into an overaroused state may struggle with topic maintenance (Belser & Sudhalter, 1995), inattention, impulsivity, lack of inhibition with speech (i.e., talking incessantly with little detail to content), poor organization of language, poor grading in the output of vocal quality, and perseveration. Additionally, if these children become so overwhelmed that they cannot cope, they will shut down. This is usually seen first in significantly decreased verbalizations, poor eye contact, and reduced interactions with people and objects in the environment. Underarousal is at the opposite end of the arousal spectrum. Some people think of this in its extreme as a lack of even registering what is going on in the environment. Affected children usually appear to be passive participants in their environment. They are slow to respond, especially to isolated or single-channel sensory input. They tend to respond better if given combined cues, such as touch and auditory stimuli coupled with visual stimuli. Underarousal is reflected in the quality of their play experience, which is then reflected in their language. They usually are slow to acquire receptive and expressive language abilities as their play interactions lack the richness needed to explore and develop schemas. Limited vocabulary development, poor social skill development, and slow processing and response time typify their language difficulties.

CASE STUDY: ANDREA

Andrea is a 4-year-old Latino girl with diagnosed self-regulation problems as well as auditory-processing and expressive language difficulties. She comes from a large, loving family, where her siblings and parents help her in a very empathetic manner with her need for constant movement and structure. When she first started combined occupational and speech/language therapy in a group setting, her attention was poor, her activity level was high, and she appeared disorganized and impulsive in her behavior and her language, which was characterized by tangential and uninhibited verbalizations as well as inattention to incoming verbal information. She was quickly overwhelmed by the amount of stimulation coming from the other children, and she tried to escape by literally "swinging from the rafters." Andrea was observed to become so overstimulated that several times she physically withdrew from the setting and seemed to lose her ability to verbally express herself until someone intervened to help her calm and reorganize.

When Andrea's treatment plan was developed, the focus was placed on keeping her arousal level within the normal range in order to help her focus and be able to work on language skill development. By paying attention to the amount and quality of stimuli present during each group activity, providing calming inputs regularly, and teaching her family how to incorporate these strategies at home. Andrea quickly began to make changes in developing more appropriate social play and language. Some strategies used in sensory-based programming for Andrea included: the use of "heavy work" to the muscles and joints through pushing, pulling, lifting, and carrying activities as active forms of calming inputs, both at home and school; having her chew two pieces of Bazooka® bubble gum to provide similar calming input to the mouth, which aided her in focusing while doing seated tasks; and engaging her in chores at home and school as a readily accessible means of incorporating heavy work throughout her day and helping her to stay focused.

CASE STUDY: JASON

Jason is a nearly 5-year-old boy who lives with his mother in a housing project in a large metropolitan area. He likes to watch television while snacking on packages of pepperoni, and he is quite overweight. His main interests revolve around food and television, as do his mother's. They rarely venture outside the home except for school or required errands. Jason is an underaroused child who is awkward socially due to his limited skills and experience. His language reflects his limited experiences; for example, he described his favorite play activity at home as performing opening and closing activities in a pretend doughnut shop. His language is very self-referent and he has difficulty knowing how to have conversations with other children. Jason's treatment plan emphasized achieving and then maintaining a higher level of arousal. By using movement activities such as (1) flying across the room on a trapeze suspended from a zip line and crashing into a pile of pillows, and (2) incorporating "superhero" play while prone on a soft sling swing attached to ceiling supports with elastic cords, Jason was "perked up." He was then able to attend and process language input and to more appropriately express himself within a group setting. Other gains observed included a noticeable change in social interaction skills and a willingness to participate in community outings.

Sensory Discrimination Related to Communication

Sensory discrimination is a major category of sensory processing, as outlined earlier in the chapter. The sensory integrative disorders outlined by Ayres were mostly clustered in this area. Though all the clusters may have an impact on language in one way or another, the most salient are outlined under the headings postural mechanisms and praxis.

The hallmark of sensory discrimination is that it is the information-gathering network for the nervous system, and through this it is our learning system. The sensory discrimination system interacts with the sensory modulation system in setting the tone for learning.

Postural Mechanisms. The development of a stable base from which to move is a critical element of coordinated motor skill and movement. It is not surprising, therefore, that stability-mobility patterns play a significant role in the smooth expression of related sensorimotor activities (i.e., ocular motor control, eye-hand coordination, articulation, upper trunk control for hand use, SSB synchrony, etc.) (Oetter et al., 1993).

CASE STUDY: AMY

Amy is a 3-year-old girl who was born prematurely. She was on oxygen and respiratory treatment until 6 months ago. She had typical oral feeding development except for needing to eat frequently in short bursts secondary to respiratory compromise. This resolved well in the first year, and following this she ate and grew well. Amy was referred to therapy because her speech was telegraphic in nature secondary to poor breath support. She was also very difficult to hear at the end of each statement due to the poor breath support. Amy's behavior could be characterized as passive and disorganized. Because of this, combined occupational therapy and speech sessions were utilized to treat her problems in both areas from a postural developmental frame of reference.

In a typical treatment session, Amy sat on a therapy ball while playing "listening lotto." The occupational therapist facilitated her movement through all ranges of rotation patterns and challenged her midline orientation in order to recruit stability with mobility in postural functions (Gilfoyle, Grady, & Moore, 1990). This was done in play, with the speech-language pathologist facilitating language production during the game. By increasing Amy's ability to meet the challenges of gravity and movement through three-dimensional space, postural skills emerged (Bly, 1983) and provided a foundation for better active control of the muscles that support respiration (Oetter et al., 1993). Last, the use of sucking and blowing toys and games completed the treatment session.

Praxis. The most simplistic definition of praxis is that it is the motor-planning process. Occupational therapists have broadened this definition to encompass sensory integrative functions within the nervous system. Speech-language pathologists have their own interpretation of dyspraxia, focused in the oral/verbal functions. It is important to know that these differences in semantics can at times be confusing. Gaining insight into each other's expertise only adds to our knowledge base and in turn strengthens our clinical and team skills. According to occupational therapy SI theory, praxis is an emergent process that is categorized into phases. Ayres put forth this idea and called the phases ideation, planning, and execution. Praxis is the process used in all skill development. Oral, verbal, and gross and fine motor planning (praxis) are the most theorized about. Ayres's theory defined the process as follows:

Ideation: Ability of the brain to conceive of an action—"What to do."

Planning: Ability to organize the plan for action—"How to do it."

Execution: Ability to carry out a sequence of action—"Just do it!"

With respect to speech-language therapy, Ayres's schema of ideation, planning, and execution are applicable to verbal and oral dyspraxia. They provide a framework for conceptualizing the disorder as well as planning intervention. When a new skill is learned, actions are thought through. Consider, for example, a toddler planning and coordinating movements in the suck/swallow/breathe synchrony while learning to sip through a straw. As the actions are repeated over and over again, they become automatic. Similarly, as new skills, such as phonological combinations, are practiced, they too become more automatic.

Marshalla (1992) summarized theories postulated by Ayres (1979) and other researchers in the areas of sensory integrative dysfunction, namely, that dyspraxia is the result of poor organization of tactile, vestibular, or proprioceptive sensations. Affected children are not able to learn from these sensory feedback loops, which are critical for accurate and precise articulation, and hence they cannot utilize this information for speech production. The use of sensory integration intervention thus becomes integral in working with the dyspraxic child.

Difficulties with praxis result in dyspraxia. Ayres (1972, 1989) devoted much of her research effort toward developing assessment tools helpful in delineating the types of dyspraxia and the neurosensory processing correlates of praxis. In the speech-language profession, dyspraxia is identified by observation of clusters of symptoms. Dodd (1995) outlined characteristics of developmental verbal dyspraxia, as noted in Table 9-2.

Delayed language onset and significant articulation deficits characterize dyspraxia. Children with speech dyspraxia may have disordered language

Table 9-2. Characteristics of Developmental Verbal Dyspraxia

From case history	*From standard speech assessment*
problems with feeding	deviant speech development
little vocal play or babbling	vowel errors
little imitation in infancy	omissions greater than other speech error types
family history of communication disorders	inconsistent errors
family history of written language disorders	increased errors with performance load
delayed language onset	metathesis
use of word token once only	inability to maintain syllabic integrity
gross/fine motor incoordination	voicing errors
body dyspraxia/body awareness in space	difficulities sequencing phonemes
"soft" neurological signs	high number of errors per word
slow progress in therapy	difficulty with articulatory complex sounds
	epenthesis
	syntagmatic errors in severe cases
	paradigmatic errors in less severe cases
	difficulty with polysyllabic words
	reduced phoneme repertoire

If routine assessment identifies a number of the above characteristics, then further assessment and observation should seek:

Specified assessment tasks	*Observations*
dyspraxia for isolated and/or sequenced oromotor movements	inconsistent oral-nasal resonance
deficits in oral perception	nasal emission
receptive-expressive language gap	equal stress and/or slow rate of speech
word-finding difficulties	poor self-monitoring
syntactic errors	variable performance between and within sessions
comprehension equals cognitive abilities	trial-and-error groping, silent posturing
difficulties with long verbal instructions	prolongations and repetition
slow diadochokinetic (DDK) rates	
difficulty sequencing in DDK tasks	

Dodd, B. 1995. *Differential diagnosis and treatment of children with speech disorder* (p. 96). Singular Publishing Group, Inc. 401 West "A" Street, Suite 325, San Diego, California 92101-7904. (1-800-521-8545). Reprinted with permission.

as well as disordered speech (Stackhouse, 1992). Some theorists hypothesize that deficits underlying dyspraxia include planning at both the linguistic and motor output levels (Dodd, 1995). A general apraxic condition affecting both speech-motor and fine-motor control might explain an association between clumsiness and developmental speech disorder (Bishop & Edmundson, 1987).

CASE STUDY: SAM

Sam is a boy aged 2;11. He possesses typical receptive language skills but significantly delayed expressive skills, consisting of the use of only 20 words. He is a "picky" eater, preferring French fries and macaroni and cheese to other food choices, which often require skilled oral motor patterns to manage. He does not verbally imitate, nor does he imitate body movements. He gropes when trying to imitate oral movements and looks awkward when trying to imitate body movements. Sam's motor style can be characterized as clumsy. He easily trips over objects simply because he becomes disorganized in the sequence of navigating through environmental space. He has trouble coordinating his movements to climb on and over things, which limits his gross motor skill repertoire. He has trouble grading his movements, so he is often very rough on objects and people. Sam's hands also are uncoordinated. He cannot manage constructional toys, and his fine motor development is delayed. Sam's praxis process is disordered. He has trouble getting started (initiating), and his poor imitation skills leave him feeling lost regarding what to do. He does not ideate well, so does not really even know what to do with toys, playground equipment, or same-age peers. His parents are very concerned about his development and have even begun to wonder if he has normal learning potential. Simply enrolling him in preschool to provide models for what to do was not enough to help him, so they pursued intervention.

Sam's treatment plan focused on treating his dyspraxia from both an occupational therapy and a speech-language pathology perspective. His two therapists consulted weekly with each other to coordinate goals. The use of a traveling therapy notebook served this purpose, as well as allowing the family to have information and input.

Sam's speech therapy sessions utilized a variety of strategies to improve his oral awareness and verbalizations. Oral exploratory play in front of a mirror was successful in helping Sam become more aware of his oral structures and how they move. This sort of activity helped him learn that his oral movements can become automatic. Increased tactile/proprioceptive awareness coupled with visual feedback created the foundation for learning sound sequences and words. Movement and rhythm were used in play to enhance speech prosody and smoothness of speech production for environmental sounds as well as word approximations. Words targeted were consonant-vowel-consonant (C-V-C) combinations that were motorically easy to produce and important to make him more communicatively powerful in his environment. The joint goals established by Sam's therapists helped his speech-language pathologist to incorporate movement activities into the speech sessions. Starter phrases such as "Ready, set, go!" were utilized by both therapists because of Sam's need for help initiating and ideating due to both speech and motor dyspraxia.

Sam's OT sessions utilized a classical SI approach in facilitating his skill development through providing the "just right" challenge in motor and somatosensory play and exploration. Having Sam use suspended equipment while engaged in fantasy play was a fun way to help him use his emerging language skills and apply them to his developing motor skills.

INTERDISCIPLINARY COLLABORATION

Occupational therapists and speech-language pathologists will find it useful to be familiar with each other's job roles and theory bases. Children with communication needs often have problems with dyspraxia or attention that would benefit from pediatric occupational therapy. Conversely, many children with sensory-processing–based difficulties have speech or language disorders needing the expertise of a speech-language pathologist.

Finding ways to collaborate is vital to excellence in service provision. Schopmeyer and Lowe (1992) presented a scheme for models of collaboration. These ideas reach to all diagnoses and disciplines. The types of combined OT/speech-language pathology treatment are:

1. *Consultative:* This is probably where most therapists begin to interact, when talking to each other about mutual children. Consultation often takes place informally. On a more formal level, regular staffings are often a forum for asking questions, sharing problems, or requesting reinforcement of certain goals by the other therapist. Consultation may be thought of as both the simplest and the most advanced form of combined treatment: Eventually, both therapists may become so familiar with each other's disciplines that problems may be addressed through verbal consultation that may have previously required observation or actual experience.

2. *Observational:* When one therapist observes another, techniques and objectives can be demonstrated that may be difficult to convey through verbal description. Scheduling of observation time often begins as an outgrowth of consultation. While observation is time-consuming for the observing therapist (who is pulled away from providing direct treatment), the benefits of seeing, rather than talking about, issues may outweigh this drawback. Moreover, the observational model does not require prior joint planning time; it can be done on the spur of the moment, when a therapist has some unexpected free time.

3. *Side-by-Side:* In this model, the occupational therapist and speech-language pathologist work together with a child or group of children but each therapist has separate goals, with equal responsibilities for different compo-

nents of the activity. There is little overlap of goals in the use of this model; rather, a common activity is used as a vehicle to address two sets of objectives. Either or both (alternating) therapists may lead the activity.

4. *Supportive:* In the supportive model, one therapist acts as a facilitator to enable the other therapist to address his or her goals more effectively. One therapist usually leads the activity, with the facilitating therapist assuming a secondary role. However, if problems occur in trying to achieve a specific outcome, the supporting therapist may temporarily step in and take the lead in order to establish a more effective learning environment.

5. *Transdisciplinary:* In this model, both the occupational therapist and the speech-language pathologist are responsible for planning the session and establishing objectives. Both share equally in providing sensorimotor and language input during the session. To be truly transdisciplinary, the two therapists should be indistinguishable to an observer.

Within each of these models there are levels and variations based on the therapist's knowledge and experience with combined treatment. It is important to know one's own limits as a transdisciplinary therapist and to recognize "red flags" (such as overstimulation) and react appropriately by seeking help. These models are presented as a means to foster a collaborative spirit among early interventionists.

SUMMARY

Sensory integration is a neurologic process as well as a primary theory in pediatric occupational therapy. SI is reciprocally dependent with communication, and both are at the heart of the child's development of play and socialization. This chapter has given an overview of the process of SI, how communication is affected by SI, and how SI is affected by communication. Case studies and models for intervention were presented to highlight the usefulness of these ideas.

REFERENCES

Adler, S. (1983). *The nonverbal child.* Springfield, Ill.: Thomas.

Affolter, F. (1991). *Perception, interaction and language.* New York: Springer-Verlag.

Alexander, R. (1987). Prespeech and feeding development. In N. McDonald (Ed.), *Treating cerebral palsy: For clinicians by clinicians* (pp. 133–152). Austin, Tex.: Pro-Ed.

Alexander, R, Boehme, R. & Cupps, B. (1994). *Normal development of functional motor skills: The first year of life.* Tucson: Therapy Skill Builders.

Ayres, A. J. (1964). Tactile functions: Their relation to hyperactive and perceptual motor behavior. *American Journal of Occupational. Therapy, 18,* 83–95.

Ayres, A.J. (1972). *Sensory integration and learning disorders.* Los Angeles: Western Psychological Services.

Ayres, A. J. (1975). Sensorimotor foundations of academic ability. In W. M. Cruickshank & D. P. Hallahan (Eds.), *Perceptual and learning disabilities in children,* (Vol. 2, pp. 301–338). Syracuse, N.Y.: Syracuse University Press.

Ayres, A. J. (1979). *Sensory integration and the child.* Los Angeles: Western Psychological Services.

Ayres, A. J. (1985). *Developmental dyspraxia and adult-onset apraxia.* Torrance, Calif.: Sensory Integration International.

Ayres, A. J. (1989). *Sensory integration and praxis tests.* Los Angeles: Western Psychological Services.

Ayres, A. J. & Mailloux, Z. (1981). Influence of sensory integration procedures on language development. *American Journal of Occupational Therapy, 35*(6), 383–389.

Belser, R., & Sudhalter, V. (1995). Arousal difficulties in males with fragile X syndrome: A preliminary report. *Developmental Brain Dysfunction, 8,* 270–279.

Bishop, D., & Edmundson, A. (1987). Specific language impairment as a maturational lag: Evidence from longitudinal data on language and motor development. *Developmental Medicine and Child Neurology, 29,* 442–459.

Bloom, L., & Lahey, M. (1978). *Language development and language disorders.* New York: Wiley.

Bly, L. (1983). *The components of normal movement during the first year of life and abnormal motor development.* Birmingham, Ala.: Pathway Press.

Culatta, B. (1978). The relationship between perceptual dysfunction and language disorders: A case report. *Journal of Communication Disorders, 11,* 51–63.

Densom, J. F., Nuthall, G. A., Bushnell, J., & Horn, J. (1989). Effectiveness of a sensory integrative therapy program for children with perceptual-motor deficits. *Journal of Learning Disabilities, 22,* 221–229.

Dodd, B. (1995). *Differential diagnosis and treatment of children with speech disorder.* San Diego: Singular Publishing.

Elman, J. L., Bates, E. A., Johnson, M. A., Karmiloff-Smith, A., Parisi, D., & Plunkett, K. (1996). *Rethinking innateness: A connectionist perspective on development.* Cambridge, Mass.: MIT Press.

Fisher, A. G., Murray, E. A., & Bundy, A. C. (1991). *Sensory integration theory and practice.* Philadelphia: Davis.

Gilfoyle, E. M., Grady, A. P., & Moore, J. C. (1990). *Children adapt.* Thorofare, N.J.: Slack.

Gordon, J. (1992). [Lecture presented at Pediatric NDT certification course]. Denver.

Greenspan, S., & Wieder, S. (1993). Regulatory disorders. In C. H. Zeanah (Ed.), *Handbook of infant mental health* (pp. 280–290). New York: Guilford.

Hebb, D. O. (1949). *The organization of behavior: A neuropsychological theory*. New York: Wiley.

Kandel, E., Schwartz, J. H., & Jessell, T. M. (1991). *Principles of neural science*. Norwalk, Conn.: Appleton & Lange.

Kandel, E., Schwartz, J. H., & Jessell, T. M. (Eds.). (1995). *Essentials of neural science and behavior*. Norwalk, Conn.: Appleton & Lange.

Keilhofner, G. (Ed.). (1995). *A model of human occupation: Theory and application*. Baltimore: Williams & Wilkins.

Kimball, J. G. (1993). Sensory integrative frame of reference. In P. Kramer & J. Hinojosa (Eds.), *Frames of reference for pediatric occupational therapy* (pp. 87–131). Baltimore: Williams & Wilkins.

Kramer, P., & Hinojosa, J. (Eds.). (1993). *Frames of reference for pediatric occupational therapy*. Baltimore: Williams & Wilkins.

Marshalla, P. (1992). *Oral motor techniques in articulation therapy*. Seattle: Innovative Concepts.

Marshalla, P. (1994). *Oral motor techniques in articulation therapy*. Conference presentation, Golden, Colo.

Miller, L. J., McIntosh, D. N., McGrath, J., Shyu, V., Lampe, M., Taylor, A., Tassone, F., Neitzel, K., Stackhouse, T., & Hagerman, R. (in press). Electrodermal reactivity in patients with Fragile X Syndrome. *American Journal of Medical Genetics.*

Moerk, E. (1977). *Pragmatic and semantic aspects of early language development*. Baltimore: University Park Press.

Montague, A. (1981). *Touching: The human significance of the skin*. New York: Harper & Row.

Morris, S. E. (1981). *The normal acquisition of oral feeding skills: Implications for assessment and treatment*. New York: Therapeutic Media.

Oetter, P., Laurel, M., & Cool, S. (1991). Unit 10. Sensorimotor foundations of communication. In Royeen, C. (Ed.), *AOTA Self Study Series: Neuroscience foundations of human performance*. Rockville, Md.: American Occupational Therapy Association (AOTA).

Oetter, P., Richter, E., & Frick, S. (1993). *M.O.R.E.: Integrating the mouth with sensory and postural functions*. (1st complete ed.). Hugo, Minn.: PDP Products.

Ottenbacher, K., & Short, M. A. (1985). Sensory integrative dysfunction in children: A review of theory and treatment. In D. Routh & M. Wolrich (Eds.), *Advances in developmental and behavioral pediatrics* (Vol. 6, pp. 287–329). Greenwich, Conn.: JAI.

Owens, R. E. (1988). *Language development: An introduction*. Columbus, Ohio.: Merrill.

Parham, L. D., & Mailloux, Z. (1996). Sensory integration. In J. Case-Smith, P. N. Pratt, & A. S. Allen (Eds.), *Occupational therapy for children* (3rd ed., pp. 307–355). St. Louis: Mosby.

Paul, R., Cohen, D. J., & Caparulo, B. K. (1983). A longitudinal study of patients with severe developmental disorders of language learning. *Journal of American Academy of Child Psychiatry, 22,* 525–534.

Pinder, G. L. (1987, January). *Developmental sequence and connections among areas of motor, oral-motor, vocalization, and cognitive development from birth through four years.* Unpublished doctoral dissertation, University of Washington, Seattle.

Pribam, K., & McGinnis, D. (1975). Arousal, activation and effort in the control of attention. *Psychological Review, 82,* 116–149.

Shopmeyer, B. B., & Lowe, F. (Eds.). (1992). *The Fragile X child.* San Diego: Singular Publishing.

Stackhouse, J. (1992). Developmental verbal apraxia: A review and critique. *European Journal of Disorders of Communication, 27,* 19–34.

Stern, D. (1985). *The interpersonal world of the infant.* New York: Basic Books.

Vygotsky, L. S. (1978). *Mind in society.* Cambridge, Mass.: Harvard University Press.

Wilbarger, P. (1991, Sept.). Planning an adequate "sensory diet"—application of sensory processing theory during the first year of life. *Zero to Three,* 7–12.

Wilbarger, P., & Wilbarger, J. (1991). *Sensory defensiveness in children 2–12: An intervention guide for parents and other caretakers.* Santa Barbara, Calif.: Avanti Education Programs.

Windeck, S. L., & Laurel, M. (1989, March). A theoretical framework combining speech-language therapy with sensory integration treatment. *Sensory Integration Special Interest Section Newsletter, 12,* 1–8. Rockville, Md.: American Occupational Therapy Association.

Wolf, L. S., & Glass, R. R. (1992). *Feeding and swallowing disorders in infancy: Assessment and management.* Tucson: Therapy Skill Builders/ Psychological Corporation.

Glossary

adaptive response—a successful response to an environmental challenge. A central tenet of sensory integration/occupational therapy treatment states that development is enhanced and facilitated through the elicitation of adaptive responses. Adaptive responses play a mechanistic role in sensory integration development.

African American English vernacular (AAEV)—a speech and language dialect spoken by many African American speakers.

aid—an external, physical book, board, chart, or device to transmit messages.

arousal—a general, rather than particular, fluctuation in central nervous system activity, as opposed to particular fluctuations related to attention. Typically moment-to-moment changes in arousal are facilitated by sensorimotor input and output in order to maintain an optimal level, which follows a classic inverted "U" performance pattern.

assessment—a broad term that covers the entire "assessment" process including screening, diagnosis, assessment for intervention planning, and evaluation of a child's progress (as used in all chapters except Chapter 4); *or* a planned process of activities and strategies specifically used to plan intervention (as defined by the Individuals with Disabilities Education Act Amendments, 1997, and Bricker and Losardo, Chapter 4).

augmentative and alternative communication (AAC)—clinical practices that focus on severe expressive communication disorders.

child-centered approaches—the clinician follows the child's lead.

clinician-based intervention—the clinician serves as the primary agent of intervention.

clinician-directed approaches—the clinician controls activities.

code switching—shifting from one language or dialect to another during a conversation.

communicative functions—the purposes for which a child communicates.

communicative means—the ways in which a child communicates, verbally (e.g., speaking, signing) or nonverbally (e.g., gesturing, facial expressions).

consultant—individual who helps consumers shape a path toward consumer-selected goals with ongoing input from the consumer.

conventional literacy—known to lay audiences as "real reading" and "real writing," conventional literacy includes reading and writing behaviors that the members of a culture have implicitly or explicitly agreed on as denoting traditional reading and writing. Conventional literacy is often used to indicate the first signs that a child has made a transition from emergent to traditional literacy.

criterion-referenced assessments—assessments that compare the child's behaviors to a predetermined level of performance or a criterion of behaviors in each domain.

cultural competence—the ability to be aware of one's own cultural limitations, respect cultural differences, and use cultural resources in intervention.

culturally-linguistically different (CLD)—one who speaks the dialect of a non-mainstream culture.

cultural sensitivity—the ability to be aware of, and appreciate, other cultures.

curriculum-based assessment (CBA)—assessment that provides a direct application of criterion-referenced assessment strategies to instructional content. Assessment and curricular content are coordinated to address the same skills and abilities. Assessment typically focuses on identifying the settings, conditions, and goals for parents and interventionists to use daily activities as a vehicle for teaching.

curriculum-based intervention—use of the child's curriculum as a vehicle for remediation and intervention.

developmental disabilities (DD)—a group of handicapping conditions that are manifested during the developmental period and are chronic in nature (e.g., cerebral palsy, mental retardation, autism).

diagnosis—the process used to determine the nature of the problem and whether a child is eligible for services.

dialect—variations of the speech and language used within a particular language.

dynamic assessment—a proactive, continuous process for purposes of planning and providing services to children with respect to their evolving abilities and needs; guided learning for the purpose of determining children's potentional for change.

dyspraxia—a disruption in any or all points of the process of praxis. Sometimes this is referred to as a problem with coordination, a difficulty with motor planning, or clumsiness; dyspraxia is a more accurate description of the condition.

ecological communication program (ECO)—a system for intervention that proposes to guide the development of interactions between children and their partners from play through conversation.

ecologically valid assessment—assessment that takes into account the influence on the child and family of physical and social factors, cultural beliefs and ideologies, and relationships with others.

emergent literacy—the reading and writing behaviors and concepts of young children that precede and develop into conventional literacy.

emergent reading—the oral production of a familiar book's text by a nonconventional reader with indications that the act is considered to be reading.

ethnographic assessment—evaluation of communicative behaviors from a cultural perspective.

evaluation—activities used to determine a child's initial and continuing eligibility, including a determination of the status of the child across developmental areas (as defined in the original Individuals with Disabilities Education Act Amendments (1997); *or* activities that provide a comparison of the child's performance before and after intervention (as defined by Bricker and Losardo, Chapter 4).

family—includes the parent-child unit that meets the child's needs, whether including one or more parents, siblings, and/or extended family.

interdisciplinary team—a team made up of parents and professionals from multiple disciplines who each have specialized knowledge in their own area and who work to integrate their assessment and/or intervention information about the child and family.

intervention—those activities and strategies used to nurture the child's development and support the family's role in that process.

late talking toddlers—toddlers who have less than a 50-word productive vocabulary and/or no multiword combinations by age 2; such children may also have comprehension delays.

linked system approach—a linked system approach attempts to link program goals, assessment procedures, curricular content, and subsequent evaluation of children's progress on target goals and objectives.

measurement processes—measurement involves at least four processes with uniquely different purposes: screening, diagnosis, program-relevant assessment, and evaluation.

milieu teaching—instruction that is conducted in a naturalistic setting but employs various operant-teaching techniques.

multidisciplinary team—a team made up of parents and professionals from multiple disciplines who each assess and provide information about the child and family.

norm-referenced tests—tests that compare the child's behaviors to those of a sample of individuals similar in age and demographic variables.

parent-based intervention—parents are trained to serve as the primary intervention agents.

partners—those who regularly interact with the child.

praxis—the central nervous system process of conceptualizing, organizing and planning, executing, and monitoring nonhabitual (motor) tasks. Sometimes the concept of praxis is reduced to the more common term, *motor planning,* although as the definition reveals, planning is only one component of praxis.

program-relevant assessment—assessment used to gather baseline information and to establish specific intervention goals and objectives.

proprioception—sensation of movement and body position through information from muscles and joint compression.

routines—predictably occurring contexts in which children find themselves engaged in the same activity with a partner or partners.

screening—a quick, economical look at a child's repertoire, which, if used, should occur prior to the other measurement processes. The purpose of screening is to decide whether a child's performance is sufficiently different from that of other children of the same chronological age to warrant more comprehensive testing.

sensory integration (SI)—the organization of sensation for use, a primary central nervous system function. Also, a frame of reference used in occupational therapy for individuals who have difficulty with this primary central nervous system function.

sensory modulation—graded responses generated by the central nervous system in order to take in appropriate levels of sensation from the environment.

specific expressive language delay—category describing late talking toddlers whose delays are restricted to productive language.

specific language impairment (SLI)—language disorder that is not associated with general cognitive delay, sensorimotor deficits, or emotional disturbance.

standard English vernacular (SEV)—speech and language used by mainstream America.

strategy—a self-discovered or taught process for using symbols, aids, and systems to enhance communication.

suck/swallow/breathe (SSB)—is a triad of primary oral motor mechanisms, the rhythmical, coordinated pattern of sucking, swallowing, and breathing. An intact SSB synchrony is critical to many elements of sensorimotor and cognitive development, including speech and language development, state regulation, postural control, feeding/eating behavior, ego development, and eye-hand coordination.

symbols—representations of basic vocabulary concepts through objects, pictures, gestures, signs, and/or icons.

system—the collective components used to enhance communication, including symbols, aids, strategies, and techniques.

tactile—type of information related to touch and pain that is transmitted through receptors in the skin.

technique—a specific means to select, access, and/or transmit a message.

traditional assessment—assessment that is typically designed around standardized measures, using a specified set of conditions and hypothetical constructs, and is focused on identifying the child's disabilities.

transdisciplinary team—a team made up of parents and professionals from one or more disciplines who have cross-disciplinary expertise, although one professional may serve as the primary interactant with the child and family.

vestibular—refers to the sensory system responsible for the detection of head position, movement, and gravity; the receptors (otoliths and semicircular canals) are located in the inner ear.

Index

Note: Page numbers in **bold type** reference non-text material

D

I

J

L